Aflatoxin B1 Occurrence, Detection and Toxicological Effects

Edited by Xi-Dai Long

Published in London, United Kingdom

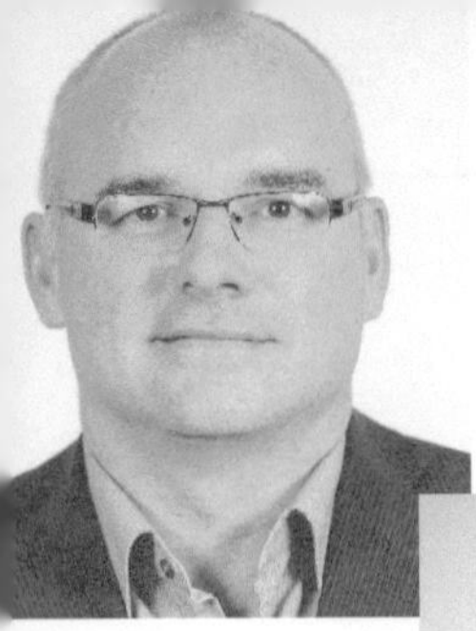
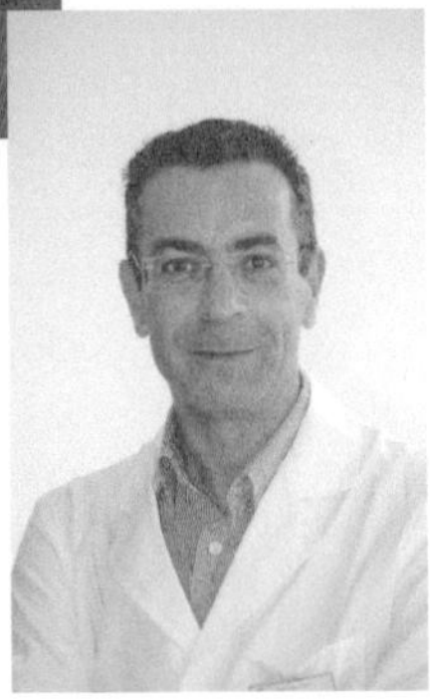
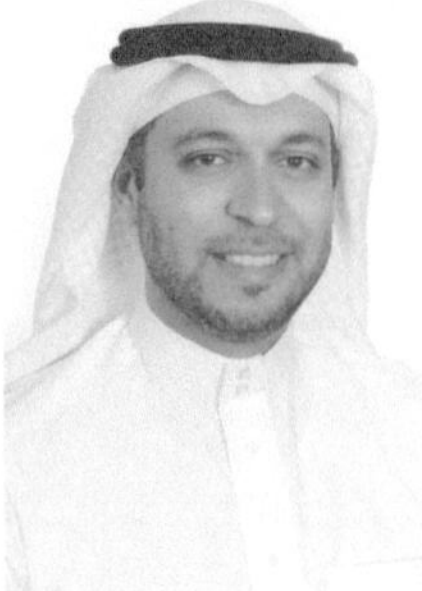
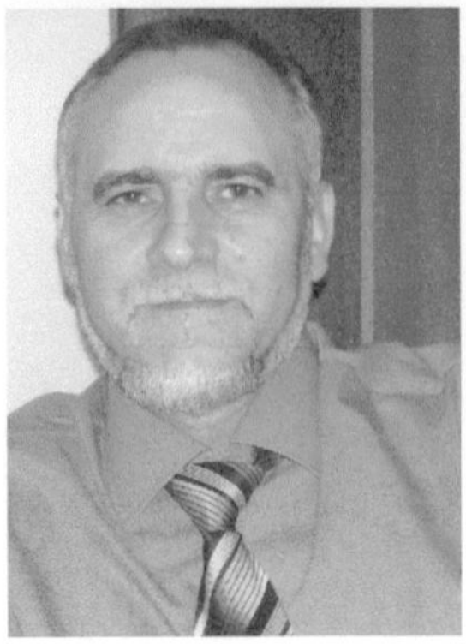
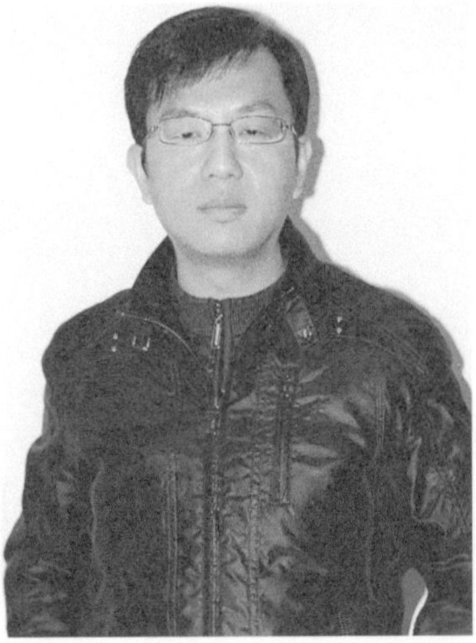
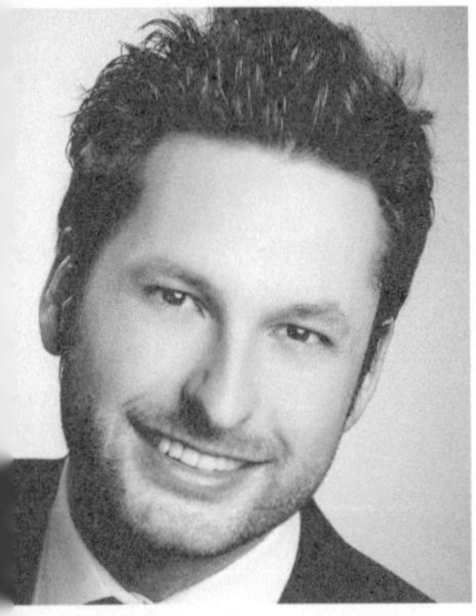
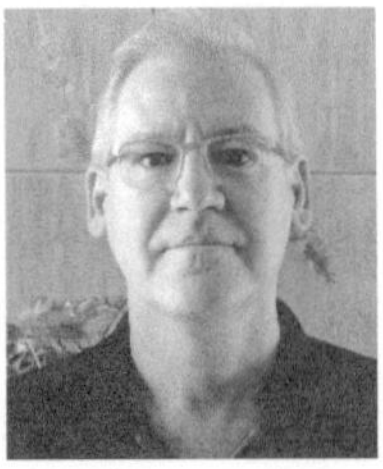

IntechOpen

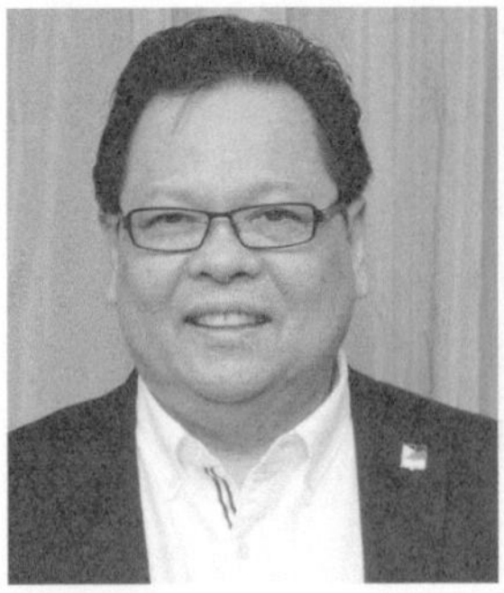
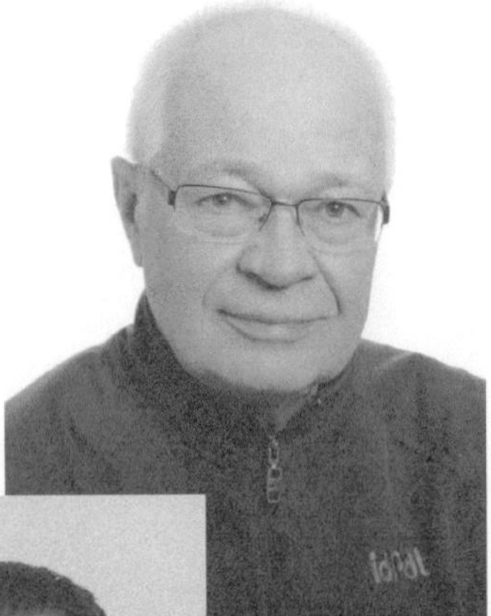
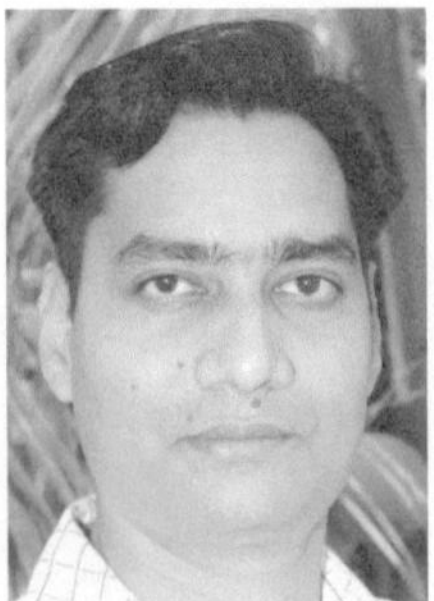
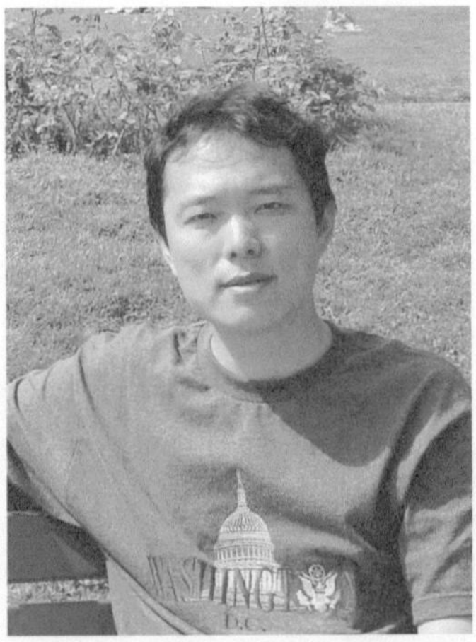
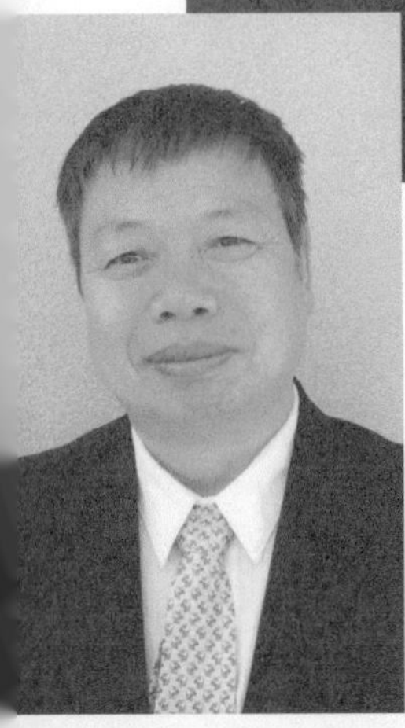
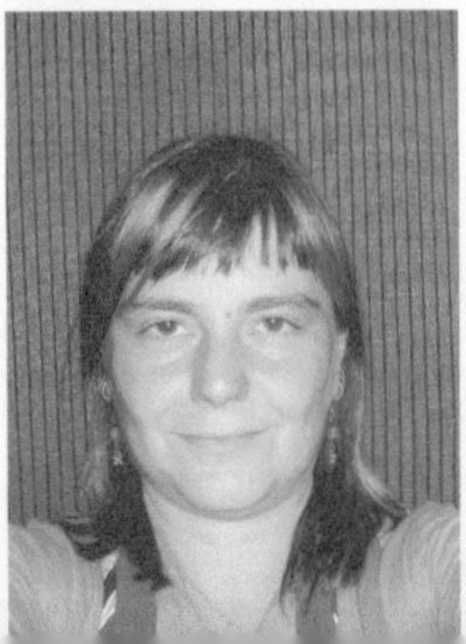

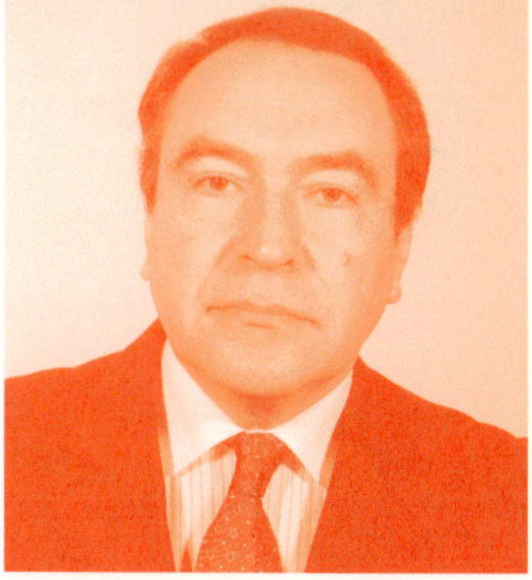
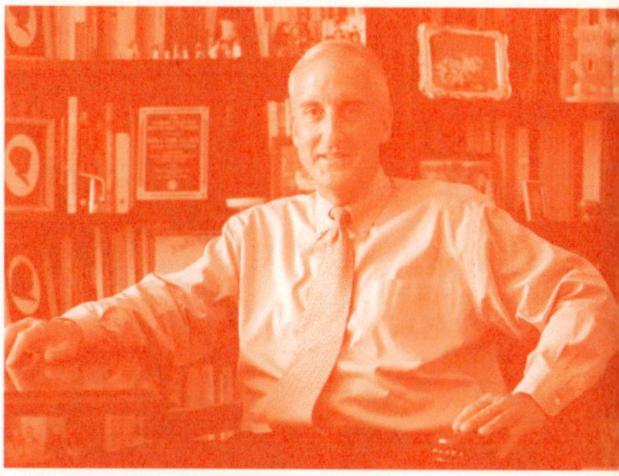
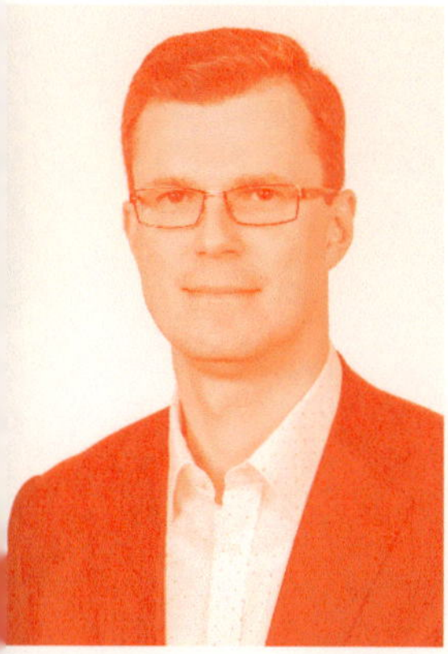
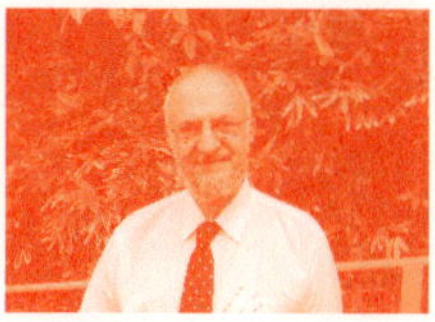
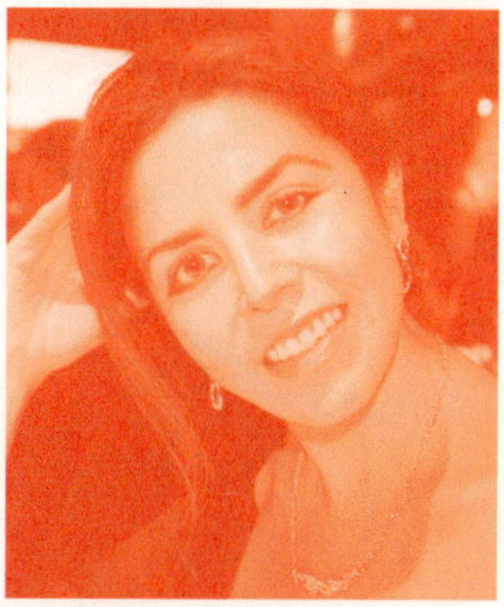

Supporting open minds since 2005

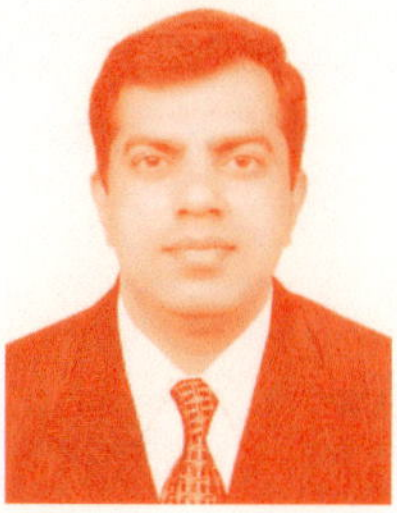
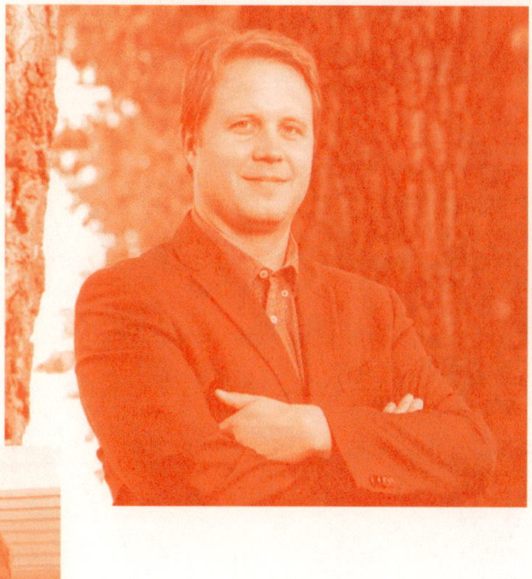
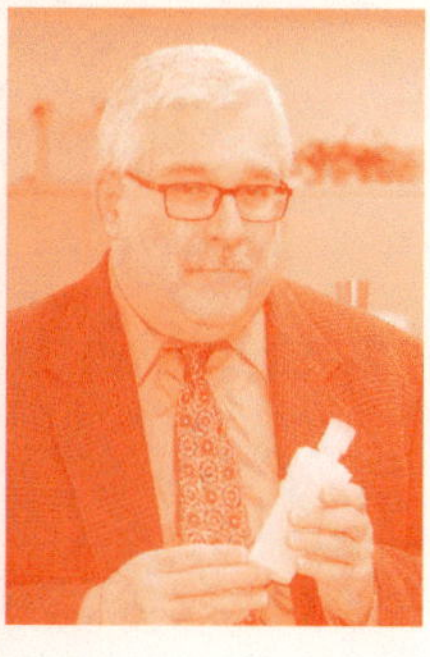
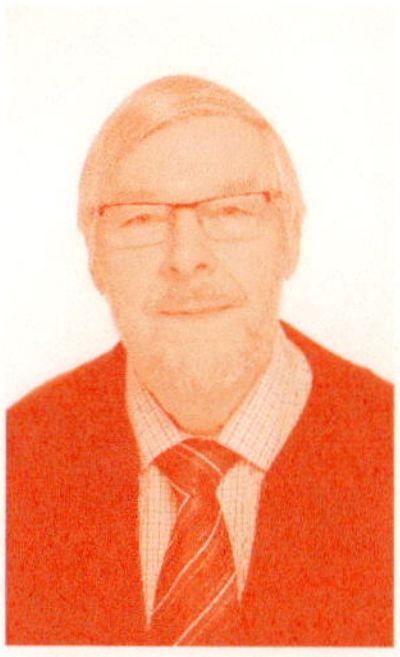
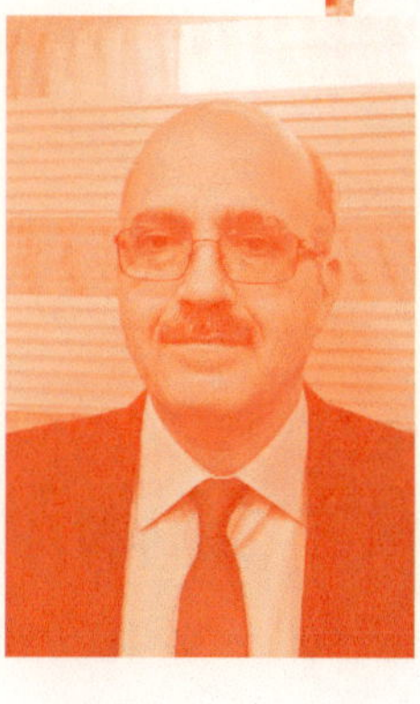
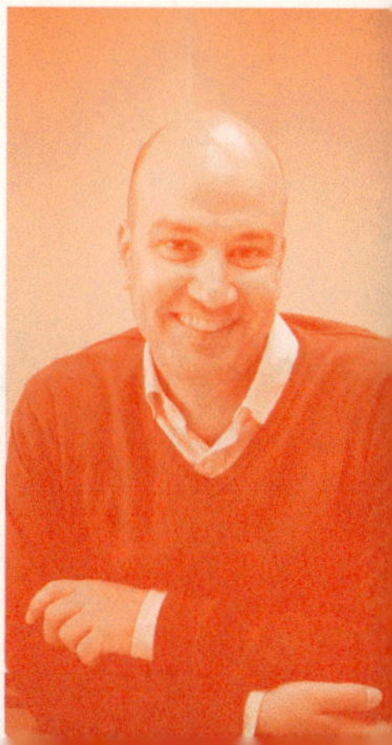
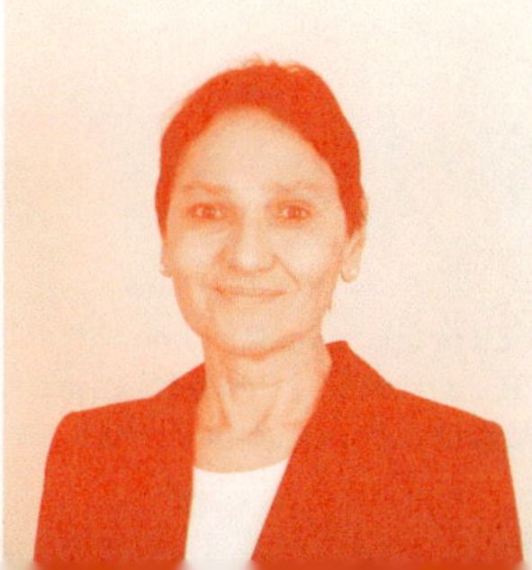

Aflatoxin B1 Occurrence, Detection and Toxicological Effects
http://dx.doi.org/10.5772/intechopen.77925
Edited by Xi-Dai Long

Part of IntechOpen Book Series: Biochemistry, Volume 14
Book Series Editor: Miroslav Blumenberg

Contributors
Jie Li, Adekunle Odunayo Adejuwon, Victoria Tsygankova, Xi-Dai Long, Yan Deng, Xue-Min Wu, Xiao-Ying Huang, Jin-Guang Yao, Qin-Qin Long, Xiao-Qin Wu, Nancy Nleya, Mulunda Mwanza, Lubanza Ngoma, Xing-Zhizi Wang, Qun-Ying Su, Joseph Lalah, Yamina Ben Miri, Djamel Djenane, Agustin Ariño, Yuhua Shan, Qian Yang

First published in London, United Kingdom, 2020 by IntechOpen
IntechOpen is the global imprint of INTECHOPEN LIMITED, registered in England and Wales, registration number: 11086078, 7th floor, 10 Lower Thames Street, London, EC3R 6AF, United Kingdom
Printed in Croatia

British Library Cataloguing-in-Publication Data
A catalogue record for this book is available from the British Library

Additional hard and PDF copies can be obtained from orders@intechopen.com

Aflatoxin B1 Occurrence, Detection and Toxicological Effects
Edited by Xi-Dai Long
p. cm.
Print ISBN 978-1-83880-255-4
Online ISBN 978-1-83880-256-1
eBook (PDF) ISBN 978-1-83880-183-0
ISSN 2632-0983

For EU product safety concerns:
IN TECH d.o.o., Prolaz Marije Krucifikse Kozulić 3, 51000 Rijeka, Croatia,
info@intechopen.com or visit our website at intechopen.com.

IntechOpen Book Series
Biochemistry
Volume 14

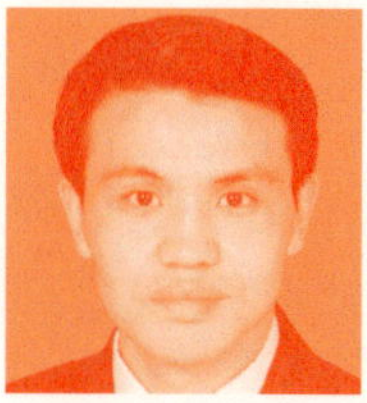

Prof. Long Xi-Dai is a lecturer at Youjiang Medical University for Nationalities and Shanghai Jiao Tong University, China. He started his teaching career at Youjiang Medical University for Nationalities, Bose, in 2004. He obtained his PhD degree in Tumor Pathology at the Shanghai Jiao Tong University, Shanghai, China. His research focuses on the analysis of aflatoxin toxification and detection, hepatocellular carcinoma genetics, molecular mechanisms, epidemiology, and tumor susceptibility. His current research interests focus on the association between aflatoxins and hepatocarcinoma. He has more than 50 publications, serves on the editorial boards of seven journals, and regularly reviews for 25 journals and five granting bodies. His achievements have been recognized by several awards and honors, including Shanghai Shu-Guang Scholar, Guangxi Specially-invited Expert, and Guangxi Zhouyue Scholar.

Editor of Volume 14:
Xi-Dai Long
Diagnostic and Research Center of Clinic-Pathology
The Affiliated Hospital of Youjiang Medical University for Nationalities, Bose, China

Book Series Editor: Miroslav Blumenberg
NYU Langone Medical Center, New York, USA

Scope of the Series

Biochemistry, the study of chemical transformations occurring within living organisms, impacts all of life sciences, from molecular crystallography and genetics, to ecology, medicine and population biology. Biochemistry studies macromolecules - proteins, nucleic acids, carbohydrates and lipids –their building blocks, structures, functions and interactions. Much of biochemistry is devoted to enzymes, proteins that catalyze chemical reactions, enzyme structures, mechanisms of action and their roles within cells. Biochemistry also studies small signaling molecules, coenzymes, inhibitors, vitamins and hormones, which play roles in the life process. Biochemical experimentation, besides coopting the methods of classical chemistry, e.g., chromatography, adopted new techniques, e.g., X-ray diffraction, electron microscopy, NMR, radioisotopes, and developed sophisticated microbial genetic tools, e.g., auxotroph mutants and their revertants, fermentation etc. More recently, biochemistry embraced the 'big data' omics systems.

Initial biochemical studies have been exclusively analytic: dissecting, purifying and examining individual components of a biological system; in exemplary words of Efraim Racker, (1913 –1991) "Don't waste clean thinking on dirty enzymes." Today however, biochemistry is becoming more agglomerative and comprehensive, setting out to integrate and describe fully a particular biological system. The 'big data' metabolomics can define the complement of small molecules, e.g., in a soil or biofilm sample; proteomics can distinguish all the proteins comprising e.g., serum; metagenomics can identify all the genes in a complex environment e.g., bovine rumen. This Biochemistry Series will address both the current research on biomolecules, and the emerging trends with great promise.

Contents

Preface XI

Section 1
Aflatoxin B1 Occurrence 1

Chapter 1 3
Aflatoxin B1: Chemistry, Environmental and Diet Sources and Potential Exposure in Human in Kenya
by Joseph Owuor Lalah, Solomon Omwoma and Dora A.O. Orony

Chapter 2 37
Aflatoxin Occurrence in Dairy Feeds: A Case of Bulawayo, Zimbabwe
by Nancy Nleya, Lubanza Ngoma and Mulunda Mwanza

Chapter 3 53
α-Amylase Production by Toxigenic Strains of *Aspergillus* and *Penicillium*
by Adekunle Odunayo Adejuwon and Victoria Anatolyivna Tsygankova

Chapter 4 75
Prevention by Essential Oils of the Occurrence and Growth of *Aspergillus flavus* and Aflatoxin B1 Production in Food Systems: Review
by Yamina Ben Miri, Azem Belasli, Djamel Djenane and Agustín Ariño

Section 2
Aflatoxin B1 Detection 93

Chapter 5 95
A New Approach for Detection of Aflatoxin B1
by Xing-Zhi-Zi Wang

Chapter 6 107
The Blood AFB1-DNA Adduct Acting as a Biomarker for Predicting the Risk and Prognosis of Primary Hepatocellular Carcinoma
by Qin-Qin Long, Xiao-Qin Wu and Jin-Guang Yao

Section 3
The Toxification Effects of Aflatoxin B1 117

Chapter 7 119
The Toxic Effects of Aflatoxin B1: An Update
by Yuhua Shan

Chapter 8 141
The Carcinogenicity of Aflatoxin B1
by Jie Li and Mengxi Liu

Chapter 9 153
X-Ray Repair Cross Complementing 4 (XRCC4) Genetic Single Nucleotide Polymorphisms and the Liver Toxicity of AFB1 in Hepatocellular Carcinoma
by Yan Deng, Xue-Min Wu, Xiao-Ying Huang and Xi-Dai Long

Section 4
The Detoxification of Aflatoxin B1 175

Chapter 10 177
Decontamination of Aflatoxin B1
by Qian Yang

Chapter 11 191
The Toxification and Detoxification Mechanisms of Aflatoxin B1 in Human: An Update
by Qun-Ying Su

Preface

Aflatoxin B1, a class-chemical carcinogen mainly produced by *Aspergillus flavus*, has noticeable toxicity because of its organophilism, mutagenic features, and carcinogenicity. Progression in understanding aflatoxin B1 has greatly improved with new techniques in genome sequencing and the development of molecular methods and tools that enable rapid molecular and genetic analyses for individual genomes. Especially, the genetics of aflatoxin B1 biosynthesis is regarded as a model to gain insight into fungal metabolism. This book reviews a number of important topics related to aflatoxin B1.

This book consists of 11 chapters, divided into four parts. The chapters are written by experts in the field of aflatoxins. Select topics are presented here to provide a snapshot of current understanding of the occurrence and metabolism of aflatoxin B1, the contamination, exposure, and detection of aflatoxin B1, and the toxicological effects and detoxification of aflatoxin.

The first part, Chapters 1–4, is devoted to the occurrence of aflatoxin B1, focusing on its chemistry, biological metabolism, and food exposure and control. In the first chapter, Joseph Owuor Lalah et al. review the chemistry, synthesis, analysis, and identification techniques, production conditions, and exposure information of aflatoxin B1 in Kenya. The second chapter by Nancy Nleya et al. illuminates aflatoxin occurrence in dairy feeds on the basis of analyses from a case in Bulawayo, Zimbabwe. Adekunle Odunayo Adejuwon et al. in the third chapter describe the potential value of aflatoxin B1-producing toxigenic strains of *Aspergillus flavus*, *Aspergillus parasiticus*, *Penicillium citrinum*, and *Penicillium rubrun*. Interestingly, their findings provide an important method for the industrial production of α-amylases. In the fourth chapter, Yamina Ben Miri et al. systematically review prevention by essential oils of the occurrence and growth of *A. flavus* and aflatoxin B1 production in food systems.

The second part of the book consists of Chapters 5 and 6 and deals with an updated view of aflatoxin B1 detection. In the fifth chapter, Xing-Zhizi Wang summarizes and evaluates the detection methods for aflatoxin B1, including enzyme-linked immunosorbent assay, high-performance liquid chromatography, and thin-layer chromatography. The sixth chapter by Qin-Qin Long et al. displays the effects of the aflatoxin B1-DNA adduct in the nucleus from peripheral blood white cells on the risk and prognosis of hepatocellular carcinoma investigated via a hospital-based case–control study. In their study, they collected relatively large samples without hepatitis virus B or C infection, including 380 patients with pathologically diagnosed hepatocellular carcinoma and 588 controls without any evidence of hepatic diseases. Their results show that the increasing amount of blood aflatoxin B1-DNA adducts significantly increase the risk and poor outcome of hepatocellular carcinoma. This is indicative of the serum aflatoxin B1-DNA adducts acting as a potential valuable detection method for aflatoxin B1.

The third part, consisting of Chapters 7–10, discusses the toxifications of aflatoxin B1 and particularly focuses on genic toxification, cytotoxicity, carcinogenicity, and liver injury. The seventh chapter by Yuhua Shan summarizes the toxicity and toxic mechanisms of aflatoxin B1 as well as detoxification of aflatoxin B1. The eighth chapter by Jie Li et al. summarizes recent literature involving aflatoxin B1's carcinogenicity, including the metabolism of aflatoxin B1 and DNA damage such as adduct formation, oxygenic damage, genic mutations, and genetic alteration. They also discuss how aflatoxin B1 results in abnormal DNA repair and reactive oxygen species depression, and explore all known biomarkers for predicting aflatoxin B1's carcinogenicity. The following chapter by Yan Deng et al. shows an important molecular mechanism: the different modificative effects of genetic single-nucleotide polymorphisms (GSNPs) in DNA repair gene XRCC4, using hospital-based clinical sample analysis. In their study, they screened a total of 143 GSNPs in the coding regions of XRCC4 and ultimately five SNPs (rs1237462915, rs28383151, rs762419679, rs766287987, and rs3734091) were confirmed to significantly alter the hepatoxic effects of aflatoxin B1. Particularly, they also found that some XRCC4 GSNPs (rs28383151, rs766287987, and rs3734091) modified the prognosis of patients with hepatocellular carcinoma.

The last part includes Chapters 10 and 11 and covers detoxification methods and corresponding mechanisms. In the eleventh chapter, Qian Yan reviews all known methods for aflatoxin B1 decontamination, including physical methods (e.g. cleaning and segregation, heating, microwave heat treatment, irradiation, electrolyzed water treatment, and pulsed light technology), chemical methods (e.g. ammonia decontamination treatment, hydrochloric acid treatment, lactic acid and citric acid treatment, and ozonation), biological methods (e.g. soil bacteria, fungi, yeasts and lactic acid bacteria, enzymes, and cold plasma technology), the sorbent additives method, and so on. In the twelfth chapter, Qun-Ying Su summarizes all significant detoxification mechanisms of aflatoxin B1 in the human body.

Together, the chapters in this book are a collection of contemporary works on aflatoxin B1 occurrence, detection, and toxification. Although not every topic in aflatoxin B1 could be reviewed or discussed in this book, I do believe that the authors have done an outstanding job and that it is helpful for readers who wish to become more familiar with the corresponding fields.

The editor wishes to acknowledge Ms. Kristina Kardum for her tireless efforts in collecting and organizing all of the manuscripts from our illustrious contributors.

Xi-Dai Long, PhD
Professor,
Diagnostic and Research Center of Clinic-Pathology,
The Affiliated Hospital of Youjiang Medical University for Nationalities,
Bose, China

Section 1

Aflatoxin B1 Occurrence

Chapter 1

Aflatoxin B1: Chemistry, Environmental and Diet Sources and Potential Exposure in Human in Kenya

Joseph Owuor Lalah, Solomon Omwoma and Dora A.O. Orony

Abstract

Cancer incidences and mortality in Kenya are increasing according to recent reports and now number among the top five causes of mortality in the country. The risk factors responsible for this increase in cancer incidences are assumed to be genetic and/or environmental in nature. The environmental factors include exposure to carcinogenic contaminants such aflatoxins (AFs). However, the exact causes of the increase in cancer incidences and prevalence in many developing countries are not fully known. Aflatoxins are known contaminants produced by the common fungi *Aspergillus flavus* and the closely related *Aspergillus parasiticus* which grow as moulds in human foods. Aflatoxin B1 (AFB1) is most common in food and is 1000 times more potent when compared with benzo(a)pyrene, the most potent carcinogenic polycyclic aromatic hydrocarbon (PAH). Aflatoxins have therefore drawn a lot of interest in research from food safety and human health point of view. In this chapter, the chemistry, synthesis, identification, toxicology and potential human health risks of AFB1 in Kenya are discussed.

Keywords: aflatoxin B1, chemistry, determination, toxicity, exposure, health risks, Kenya

1. AFB1 chemistry

The aflatoxins were discovered in a toxic peanut meal after causing 'turkey X' disease, which killed large numbers of turkey poults, ducks, young pheasants and chicks in the UK in the early 1960s [1], and more than 100,000 young turkeys in poultry farms were killed [2]. The peanut meal was highly toxic, and the toxin-producing fungi was identified as *Aspergillus flavus* hence the name of the toxin, aflatoxin [2]. Extracts of the feed later induced the now known toxic symptoms in experimental animals, and purified metabolites with properties identical to aflatoxins B1 and G1 (AFB1 and AFG1) were later isolated from the *Aspergillus flavus* cultures [1, 3, 4].

Structural elucidation of aflatoxins was accomplished and confirmed by total synthesis in 1963 [4]. There are four major aflatoxins B1, B2, G1 and G2 plus two additional toxic metabolic products M1 and M2 that are of significance as direct contaminants of foods and feeds and whose structures have been elucidated [3, 4].

These toxins have similar structures and form a unique group of highly oxygenated, naturally occurring heterocyclic compounds [5]. Their structures and molecular formulae are shown in **Figure 1**. *Aspergillus flavus* typically produces aflatoxin B1, which is the most potent and the most frequently identified in aflatoxin contaminations, and aflatoxin B2, whereas *Aspergillus parasiticus* produces aflatoxin G1 and aflatoxin G2 as well as aflatoxin B1 and aflatoxin B2. Four other aflatoxins M1, M2, B2A and G2A [3, 6], which are produced in minor amounts, were subsequently isolated from cultures of *Aspergillus flavus* and *Aspergillus parasiticus*. Aflatoxins M1 and M2, which are found in milk of animals that have consumed feeds contaminated with AFB1, are the hydroxylated metabolites of aflatoxins B1 and B2, respectively [3, 7]. Aflatoxins are, in essence, known as a group of mycotoxins which are produced primarily by some strains of *Aspergillus flavus* and by most strains of *Aspergillus parasiticus*, plus related species of *Aspergillus niger*, among others [8].

Aflatoxins are just a subset of class of mycotoxins which are fungal metabolites rampant and invisible in the environment and have caused severe effects on food security and safety especially within sub-Saharan African (SSA) societies [9]. This class of mycotoxins include *Fusarium* mycotoxins which have been found in oesophageal cancer-prone areas of South Africa [10], aflatoxins, fumonisins and ochratoxin A which have all been found to be rampant across West, East and Central Africa [11, 12]. Aflatoxins have become the most common and ubiquitous food contaminants produced by the common fungi *Aspergillus flavus* and the closely related *Aspergillus parasiticus*.

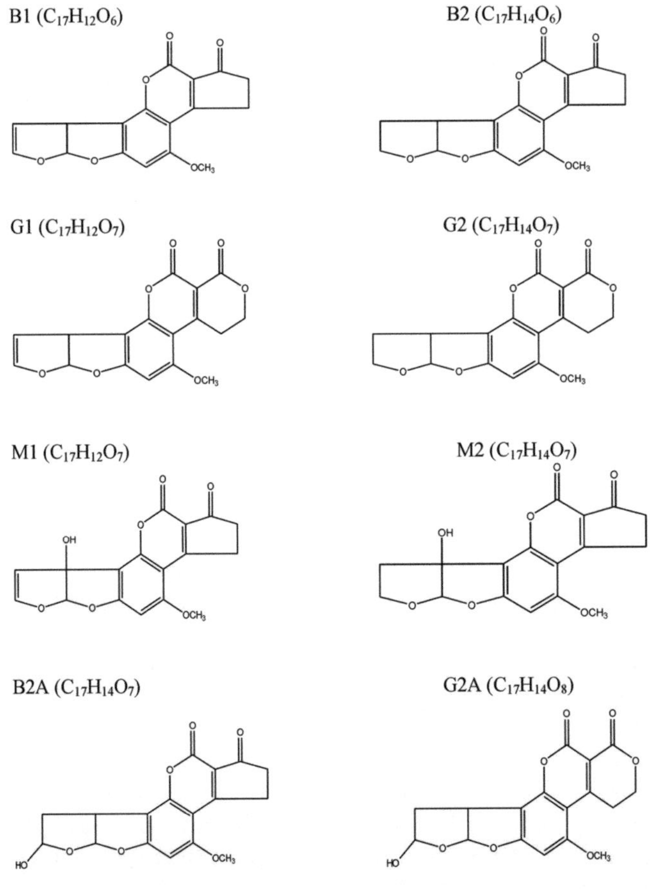

Figure 1.
Chemical structures of aflatoxin B1 and other related aflatoxin metabolites [3, 6].

Aflatoxin B1 (AFB1) is a secondary metabolite produced by *Aspergillus flavus* and *Aspergillus parasiticus* when environmental factors are favourable [13, 14]. It has also been characterized as a biological toxin. Biological toxins are defined as toxic substances produced by microorganisms, animals and plants that have the capability of causing harmful effects when inhaled, ingested, injected or absorbed (medical dictionary). Referring to **Figure 1**, all aflatoxins are heterocyclic compounds which have a common benzene ring, with slight variations only in terms of the presence of double bonds and ketonic groups and the metabolites having hydroxy groups, with hydroxylation positions varying from one metabolite to another. These structures indicate slight aqueous solubility and ease of epoxidation reaction, respectively, which are considered to influence both their excretion and toxicity. AFB1 which is the most prevalent and most potent, a human health hazard globally, has a peculiar double bond in the cyclic ring which is also observed in G1 and M1. For activation, AFB1 requires epoxidation to aflatoxin B1 2,3-epoxide. The microsomal cytochrome P450 (CYP450) monoxygenases biotransform the toxin to the less toxic metabolites aflatoxins M1 and G1 [5]. Aflatoxins are highly oxygenated and naturally occurring heterocyclic compounds [4] which have been separated based on their fluorescence under UV light and the presence or lack of a double bond at the 8, 9 carbons. Aflatoxins B1 and G1 have a double bond at the 8, 9 carbons, which allows for formation of an epoxide, a more toxic form of AFB1 and AFG1, while AFB2 and AFG2 do not. Aflatoxins B2 and G2 were established as the dihydroxy derivatives of B1 and G1, respectively. Whereas, aflatoxin M1 (AFM1) is 4-hydroxy aflatoxin B1, aflatoxin M2 is 4-dihydroxy aflatoxin B2 [5]. Hydrogenation of B1 and G1 yields B2 and G2, respectively.

The important physico-chemical properties of AFB1 are shown in **Table 1**. It is odourless, tasteless and colourless. It is difficult to detect sensorically, and therefore it poses a real challenge to food handlers, consumers and regulators who are in a bid to control or eradicate it [15–17]. AFB1 exists as colourless to pale yellow crystals or white powder [18]. Aflatoxins are densely fluorescent; B refers to blue fluorescence, while

Physico-chemical property	
IUPAC name	2,3,6a,9a-Tetrahydro-4-methoxycyclopenta[c] Furo[3′,2′:4,5]furo[2,3-*h*][l] benzopyran-1,11-dione
MW	312.277 g/mol
mp	268–269°C
Physical state	Colourless pale yellow crystalline to solid or white powder; odorless
Specific Optical rotation	−558 °/D at 25°C (0.1 M in chloroform) or −480 °/D at 25°C (0.1 M in dimethyl formamide)
Vapour pressure	2.65×10^{-10} mmHg at 25°C
Water solubility	16.14 mg/l at 25°C; decreases at low temperature; generally soluble in water and polar solvents
Stability	Stable until melting point; decomposed by UV irradiation in water/chloroform
Log K_{ow}	1.23
BCF (fish)	3
Koc (soil)	Ranges within 682–2.317×10^{-4}
Henry's law constant	1.4×10^{-13} atm m^3/mol at 25°C
Fluorescence emission	Densely fluorescent blue (λmax = 450 nm)
UV absorption	Absorbs at 223, 265 and 362 nm
Mass spectrum	Identified by LC–MS; ionization ESI; precursor-type $[M + H]^+$; m/z 313.071

Table 1.
Physico-chemical properties of AFB1.

G signifies green fluorescence. AFB1 exhibits a blue fluorescence with a fluorescence emission spectrum maximum of 425 nm and has UV maximum absorbance values at 223, 265 and 362 nm (in ethanol). It strongly absorbs UV light and is decomposed by it when dissolved in water or chloroform or when it is in form of solid films. AFBI has a Henry's law constant value of 1.40×10^{-13} atm m^3/mol at 25°C and a vapour pressure of 2.65×10^{-10} mmHg at 25°C. These properties would enable it to be less volatile and therefore has become very ubiquitous in the environment, becoming distributed in air, water and soil [15, 18]. It therefore can spread easily on the farm or in stores causing heavy damage to agricultural food crops and stored grains, respectively.

The vapour pressure of AFB1 indicates that AFB1 will tend to exist solely in particulate phase in the atmosphere if released into air, according to a model of gas/particle partitioning of semivolatile organic compounds [19]. The particulate bound AFB1 will then tend to be removed from the atmosphere by wet and dry deposition. Since it absorbs UV light, it is susceptible to direct photolysis by sunlight. If released to soil, AFB1 is expected to have low mobility based on its K_{oc} value which ranges from 682 to 2.3×10^4 and Freundlich adsorption coefficients, ranging from 17 to 238 mg/kg in different soil types. Volatilization from moist soils or water surfaces is not expected to be an important fate process based on its Henry's law constant value of 1.4×10^{-13} atm-cm/mol. It is also not expected to volatilize much from dry soil surfaces based on its vapour pressure which is very low. The K_{oc} of AFB1 indicates that it is expected to adsorb to soil and sediment. However, based on its K_{ow} and BCF values, AFB1 would tend to have a relatively moderate potential for bioconcentration in aquatic organisms and animal adipose tissue. Perhaps this explains why it is rapidly absorbed in the stomach and intestines and why it is present in the blood, kidney and liver where it imparts its toxicity. In the water environment, AFB1 can undergo hydrolysis as it contains a cyclic ester functional group and the rates of hydrolysis are similar to those of non-cyclic esters, ranging from months to a year under normal environmental conditions (i.e. pH 5–9) [19]. However, ring strain and steric hindrance have been reported to prevent its ease of hydrolysis, and therefore the extent of hydrolysis is unexpectedly low [18]. AFB1 biodegradation in soil and water has been studied, and it has been found that biodegradation may not be a very important environmental fate process. For example, after incubation for 120 days in silt loam, clay loam and sandy loam soil types, respectively, only 8.1, 4.9 and 1.4% complete mineralization to CO_2 was achieved [19]. Biodegradation in various soils with different pHs (ranging 5.8–7.3), organic carbon (OC) (ranging 0.46–2.82%) and cation exchange capacity (CEC) (ranging 11.7–18) showed very low concentrations of metabolites B2 and G2 after 1 day in a 20-day experiment, and the TLC results indicated that adsorption onto soil prevented AFB1 decomposition.

Biotransformation of aflatoxins has been studied and found to occur via four main routes [19–23]: (i) hydroxylation of carbon atom at junction of the two fused furan rings, aflatoxin B1 is converted into AFM1, and this occurs to some extent in the mammalian liver [19, 20]; (ii) oxidative o-demethylation of single aromatic methoxy-substituent gives aflatoxin P1 [19]; (iii) hydration of vinyl double bond would afford hemiacetals, and aflatoxin B1 has been converted to into hemiacetal AFB2A in pig, mouse and avian livers through this route [19, 22] and (iv) reduction of cyclopentenone ring, dihydroaflatoxicol, but this biotransformation seems to be confined to avian species and not mammals [19]. While the hydroxylated metabolite AFM1 is the product of metabolism of AFB1 and AFB2, G1 and G2 were established as dihydroxylated derivatives of B1 and B2, respectively. AFM1 is 4-hydroxy aflatoxin B1 and AFM2 is 4-hydroxy aflatoxin B2. The order of acute and chronic toxicity is B1 > FG1 > B2 > G2 [20].

Extensive studies on reactions of aflatoxins to various physico-chemical conditions and reagents have been conducted because of possible application of such reactions in detoxification of materials contaminated with aflatoxins [24]. In dry state, aflatoxins are heat stable up to melting point. However, in the presence of moisture and elevated temperatures, aflatoxins are destroyed to certain extents over a period of time. Such destructions of aflatoxins have been found to occur in oil seeds, meals and roasted peanuts or in aqueous solution at pH 7 [15–17]. It is postulated that such treatments can lead to the opening of the lactose ring, with possible destruction of decarboxylation, at elevated temperature [21]. In alkaline solution, hydrolysis of the lactose ring occurs, but this hydrolysis appears reversible, since it has also been shown that recyclization occurs following acidification of basic solutions containing aflatoxin [21, 24]. At a temperature of 100°C, lactose ring opening can occur, followed by a decarboxylation reaction [21]; and this reaction can further lead to a loss of the methoxy group from the aromatic ring [22]. In the presence of mineral acids, aflatoxins B1 and G1 are converted to aflatoxins B2A and G2A, respectively, due to acid-catalyzed insertion of water molecules across the double bonds in the furan ring, leading to hydroxylation (see **Figure 1** chemical structures). In the presence of acetic and hydrochloric acids, the reaction of AFB1 and AFG1, respectively, gives the acetoxyl derivatives, with acetoxyl groups attached on the benzene rings [22]. Similar adducts of aflatoxins B1 and G1 are formed with methanoic acid-thionyl chloride, acetic acid-thionyl chloride and trifluoroacetic acid [22]. Reactions with oxidizing agents, such as sodium hypochlorite, potassium permanganate, chlorine, hydrogen peroxide, ozone and sodium perborate, change the aflatoxin molecule in some way as indicated by loss of fluorescences although the mechanisms of these reactions are still uncertain as the products remain unidentified in most cases [25]. Hydrogenation of aflatoxins B1 and G1 yields aflatoxins B2 and G2, respectively. If further reduced by 3 mol of hydrogen, aflatoxin B1 yields tetrahydroxyl aflatoxin, while reduction of aflatoxins B1 and B2 with sodium borohydride yields aflatoxins RB1 and RB2, respectively. The RB1 and RB2 arise because of the opening of the lactose ring followed by reduction of the acid group and the keto group in the cyclopentane ring. However, it should be noted that breakdown of aflatoxins by various means does not guarantee safety of the contaminated substance. At times this breakdown is reversible or may lead to another form of aflatoxin. Besides, reaction products have not been subjected to detailed examination, including length of time the reactions take place [25]. Researchers have just concluded that the decomposition is not complete based on trials with food samples [26].

In general, the aflatoxins have been considered as difuranocoumarins, which are highly substituted coumarin derivatives containing a fused dihydrofurofuran moiety [1, 3, 4]. In particular, AFB1 is characterized by the fusion of a cyclopentenone ring to the lactone ring of the coumarin structure (**Figure 1**) and by strong fluorescence emission in the blue region (hence the designation B) when exposed to ultraviolet light [1, 3, 4]. Aflatoxins Bs strongly emit blue colour when they absorb UV light, and aflatoxins Gs strongly emit green colour when they absorb UV light. AFM1 is the principal hydroxylated metabolite of AFB1 and is produced upon the action of cytochrome P450 1A2 (CYP1A2) [27, 28]. It is strongly fluorescent, emitting blue-violet light. Specifically, AFB1 has similar chemical properties to other metabolites which include its slight solubility in water and polar organic solvents and less solubility in nonpolar solvents [23]. It has strong thermal stability, even at high temperature (>100°C), and this prevents it from being thermally degraded completely during food manufacturing, for example, when milk and dairy products are processed, since pasteurization and other thermal treatment methods alone are ineffective [29, 30]. Other chemical properties of AFB1, such as its instability to UV light or extreme pH conditions (<3 or >10) and reactivity of lactone moiety in the presence of ammonia or hypochlorite, have been useful in the development of methods for decontamination of feed and food [29, 30]. Several physical treatment methods like exposure to microwaves, gamma rays, X-rays and ultraviolet light have been investigated, but inconsistency of the results has discouraged their use, especially for heavily contaminated samples [31]. At present, ammoniation [32] and adsorption on clays or organic adsorbents [29] have commonly been used to achieve a good level of decontamination without disruption of the nutritional properties or safety of feed.

Biological methods of detoxification of mycotoxins are of two different types: the first being via enzymatic degradation and the second via sorption. In enzymatic biochemical processes, live microorganisms can biodegrade and mineralize the mycotoxins completely to CO_2 or absorb them by attaching them to their cells by active interaction and accumulation and thereby reducing them from the media. Dead organisms can adsorb mycotoxins, and they can be used to make biofilters for fluid decontamination of products, where the aflatoxins are left on the filter and the products become subsequently decontaminated, or as probiotics to bind and remove mycotoxins from the human intestine [15, 33]. Enzymatic degradation can be complete mineralization to CO_2, in which either extracellular or intracellular enzymes and various species of bacteria have been identified including *Pseudomonas*, *Bacillus* and *Lactobacillus* and used to inhibit toxicity or production of aflatoxins by *Aspergillus*. A large number of microorganisms (approximately 1000) have been screened for this purpose, but only *Lactobacillus* have been adopted [34, 35]. AFB1 and AFM1 have been shown to have a strong binding ability to other molecules, and recently research has been focusing on the AFB1-binding capacity to certain metabolites, for example, different strains of *Lactobacillus* in milk for aflatoxin decontamination in different products such as yoghurt [34, 36, 37].

Various chemical treatment processes have been tried, including sodium hypochlorite (NaOCl), potassium permanganate ($KMnO_4$), hydrogen peroxide (H_2O_2), sodium bicarbonate, sodium chloride and sodium borohydride ($NaHBO_3$) a well-known reducing agent, to detoxify or decompose aflatoxins in various foods [16, 38, 39]. These reagents can be used, and, for example, formaldehyde and NH_3 were found to neutralize AFB1, while $NaSO_4$ was found to be less efficient in neutralizing AFB1 [38]. However, these reactions have to be optimized in terms of quantities needed and reaction time as well as temperature and pressure conditions required. Different cooking methods have also been tried to remove aflatoxins from foods [16, 17, 38, 40]. Normal cooking of rice was found to destroy only 49% AFB1 [16, 17]. In other experiments to study the reduction of aflatoxins in various products, boiling of maize in traditional cooking used in Kenya destroys 11–17.6% AFB1 and AFG2 [40], while in beer making 18–27% AFB1 still remain [38] and in bread making 25% still remain [26]. Kirui [39], in assessing the levels of aflatoxins that were left after various treatments following physico-chemical and traditional cooking methods for maize and maize products, found that boiling maize reduced total aflatoxin level from 83 to 7 ppb, dry decortication reduced the level from 51.3 to 9.6 ppb, boiling with Magadi soda (food softener) reduced the level from 59 to 13.4 ppb, solar irradiation (18 h) reduced the level from 60.8 to 13.7 ppb and UV irradiation (18 h) reduced the level from 81.7 to 61.4 ppb. He found that only dry decortication method, which involves boiling with Magadi soda followed by washing with water and boiling, respectively, reduced the levels significantly but not completely below the maximum limits. Alkali treatment with inorganic (e.g. boiling with NaCl) and organic bases were reported to be effective and economically feasible [17]. Occupational exposure to AFB1 has been reported to occur through inhalation and dermal contact at work places where commodities such as peanuts, grains, linseed oil or animal feeds are produced, stored or used. An average AFB1 exposure of 64 ng/d-kg body weight was reported for Danish workers in the animal feed production industry. General population may most likely be exposed to AFB1 via ingestion of contaminated food [18].

2. Synthesis of aflatoxin B1

The biosynthetic pathway of AFB1 has been explained by researchers. It is derived from both a dedicated fatty acid synthase (FAS) and a polyketide synthase (PKS) which occur in the mould, together known as norsolorinic acid synthases. The biosynthetic pathway has been described by Singh and Hsich [41], Yu et al. [42] and Dewick [43], among others, and, an outline of the method can be found in Wikipedia. The process begins with a FAS-aided synthesis of hexanoic acid, which is the starter unit for the iterative type I PKS. A PKS catalyzes addition of seven malonyl-CoA molecules to the hexanoic acid to form a C20 polyketide compound. The polyketide folds through a cyclization process induced by a PKS to form an anthraquinone norsolorinic acid, and a reductase enzyme then catalyzes the reduction of the ketone on the norsolorinic acid side chain to yield an intermediate, an averantin [41–43]. From here, various processes which are assisted with different enzymes including hydroxylases, dehydrogenases (for oxygenation and cyclization), CYP450 oxidases, esterases, reductases, methyl transferases and oxidoreductases occur, leading to different intermediates. The pathway for AFB1 biosynthesis is very complicated, and some of the enzymes and intermediates involved continue to be elucidated and characterized [43].

Under favorable moulding conditions, *Aspergillus flavus* spores germinate by attaching their mycelium in a food substrate and secreting enzymes which break down nutrients into simpler compounds capable of digestion. During digestion, *Aspergillus flavus* then produces, as described in the foregoing paragraph, secondary metabolites, including AFB1, meant to give the fungi a competitive edge against other microorganisms [44].

For research and other purposes, aflatoxins can be produced in small quantities by fermentation of *Aspergillus flavus* or *Aspergillus parasiticus* on solid substrates or media [45]. It is extracted by solvents and purified by chromatography [45]. AFB1 and other aflatoxins have been produced through this method by many chemical companies including Sigma-Aldrich, among others. While doing the purification, it is important to note that *Aspergillus flavus* produces only B aflatoxins and sometimes the mycotoxin cyclopiazonic acid (CPA), while *Aspergillus parasiticus* produces both B and G aflatoxins but not CPA. Various mutants of *Aspergillus flavus* have varying relative stability ratios of B2/B1 [45, 46]. Ada and Matcha [46] described a method for aflatoxin production by fermentation in which an *Aspergillus flavus* strain isolated from groundnut, referred to as *Aspergillus flavus* strain AJ, was used. The *Aspergillus flavus* strain AJ was found to be very stable and consistently yielded higher levels of aflatoxins, especially AFB1, after transfers [46]. In their preparation Ada and Matcha [46] used inoculums prepared by inoculating tubes (1.5 × 15 cm) of potato-dextrose-agar with spores of the AJ. This strain was used to produce an aflatoxin stain AJ2010. The potato-dextrose-agar gel was prepared by adding 20 g dextrose, 20 mg NaCl and 1 g of agar in 100 ml distilled in a conical flask, adjusting and maintaining the mixture at pH 7. The mixture was kept momentarily at 121°C in an autoclave and then platted in a laminar flow [46, 47]. The inoculated slants were then incubated for 7–21 days at 28°C after which the cultures had a heavy crop of green *conidia*, and the spores were scraped loose with a loop. The slants were shaken to give a uniform suspension of spores, and the spore suspension (0.5 ml) was used to inoculate each of 100 g of the substrate (groundnut), a fish feed. Fermentation which involved the growth of *A. flavus* on the feed (100 g) at high moisture levels to produce a pale green aflatoxin substrate was carried out by mixing 25 ml distilled water with 50 g of fish feed in an Erlenmeyer flask. The mixture was allowed to stand for 1 h with frequent shaking, and then the flasks were autoclaved at 15 psi for 15 min before cooling and inoculation, keeping the flasks at 28°C and blending on a shaker at 188 rev/min. The flasks were removed, and the feed was prevented from binding with the produced mould mycelium by shaking vigorously. The product could be used for experiments directly or for extraction of a concentrate of aflatoxins using 80% methanol as explained by Nelson et al. [48] and Ada and Matcha [46, 48].

3. Analysis and identification of aflatoxin B1

Several sampling and analytical methods which include thin-layer chromatography (TLC), high-performance liquid chromatography (HLPC), mass spectrometry and enzyme-linked immunosorbent assay (ELISA), among others, have been used to analyse aflatoxin B1 in various contaminated foods [49]. According to the Food and Agriculture Organization, the worldwide maximum tolerated levels of aflatoxin B1 were reported to be in the range of 1–20 μg/kg in human foods and 5–50 μg/kg in dietary cattle feeds in 2003 [50]. Apart from these limits, the WHO, EU, USFDA and Kenya Bureau of Standards (KEBS) have set international and national maximum limits for a specific aflatoxin metabolite (e.g. AFB1) level, as well as a total concentration which involves the summation of concentrations of all detected metabolites (AFB1, AFB2, AFG1, AFG2 and AFM1) in a sample. It is therefore important to optimize and interpret standard procedures for extraction, detection and quantitation of aflatoxins in a sample. A review of the methods that have been used is presented in the following paragraphs.

Various researchers, including analysts, food specialists and health workers, have been involved in the analysis of aflatoxins including AFB1 in various materials including samples of human specimens, animal tissues, food, grains, cereals and legumes. Aflatoxins, AFB1 included, have been characterized by nuclear magnetic resonance (NMR) and liquid chromatography-mass spectrometry (LC–MS), and their mass spectral data are available in LC–MS libraries making it possible to screen samples rapidly. In addition, retention times and column flow-through patterns for aflatoxins combined with high-purity reference standards can be used in HPLC and other analytical techniques. Aflatoxins B1, B2, G1 and G2 have been determined quantitatively by HPLC with a fluorimetric detector using toluene as a mobile phase [51]. This method is applicable to food and feed extracts. Several AOAC official methods have been used to analyze AFB1 [1, 52]. These methods include ELISA, TLC and HPLC. TLC and fluorescence detection methods sometimes have reported high detection limits and are not used frequently nowadays for forensic purposes despite their popularity in the past. The methods for determination of aflatoxins in food samples and cereals for animal consumption can be validated as explained in the EC No. 882/2004 and EC No. 401/2006 methods, demonstrating their conformity with these methods, in terms of sensitivity, linearity, selectivity and precision [53].For mass spectral data, tandem mass spectrometry data containing a METLIN-tested metabolite database generated independently by the Scripps Center for Mass Spectrometry and Metabolics for identification of metabolites are available for reference in pdf. This product is available in Sigma-Aldrich. Other libraries are available for referencing including a Sigma-Aldrich database which presents HPLC Analysis of Aflatoxin Analogs on Ascentis® C18; a Sigma-Aldrich LC/MS/MS Analysis of μL Mycotoxins on Ascentis® Express Phenyl-Hexyl column and a Sigma-Aldrich UHPLC–MS/MS Analysis of μL Mycotoxins on Titan™ C18.

A high-performance liquid chromatographic method with online post-column photochemical derivatization and fluorimetric detection was used for simultaneous separation and quantitative determination of AFB1 and other metabolites in foodstuffs and feed material [53]. In one study, the chromatographic separation was accomplished by using a C18 column and analytes were eluted with an isocratic mobile phase consisting of water/methanol/acetonitrile [52]. In this method sample preparation requires simple extraction of aflatoxins with a mixture of water and methanol followed by a clean-up and a chromatographic separation step by immunoaffinity column and then detection [53]. Efficient analysis of aflatoxins B1, B2, G1 and G2 has also been achieved by matrix-assisted laser desorption/ionization time-of-flight mass spectrometry, using a UV-absorbing ionic liquid matrix with addition of NaCl to obtain matrix-free mass spectra, which enhances sensitivity via Na^+ cationization [53]. Using ionic alpha-cyano-4-hydroxycinnamic acid (Et3N-alpha-CHCA) as the matrix, the matrix-free mass spectra in the m/z range of interest were acquired, and the B1, B2, G1 and G2 aflatoxins were readily detected with very low detection limits [53]. This technique is fast and requires minimal sample preparation (just mixing the liquid matrix with methanol extract), and no derivatization nor chromatographic separation is required. The method was reported to be suitable for rapid screening of aflatoxins including AFB1 in a wide array of major crops which are often subjected to huge world commercial trades such as peanuts, maize and rice, as well as to monitor bioterrorism threats by mycotoxin poisoning [53].

Analysis of aflatoxins in clinical laboratory procedures is also often done routinely by analyzing AFB1 in blood and urine. This has been done by HPLC with various columns and a fluorescence detector as reported by Seo et al. [54]. Aflatoxin B1 recoveries ranged from 33 to 95%, for spiked human serum samples following extraction using hexane chloroform, chloroform extraction and clean-up with pentane on a silica gel column or acetone-ferric gel-chloroform extraction and clean-up with pentane on a silica gel column [55]. This reverse phase HPLC procedure was also used successfully for aflatoxins and metabolites in animal tissues, in a process involving trifluoroacetic acid-catalyzed conversion of aflatoxin B1 to a fluorescent derivative B2 [55]. Human urine and methanol extracted from the kidney, liver, brain tissues and sputum have been analysed using competitive ELISA methods with immunoaffinity columns and fluorometry, with concentrations for urine, sputum and tissue biopsies found to range from 1.0 to 5.0 ppb, with negative control patients showing no detectable mycotoxins in their fluids or tissues [56]. This study confirmed that AFB1 and other aflatoxins can be detected in body fluids and human tissues from patients exposed to mycotoxin-producing moulds in the environment and indicated which tissues or body fluids are most likely to give positive results. A procedure involving salting-out-assisted liquid/liquid extraction for multi-mycotoxin biomarkers and subsequent analysis using high-performance liquid chromatography-tandem mass spectrometry, for pig urine, has also been reported [53].

Radioimmunoassays that can detect levels as low as 0.27 pmol (0.06 ng) of AFB1 have been used to analyse crude extracts of corn and peanut butter with just traces of aflatoxins, and in these foodstuffs, as little as 1 μg aflatoxin/kg has been measured by this technique [57]. Detection limits for radioimmunoassay techniques vary ranging from 1 up to 5 μg/kg in various matrices including corn, peanut butter, cottonseed products, groundnuts and groundnut products and other cereals [1].

Recently, a comprehensive technique involving detection and quantification of aflatoxins using an AflaTest method has been described by William and George [58] and Orony et al. [59]. In this method, the presence of aflatoxins was tested in a screening step by TLC using the solvents hexane, petroleum ether, chloroform, acetone and toluene (10:10:60:10:10), and fluorescent spots were checked under UV light [59]. An AflaTest affinity column is an immunoaffinity column bound with specific antibodies of aflatoxin. When a sample is passed through, the aflatoxins become bound to the antibodies in the column [58]. A volume of 1 ml of the extract was diluted with distilled water and mixed well before filtering through a glass microfiber filter, and an aliquot of the filtrate was pipetted and passed through the AflaTest affinity column [59]. The column was cleaned twice with distilled water to remove the immunoaffinity impurities, and then aflatoxins were eluted from the column with HPLC-grade methanol and collected in a cuvette. A known volume of a developer solution (bromine solution in distilled water (5:45 vol/vol)) was added to the eluate, and then aflatoxin content was determined in the mixture using a fluorometer after a short period of 1 min. The fluorometer can have an inbuilt aflatoxin calibration standard, and it detects the intensity of the fluorescence which is determined by the amount of total aflatoxin present in the sample, and then a digital read out is obtained [59]. The limit of detection of the aflatoxins in this method was very low, about 0.05 μg/kg. Samples analysed using this method included fresh, smoked and grilled fish.

Wasike [60] used an ELISA method, which is recommended by the FAO for rapid screening of agricultural produce such as grains and involves several steps including the following: *coating* where the polystyrene plates are treated with a standard solution of either an antigen or antibody of the aflatoxin, *blocking* where unrelated protein-based solution is used to cover all the unbound sites on the plate, *detection* where enzyme-conjugated antibody or antigen binds specifically to the target antigen or antibody and *read out of results* in which the substrate (extract) is added and the signal produced by the enzyme-substrate reaction (binding) is measured [50]. The measurement can be done for total aflatoxin or single metabolite (e.g. AFB1), respectively, by UV–VIS using a calibration standard, prepared by pure analytical grade (>95% purity) AFB1 obtained from suppliers. Quantitation is based on absorbance readings (at 450 nm) versus concentrations of known standards. Several recommended quality assurance procedures were followed as described by [50]. A number of laboratories in developing countries including Kenya, where aflatoxin contamination is highly prevalent, have received training and funding to establish their own laboratories which are equipped with necessary instrumentation from the FAO to enable them to achieve rapid screening of samples using this ELISA method [50]. The FAO [50] procedure is simple, and for grains such as maize, 1 kg of the sample is weighed and milled using an electric grinder (mill). About 2 g of the ground sample is weighed into a screw-cap glass vial. This is then followed by addition of 10 ml methanol/distilled water (in the ratio of 70:30 v/v) and mixing for 10 min at room temperature using a shaker. The entire extract is filtered using a Whatman filter paper No. 1. Then 100 μl of filtrate is diluted with 600 μl distilled water of which 50 μl is employed as the substrate per well in the assay [50]. An aflatoxin test kit containing standard solutions of microtiter plate with 96 wells coated with capture antibodies; aflatoxin standard with ranges of concentrations of aflatoxin B1; a conjugate (6 ml)—peroxidase-conjugated aflatoxin B1—ready for use; anti-aflatoxin monoclonal antibodies (6 ml); Red Chromogen Pro (10 ml), a substrate/chromogen solution stained red and a 1 N sulphuric acid stop solution (14 ml) which converts the reactants from blue to yellow colour is provided [60]. A buffer salt (washing buffer pH 7.4) and distilled water and 70% methanol solution (70:30 vol/vol, methanol/distilled water), respectively, are prepared and made available for extraction of ground/homogenized material.

Nduti et al. [26] recently analysed aflatoxin B1 in cereals and other agricultural produce including sun-dried grains of maize and millet, maize flour and millet flour samples by PCR, a modified procedure similar to the ELISA methods reported by other researchers [50, 58, 59, 61]. The samples were transported immediately after sampling in cool boxes to an ISO 1705 accredited by Kenya Bureau of Standards laboratory and stored at −20°C until analysis was started. After grinding in a blender, known masses were weighed into disinfected beakers for extraction with a known volume of 70% methanol (in deionized water) by stirring. This was followed by filtering into a disinfected conical flask using Whatman filter paper No. 1. The residue on the filter paper was discarded and the filtrate preserved in the beaker for analysis. For analysis of aflatoxins, a known volume of a conjugate was introduced into the microwells using a micropipette, and then small aliquots of the filtrate were added [26]. A sample of 20 ppb of aflatoxin was put into one of the microwells as a control. After, 100 μl of the sample plus conjugate mixture was transferred to antibody-coated microwells and the mixtures incubated for 15 min. The method of Leszczynka et al. [61] was modified by using a specific conjugate mixture, thus eliminating the need for wells pre-washed with phosphate buffer solution (PBS). The PBS cleans the unbound proteins but also reduces sensitivity at the enzyme reaction site [62]. After incubation, the contents of the microwells were discarded and the microwells washed at least five times with distilled water to remove the nontoxin reactants [26]. After draining the water, an aliquot of the substrate solution was put into each of the microwells before incubation for another 5 min. The free and peroxidise-combined aflatoxins compete for the sites with mouse antibodies that are immobilized on the plates. The reaction in this process results in a colour change from a clear to a blue colouration, whose intensity indicates the aflatoxin content. A deeper colour indicates more reaction and binding with the substrate and less aflatoxin concentration in the sample. To stop the reaction, an acidic stop solution was added, which resulted in colour changes from blue to yellow, depending on the aflatoxin levels [26]. The resultant solutions in the microwells were fed into a microtiter plate PCR reader where the optical density of each microwell was read using a 450 nm filter, and the amount of total aflatoxin present in each sample was determined quantitatively online and recorded on a computer [26].

The maximum levels (MLs) are established in various countries in Europe and the USA using various standard ELISA-based procedures [63]. For aflatoxin B1, the 5121AFB method and its kit provide a competitive enzyme immunoassay based on antibodies directed against anti-aflatoxin B1 [63]. The kit includes 96 wells 12 × 8 break-apart. The conjugate is aflatoxin-horseradish peroxidase. Rapid sample preparation procedures for cereals, rice, eggs, nut, honey, mashed fruits edible oils and feed are included in the kit manual. Antibody cross-reactivity includes aflatoxin B1 (100%), aflatoxin B2 (20%), aflatoxin G1 (17%) and aflatoxin G2 (4%). These standard procedures involve conjugate and standard/sample being pipetted into the wells and incubated for 1 h at 37°C. After washing, the ready-to-use substrate is added and incubated for 30 min at 20–25°C. The reaction is stopped and the absorbance read in a UV spectrophotometer at 450 nm. A EuroProxima software converts the measured optical density into concentration of the metabolite in the starting material. The assay limits of detections (LOD) (in ppb), calculated as Xn + 3SD as determined under optimal conditions, are cereals (0.5), rice (0.4), eggs (0.2), nuts (0.75), honey (0.2), mashed fruits (0.6), edible oils (1.0) and feed (1.0). The calibration standard concentrations ranged within 0, 0.0157, 0.0313, 0.0625, 0.125, 0.25 and 0.5 ng/ml [63].

Direct evidence for human exposure to AFs by ingestion or another route has been found in a number of countries by identifying AFs or their metabolites in human biological samples [46, 64]. Thus, it is becoming a significantly important issue for health of adults and people who are directly exposed to food contaminated with AFs [46, 64, 65]. Analyses of human specimen samples have to be done sometimes both for forensic and research purposes. In one analytical procedure [56], 100 mg of kidney sample was added to 1 ml tubes containing 1 ml 50% methanol before incubation for 5 min, until it completely dissolved. After, the suspensions were centrifuged at 10,000 rpm for 10 min and the upper layers (800 μl) collected into 2 ml glass tubes, before taking 5 μl for analysis using a UHPLC Q-Orbitrap, with triplicate measurements for each aliquot. Metabolites were separated in a UHPLC system (Dionex UltiMate 3000) equipped with a Waters column (Acquity BEH C18 1.7 μm, 2.1 × 50 mm) incubated at 40°C. The mobile phases were made up of water containing 0.1% formic acid and 2 mM ammonium formate (solvent a) and acetonitrile (solvent b), as explained [56]. The Q Exactive instrument, equipped with thermoelectrospray ionization in positive and negative switching modes, was utilized to detect the aflatoxins in the above samples, and the system was calibrated and controlled by a software (Xcalibur 3.1 and Q Exactive Tune) [56]. The UHPLC Q-Orbitrap analysis can produce large amounts of raw data using TraceFinder software [56]. In addition, kidney tissue was isolated and fixed in 4% paraformaldehyde for 48 h, before paraffin embedding and sectioning using a microtome (Leica, Germany); and the sections were stained, and the histopathology was assessed under a light microscope (Olympus, Japan), with photographs being taken at 200× magnification, for confirmation of aflatoxin exposure [56]. Blood samples were centrifuged to collect serum (15 min at 3000 rpm and 4°C) for measurement of biochemical parameters, including creatinine, urea, uric acid, malondialdehyde, superoxide dismutase and total antioxidant capacity, which were undertaken using ELISA kits [56].

In another analytical method for AFB1, ELISA, TLC and HPLC were validated and used for identification of aflatoxin B1 (AFB1) in contaminated fish feed, media and fish serum samples [46, 48, 66–69, 122]. The analysis and identification of AFB1 was achieved using a DOA-ELISA test kit, followed by TLC with retention factors of 0.81, 0.79, 0.81 and 0.80 for AFB1-contaminated fish feed, media and serum samples, respectively, co-chromatographed with an AFB1 reference standard. HPLC results showed that the AFB1 levels in contaminated fish feed, media and serum samples were 2.6, 2.6 and 2.7 ng/ml, respectively. The concentrations of AFB1 were almost similar for all the three samples but slightly higher in the fish serum sample which had 2.7 ng/ml; and it was therefore concluded that because of its accuracy and sensitivity when compared with routine methods of AFB1 analysis, fish serum provides a sensitive specimen for AFB1 analysis in fish. This TLC-HPLC method was strongly recommended for monitoring AFB1 contamination in feed stuffs, especially in fisheries where the feed is under continuous exposure to moisture. The method is highly recommended in aquaculture and fisheries to screen the mycotoxins in fish feed as it gives a measure of bioaccumulation of these toxins in fish serum which can be correlated well with toxic effects on different environments like in vitro and in vivo to help in ensuring safety and measuring AFB1 tolerance. In one study [46], detailed methods for fermentation using an inoculated *Aspergillus flavus* strain isolated from groundnut to produce aflatoxins which were used to validate the analysis by TLC, HPLC and ELISA were presented.

Direct determination of urinary mycotoxins is a better approach to assess individual's exposure than the indirect estimation from average dietary intakes [70]. In a study by Fouad et al. [70], a new analytical method was developed and validated for simultaneous analysis of aflatoxins including AFB1 in urine based on ELISA. Like other ELISA methods so far described, the phenomenon of fluorescence quenching of an antibody by a specific ligand was applied in developing the technique for detection of mycotoxins, such as aflatoxin B1, ochratoxin A and zearalenone where loss of absorbance corresponds to inverse of concentration of aflatoxins [71].

Detecting aflatoxicosis in humans and animals is difficult due to variations in clinical signs and the presence of other factors such as suppression of the immune system caused by an infectious disease [72]. Of the two techniques most often used to detect levels of aflatoxins in humans, the first one involves measurement of the metabolite in urine (which however is only present for 24 h after exposure), and the second one involves measuring the level of aflatoxin-contaminated nuts, an AFB-albumin compound in the blood serum, providing information on exposure over weeks or months [72]. These biomarker measurements are important in investigating outbreaks where aflatoxin contamination is suspected. A variety of methods for detection of aflatoxins in food and feed that are highly specific, useful and practical have so far been discussed and are available for different needs. Methods are therefore available for different needs, ranging from techniques/methods for regulatory control in official laboratories (such as high-performance liquid chromatography-mass spectrometry (HPLC–MS)) [73, 74] to rapid test kits for factories and grain silos such as enzyme-linked immunosorbent assay (ELISA) [50, 73]. Potential novel aflatoxin detection systems, based on emerging technologies, include dipstick kits, hyperspectral imaging, electronic noses, molecularly imprinted polymers and aptamer-based biosensors (small organic molecules that can bind specific target molecules). The latter technologies may have relevance in remote areas because of their stability, ease of production and use. Sampling procedures for aflatoxin monitoring in export and import produce are problematic because moulds and aflatoxins are not evenly distributed throughout bulk shipments and batches of stored grain, and appropriate sampling is critical to get a representative result. Protocols for sampling procedures have been developed, in particular in the context of regulatory control. For instance, in setting maximum levels for aflatoxins, the Codex Alimentarius Commission has specified the protocols to be used for peanuts, almonds, Brazil nuts, hazelnuts, dried figs and pistachios intended for further processing and for ready-to-eat products [75]. The FAO of the United Nations [50] has developed a mycotoxin sampling tool which is available online. Recommended sampling methods are difficult to achieve, especially for subsistence farmers in rural areas who do not produce enough grain to spare the quantities needed for accurate testing. Thus, there is a need to develop rapid, low-cost, low-technology and accurate detection methods for aflatoxins to improve surveillance and control in rural areas. Organizations, such as the Partnership for Aflatoxin Control in Africa and the World Food Programme, are addressing these issues. The World Food Programme has instituted a Purchase-for-Progress Programme to ensure grain quality by creating a blue box, which contains test kits for grain quality, including aflatoxins [76]. Some of the problems encountered in sampling in Kenya have been discussed [76].

The main concern in aflatoxins exposure is that once they are formed, they are heat stable so that neither cooking nor freezing can destroy them completely and they therefore remain in food indefinitely and can cause sublethal effects in the body of humans and animals [15–17, 26, 29, 36, 38, 39]. When given a sample of food or a specimen such as human milk for a forensic test, it is possible to predict which particular aflatoxin is suspected depending on the type of food, feed or specimen. There is potential increase in consumers' health risks if higher levels of aflatoxins are permitted for various crops and other products. For example, increasing the current MLs from 4 μg/kg total aflatoxin to say 8 or 10 μg/kg for nuts such as cashew nuts, almonds and hazelnuts would have minor effects on the estimated dietary exposure, on the risk of cancer and the calculated margin of exposure, but due to carcinogenicity and genotoxicity limits, the MLs should be kept very low. The development of new methods for detecting and quantifying traces of aflatoxins and their metabolites in various matrices in future will influence not only the MLs but also reduce their lethality following human exposure.

Highlights on how changes in temperature, humidity, rainfall and carbon dioxide production due to climate change impact on fungal behaviour and consequently mycotoxin production have been investigated by researchers in Europe. Climate change has been reported as a driver for emerging food and feed safety issues worldwide, and the expected impact on the presence of mycotoxins in food and feed is of great concern [77]. AFB1 has the highest acute and chronic toxicity of all mycotoxins; hence, the maximal concentration in agricultural food and feed products and their commodities is regulated worldwide [77]. In this regard, the methods of analysis and detection, the structures and characteristics of aflatoxins and modelling of their maximum levels in various produce are expected to change in the future with changes in climate

4. Conditions for production of aflatoxin B1

The different species of *Aspergillus* require different conditions for optimal growth. The optimal temperature for *A. flavus* and *A. parasiticus* fungal growth and aflatoxin production is 35 and 33°C, respectively, and neither *Aspergillus* species produces aflatoxins when developed below 7.5 nor above 40°C [78]. Some researchers have reported ideal temperatures between 20 and 35°C and ideal relative humidity of more than 85% as optimal for growth of *Aspergillus* species and aflatoxin production [79]. According to other reports, usually the most important variables are the moisture content of the substrate and the relative humidity of the surroundings [80]. The moulds live in soil, surviving off dead plant and animal matter, but spread through the air via airborne *conidia* [26]. The moulds are often found in the outdoor and indoor air, in water, on food items, and in dust [81]. *Aspergillus flavus* and *Aspergillus parasiticus* are closely related and grow as saprophytes on plant debris of many crop plants left on and in the soil. They belong to the *Trichocomaceae* family and have a worldwide distribution but are commonly found in tropical climates with extreme ranges of rainfall, temperature and humidity [81]. Members of *Aspergillus* genus are characterized by production of nonseptate conidiophore which is quite distinct from septate hyphae; they are swollen at the tip to form a vesicle in which specialized spore-producing cells (phialides or sterigmata) are found. These specialized cells are either uniseriate or are short growths of biseriate metulae [81]. Colonies of *Aspergillus flavus* are green-yellow to yellow-green or green on Czapek's agar. They normally have biseriate sterigmata and reddish brown sclerotia. The conidia are coarse roughened and vary in size and are oval to spherical in shape. Colonies of *A. parasiticus* are dark green on Czapek's agar and remain green with age, and their sterigmata are uniseriate and usually have no sclerotia. Unlike *A. flavus*, the colonies of *A. parasiticus* are uniform in size and shape [81].

Improper farming practices have led to an increase in mould growth and aflatoxin contamination in crops and animals. Improper feeding habits such as feeding animals with spoilt maize, feeding mouldy human food to animals and blending of mouldy cattle feed with a fresh batch are some of the bad practices found in Kenya [26]. In common agricultural practice the rotten maize cobs are separated from the good maize cobs which are later shelled and milled. The rotten maize grains are used, by mixing one bag of clean grains and two bags of rotten grains, to make animal feeds [25]. This practice of dilution does not drastically reduce the amount of aflatoxin contamination in animal feeds, and hence, commercial feeds in Kenya have been found to be contaminated with aflatoxin B1 and milk with aflatoxin M1 [82]. The eastern part of Kenya has been found to have more cases of historical occurrences of aflatoxin contamination, while the central and western parts have shown increased risk of aflatoxin contamination [83]. Transferring of seeds, crops, animal feeds and animals from one region to another can also introduce *Aspergillus* in areas where it not was found originally.

Aflatoxins often occur in crops in the field before harvest and are usually associated with drought stress [79]. Poor storage conditions, especially during rainy seasons, can increase concentration of aflatoxins in produce [26]. They occur mainly in hot and humid regions where high temperature and humidity are optimal for mould's growth and toxin production [26]. The growth of fungi is caused by a number of factors which provide an ideal environment that promotes the growth [83]. The conditions that must all be prevailing for fungal growth to occur in Kenya include relative humidity above 70%, temperatures of over 30°C for a period of a few days to a week and stress to the affected plant, such as drought, flood or insect infestation. Furthermore, there must be high moisture content of crop (20% or higher) [24]. The prevailing climatic conditions in Kenya, which include drought, erratic rainfall, high temperatures ranging between 20 and 35°C and high humidity (40–89%), provide a favourable environment for growth of mould and production of aflatoxins [84]. Mould usually does not grow in properly dried and stored foods, and therefore efficient drying of commodities and maintenance of the dry state, or proper storage, are an effective measure against mould growth and production of mycotoxins [25]. Therefore, to minimize the health risk from mycotoxins, people are advised to inspect whole grains (especially corn, sorghum, wheat, rice), dried figs and nuts such as peanuts, pistachio, almond, walnut, coconut, Brazil nuts and hazelnuts, which are all regularly contaminated with aflatoxins for evidence of mould, and discard any that look mouldy, discoloured or shrivelled [11]. They are also required to avoid damage of grains before and during drying and in storage, as damaged grain is more prone to invasion of moulds and therefore mycotoxin contamination [24].

Researchers have reported on *Aspergillus* growth in maize and millet and contamination of agricultural soils in Kenya and the conditions and mechanisms that encourage their growth, which include (i) contamination of grains when they come into contact with *Aspergillus* fungal spores in soils, (ii) transfer of spores onto maize cobs when still on the plant by wind, (iii) high tropical temperatures existing in maize and millet growing regions, (iv) changes in seasons from wet to dry with hot and humid or damp conditions providing most favourable conditions, (v) insect pest damage causing 'open wounds' on seeds/grains, (vi) mistiming of ideal harvest periods, (vii) failure to separate damaged cobs from good cobs and (viii) intensional mixing of bad grains with good grains with intention of lowering aflatoxin levels [26, 60]. The lack of adherence to handling procedures such as adequate drying period, maintaining required moisture levels, the lack of optimal ventilation and temperature during storage, failure by national cereal board to purchase the grains from farmers on time and failure of the board to follow regulations such as performing analysis on moisture and aflatoxin presence in the products to ensure levels conform the required maximum level standards during their purchase [76] have also been cited as factors which encourage moulding and aflatoxin contamination in maize. The growth of moulds is also dependent on the type of crops and their nutrient content [26]. Mould growth in maize is very common, especially in warm humid climates, because it is a good substrate for mould growth, especially those species that produce aflatoxins [78, 79]. The high carbohydrate content provides the two carbon precursors for mycotoxin synthesis [79]. Other cereals such as millet, rice and sorghum and legumes also face the same threat from aflatoxin production and contamination in Kenya.

Biodegradation and metabolism of AFB1 can also generate aflatoxin metabolites in animals, human and the environment. Aflatoxin M1 (AFM1) is a product of aflatoxin B1 (AFB1) metabolism and is found in milk in areas of high aflatoxin exposure [26]. Subsequently humans may be exposed to this aflatoxin through milk and milk products, including breast milk, especially in areas where poor-quality grain is used for animal feed. The principal hydroxylated AFB1 metabolite present in most milk of cows fed with a diet contaminated with AFB1 is aflatoxin M1. Aflatoxin M1 is usually excreted after 12 h in milk and urine when animal feed contaminated with aflatoxin is administered to the animals [22]. The hydroxylated metabolite is formed as a result of biotransformation of AFB1 and AFB2 by hepatic microsomal mixed-function oxidase (MFO) system. Improper farming practices described earlier have led to an increase in risk of contamination. Commercial feeds have been found to be contaminated with aflatoxin B1 and milk with aflatoxin M1 [82]. Metabolites B2 and G2 have also been produced and detected in soil through biodegradation processes [24]. Food crops can become contaminated both before and after harvesting [24]. Preharvest contamination with aflatoxins is mainly common to grains such as maize, millet, cottonseed, peanuts and tree nuts. Postharvest contamination can be found in a variety of other crops such as coffee, rice and spices. Improper storage under conditions that favour mould growth can lead to levels of contamination much higher than those found in the field [22]. Apart from grains, postharvest production of *Aspergillus* species has resulted in aflatoxin production in other food types such as sun-dried fish in Kenya and other African countries due to poor handling and storage conditions [59, 85].

While toxicity of aflatoxin metabolites are now well recognized, it is not often known that *Aspergillus flavus* fungi itself also exerts pathogenic effects through aspergillosis or infection with the mould, which largely occurs in the lungs, skin and other organs of immune-compromised patients [65].

5. Toxicity and metabolism of aflatoxin B1

Aflatoxins are very toxic to mammals with the LD_{50} (oral, rat) being 4.8 mg/kg body weight for AFB1 reported and also to domestic animals with AFB1 LD_{50} (oral) values of 0.5 (dogs), 0.62 (pigs), 2 (guinea pigs) and 6.3 mg/kg (chicken) [86, 87]. They are known human carcinogens, and there is sufficient evidence for carcinogenicity of AFB1 in animals and human based on in vivo and in vitro studies that have been done [86, 87]. AFB1 has also been shown to be a potent mutagen and covalently binds to DNA, RNA and proteins in the liver. It is activated in the liver cells and induces principally G to T mutations [88]. DNA damage response which acts as an antitumor mechanism against genotoxic agents has confirmed that AFB1 is genotoxic. Genotoxicity studies of AFB1 on human embryo and adult liver cells in vitro have demonstrated the order of toxicity as B1 > G1 > G2 > B2 [86, 87]. Although AFB1 is a potent liver carcinogen in animals, in epidemiological studies done in Africa, it has been difficult to ascribe the incidence of human liver cancers solely to AFB1 because of concurrent exposure to other potentially causative agents (e.g. liver parasitism, hepatitis B virus, other mycotoxins as well as other carcinogenic environmental and food contaminants) that may be enhancing factors for liver damage and replication [89]. However, AFB1 binding to DNA and consequent interference with host genomes have been established and confirmed by mechanistic and inhibition studies [90]. Previously, some epidemiological studies were conducted on cancer patients aimed at evaluating the effects of AFB1 and AFM1 exposure on cancer cells in order to verify the correlation between toxin exposure and cancer cell proliferation and invasion [64].

The International Agency for Research on Cancer (IARC) has classified AFB1 and AFM1 as human carcinogens belonging to Group 1 and Group 2B, respectively, with formation of DNA adducts identified [25, 45]. Aflatoxins play a causative role in 5–28% of hepatocellular carcinoma (HCC) worldwide [91]. Marchese et al. [64] have recently reviewed the chemistry and metabolism of AFB1 and AFM1 and their involvement in cancer development. They summarized the activation pathways of AFB1 and AFM1 and stated that AFB1 epoxidation is the key step in the genotoxic process and thus in the carcinogenesis, whereby the high affinity of the epoxide intermediate for purine bases of DNA was shown to lead to formation of AFB1-N7-Gua adduct that promoted mutations in nucleotide sequence. AFB1 is mainly metabolized in the liver upon action of the microsomal mixed-function oxidase (MFO) enzymes belonging to the superfamily of CYP450. It is converted into the reactive 8,9-epoxide in a process mediated by these oxidases. The epoxide exists as two stereoisomers, exo and endo, with the former being the toxic species responsible for AFB1 genotoxicity [92]. The exo-8,9-epoxide has a high binding affinity towards DNA, forming the 8,9-dihydro-8-(N7-guanyl)-9-hydroxy-AFB1 (AFB1-N7-Gua) adduct, thus leading to DNA mutations [64]. Epoxide formation is also involved in other metabolic pathways, including (i) conjugation with glutathione (GSH) catalyzed by glutathione-S-transferase (GST) with subsequent excretion as AFB-mercapturate, a pathway which is vital for the detoxification of AFB1 as a carcinogen, even though a depletion of GHS was also reported to lead to high levels of reactive oxygen species (ROS) causing oxidative damage [93]; (ii) enzymatic and non-enzymatic conversion to AFB1-8,9-dihydrodiol, which can further be converted into a dialdehyde form, and an aflatoxin dialdehyde subsequently which can get excreted through urine as dialcohol upon action of aflatoxin aldehyde reductase (AFAR) or can bind proteins, like albumin [92] and (iii) binding to other macromolecules like proteins or RNA, causing inhibition of proteins, DNA and RNA synthesis and dysregulation of normal cellular functions [94]. Microsomal biotransformation of AFB1 also includes hydroxylation of the toxin, leading to the formation of more polar and less toxic metabolites, including mainly AFM1 and aflatoxin Q1 (AFQ1). Different studies tried to assess the role of the CYP450 enzymes which are responsible for detoxification and formation of carcinogenic metabolites. CYP1A2 and CYP3A4 strains were found to be capable of activating AFB1 and the most active isoenzymes of the CYP450 family to do this [28]. It has been reported that CYP3A4 is responsible for the formation of AFB1-exo-8,9-epoxide and trace amounts of AFQ1, whereas CYP1A2 leads to both exo- and endo-8,9-epoxide and eventually to the hydroxylated AFM1 metabolite [27]. The other two isoenzymes that use AFB1 as a substrate to a minor extent are CYP3A7, expressed in the human foetal liver, and CYP3A5 [27]. Other mechanisms of AFB1 toxicity include formation of intracellular reactive oxygen species which cause oxidative damage, resulting in AFB1 inducing cytotoxicity; and studies have demonstrated oxidative stress-induced toxic changes in the liver related to AFB1 toxicity [90, 95] oxidative stress-induced apoptosis through a mitochondrial signal pathway which has been reported [96]. AFB1 has caused oxidative and nitrosative hepatoxicity in rat and chick hepatocytes [90]. The predominant mutation caused by AFB1-N7-Gua adduct has been identified, and the sites of mutation and selectivity towards guanine bases have been elucidated [64]. These mutation studies have confirmed the links with a great number of epidemiological data on hepatocellular carcinoma (HCC) patients from regions of high aflatoxin exposure, strengthening the association between HCC incidence and aflatoxin exposure [97]. Research on human exposure to AFB1 through diet and analysis of liver and plasma metabolites have demonstrated hepatocarcinogenesis, with plasma concentrations showing that absorption and metabolism of AFB1 are rapid in human.

It has been noted that AFM1 is primarily considered a detoxification product of AFB1 metabolism, showing only 10% of mutagenicity compared to its precursor [92], and its metabolic fate is similar to that of AFB1, with the difference that AFM1 presents a poorer substrate for epoxidation, thus explaining the differences in genotoxic potencies. It has also been reported that CYP450 activation is not required for AFM1 to exert cytotoxic effects [92]. Apart from the principal biotransformation pathway involving CYP450, other activation mechanisms have been reported for aflatoxins. In fact, epoxidation catalyzed by prostaglandin H (PGH) synthase has been described by Battista et al. [98], whereas Weng et al. [99] have recently reported a mechanism in which lipid peroxidase (LPO) is the main enzyme responsible for AFB1-induced carcinogenesis, triggered by production of cyclic-methyl-hydroxy-1 and N2-propano-dG (meth-OH-PdG) adduct and/or inhibition of DNA repair.

Aflatoxicosis

Human intoxication by aflatoxins may occur via contact, ingestion and inhalation; and they can affect the liver, kidney, stomach and lungs, salivary glands, colon and skin [91]. Once ingestion of aflatoxin B1 has taken place, the gastrointestinal tract rapidly absorbs it with other aflatoxins, and the circulatory system transports them to the liver [100]. Approximately 1–3% of the ingested aflatoxins irreversibly bind to proteins and DNA bases to form adducts such as aflatoxin B1-lysine in albumin [101]. Disruption of protein and DNA bases in hepatocytes disrupts their functions and causes liver toxicity [101]. This results into chronic exposure which is defined as the ingestion of very small doses of aflatoxins in a long period of time [101]. Ingestion of higher doses of aflatoxins can result in what is called acute aflatoxicosis [100]. The order of potency for acute and chronic toxicity is B1 > G1 > B2 > G2 [20]. AFB1 may not itself be toxic, but it is metabolized to produce more toxic metabolites, and its subsequent metabolism determines both the acute and chronic toxicity.

Bankole and Adebanjo [11] have defined aflatoxicosis as poisoning which results from ingestion of aflatoxins in contaminated foods in human and feeds in animals and manifests as chronic or acute aflatoxicosis. The term is therefore not restricted to human poisoning only but can be used to describe aflatoxin poisoning in other organisms including domestic animals, birds, fish and other organisms. Chronic aflatoxicosis results from ingestion of low to moderate levels of aflatoxins. Chronic dietary exposure to aflatoxins is a major factor for hepatocellular carcinoma [11]. Common subclinical symptoms are seen through impaired food conversion and slow rate of growth with or without production of an overt aflatoxin syndrome and liver cancer [11]. Ingestion of higher doses of aflatoxin can result in an acute aflatoxicosis which manifests as hepatotoxicity with symptoms of liver damage, hemorrhage and alteration of food digestion or, in severe cases, liver failure and death (which occurs in 25% of cases of acute poisoning) [81]. No animal species is resistant to the acute toxic effects of aflatoxins [11]. The biological effects of aflatoxin can be grouped into four general categories: acute and chronic liver damage, reduced growth rate, impairment of immunologic and innate defense mechanisms and carcinogenic and teratogenic effects, respectively, and different animal species respond differently. Aflatoxicosis can be influenced by environmental factors as well as by levels ingested, duration of exposure, age health, nutritional status and diet [81]. Aflatoxin B1 is a very potent carcinogen in many species including primates, birds, fish and rodents. In each species, the liver is the primary target organ of aflatoxin toxicity and carcinogenicity in acute injury [81].

Early symptoms of hepatoxicity from aflatoxicosis can manifest as anorexia, malaise and low-grade fever, which can progress to potentially lethal acute hepatitis with vomiting, abdominal pain, hepatitis and death [25]. Symptoms of AFB1 also include yellow eyes, swollen legs, vomiting, abdominal pain and bleeding. The health impact of aflatoxin exposure in animals mainly depends on dosage and response to the epidemic, and low dosages produce nutritional interference and immunological suppression, while high doses lead to acute illness and death [81]. Aflatoxins have been detected in the blood of pregnant women, umbilical cord blood and breast milk in African countries, with significant seasonal variations [24]. Levels of aflatoxins detected in the umbilical cord blood at birth are among the highest levels ever recorded in human tissues and fluids [24], and therefore mother-to-child transfer impacts are expected to be significant. Aflatoxins have been suggested as an aetiological factor in encephalopathy and fatty tissue degeneration of viscera, similar to Reye syndrome, which is common in countries with a hot and humid climate [101], an indication that exposure can lead to symptoms such as memory loss and dementia. Aflatoxins have been found in blood during the acute phase of the disease and in the liver of affected children [24]. In recent studies, aflatoxins have been found in the brains and lungs of children who have died from kwashiorkor and those who had died from various other diseases [21].

Outbreaks of acute aflatoxicosis from highly contaminated food have been documented in Kenya, India and Thailand [104]. In April 2004, an outbreak of an acute hepatotoxicity was identified among people living in Makueni, Kitui, Machakos and Thika Counties, and epidemiological investigation determined that the outbreak was as a result of aflatoxin poisoning from ingestion of contaminated maize [105]. In July 2004, 317 cases and 150 deaths had occurred, making this one of the largest

Year	Those affected	Numbers affected	Sources of toxin	Observed effects
1977	Poultry and dogs	Unspecified	Contaminated maize	Death
1981	Human	12	Contaminated maize	Death
1984/1985	Human	Unspecified	Contaminated maize	Death
1988	Human	3	Contaminated maize	Death and acute symptoms
2001	Human	29	Contaminated maize	16 deaths and acute symptoms
2002	Poultry and dogs	Large numbers	Contaminated maize	Death
2003	Human	6	Contaminated maize	6 deaths
2004	Human	331 (500*)	Contaminated maize	125 deaths and acute symptoms
2005	Human	75	Contaminated maize	32 deaths and acute symptoms
2006	Human	20	Contaminated maize	10 deaths and acute symptoms
2007	Human	4	Contaminated maize	2 deaths and acute symptoms
2008	Human	5	Contaminated maize	2 deaths and acute symptoms
2010	Human and dogs	Unspecified	Contaminated maize	Unconfirmed dog deaths; drop in prices

*Source of Information: Nduti [102]. *Ngindu et al. [103].*

Table 2.
Aflatoxicosis cases in Kenya since 1977.

and most severe outbreaks of acute aflatoxicosis documented worldwide [106]. In 1981, an outbreak of aflatoxicosis from contaminated maize occurred in Makueni County and other parts of Kenya which reported 500 acute illnesses and 200 deaths [103]. In both 1981 and 2004, drought and food shortages were followed by unreasonable rains during harvest which probably favoured the growth of aflatoxigenic *Aspergillus* in household maize [107]. From the above cases, it is clear that aflatoxin food poisoning is a common phenomenon in eastern parts of Kenya and occurs on cereals commonly used by many communities as staple food. These cereals can be stored in processed and non-processed form. A summary of aflatoxicosis occurrences in Kenya is presented in **Table 2**.

6. Sources of AFB1 and exposure in Kenya

Dietary exposure varies greatly from country to country, and estimates of dietary exposure indicate clear differences between developed and developing countries [25]. In developed countries, mean aflatoxin dietary exposures are generally less than 1 ng/kg body weight per day, compared with some sub-Saharan African countries where mean exposure exceeds 100 ng/kg body weight [24]. The Center for Disease

Control and Prevention [108] has estimated that 4.5 billion people are exposed to aflatoxins worldwide, with the risks varying from country to country. In other reports, aflatoxin exposure in Africa ranged from 10 to 180 ng/kg body weight/ day, while exposures in Europe and North America ranged from 0 to 4 and from 0.26 to 1, respectively [108]. A study done in Kenya has shown that populations from all economic strata have aflatoxin exposure [22]. The level of aflatoxin B1—the most toxic of the aflatoxins—in blood serum in individuals was found to be similar across the rich and poor, with the highest burden among the middle wealth quintile [22]. Climate changes have been reported to play a major role and would likely lead to increased occurrences of aflatoxins and other mycotoxins (and possibly their increased co-occurrence) in Kenya and other countries [22]. It has been reported that the tropical and subtropical regions of the world including sub-Saharan Africa and parts of Southern Asia are highly likely to continue experiencing aflatoxin-related contamination issues due to high temperature and humidity conditions, particularly damp conditions during the rainy seasons, and drought being experienced in these countries as these conditions increase crop susceptibility to aflatoxin contamination [25]. In another study, it was found that there was a low awareness and understanding of the dangers of mycotoxins in food and certain practices among farmers in Kenya could therefore increase the risk for exposure [76]. Gender analysis revealed that groups having knowledge were not always responsible for risk mitigation [83]. In a study conducted in the major farming regions in Kenya, it was found that 67% of the urban smallholder dairy farmers had no knowledge that milk could be contaminated with aflatoxin M1 and none knew how they could mitigate against this exposure [24, 109].

Bankole and Adebanjo [11] mapped Kenya into aflatoxicosis risky areas taking into consideration humidity, temperature, rainfall, dairy cattle density, feed resources, farming systems and consumption of maize and milk. The eastern parts of the country had more cases of historical occurrences of aflatoxin contamination, while the central and western parts showed increased risk of aflatoxin contamination [83]. In Kenya AFB1 and other metabolites have been analysed and detected in animal commercial feeds, grains, flour and cooked diets. Among researchers, aflatoxin analysis in human and cattle feed is one of the most common research topics especially by graduate students in the national universities, although research into its human health impacts has received less attention. In a study done in 2008, it was reported that most people in Kenya were exposed to low-level doses of a wide spectrum of fungal poisoning through regular consumption of cereals such as maize and cereal products [76]. For example, an average Kenyan eats maize products at the rate of 0.4 kg/person/day such that even the lowest amount of exposure can result in a cumulative exposure likely to cause health effects [76]. Maize is the staple food (accounting for more than 75% total cereal area) and is mainly grown by small holder farmers who together with their families account for 70% of the Kenyan population [76].

In a survey done in 2001, samples of agricultural produce including grains and flour obtained from ordinary grocery stores, kiosks, supermarkets and open-air markets in Nairobi and other towns in Kenya were found to be contaminated with moulds that produce aflatoxins among other mycotoxins [26]. Recently, the mean concentration levels of aflatoxins in dry maize grains in Kenya, as analysed by ELISA method, range from 2.51 to 17.4 ppb (dry weight) in samples taken from Western, Nairobi and Eastern provinces of Kenya [26, 60, 110]. Analysis of sun-dried maize, millet, flour and fish samples from different regions in Kenya found that, in general, there are aflatoxins including AFB1 in these products, even though at lower concentrations compared with standard maximum allowed levels by the WHO, FAO, EU and KEBS [26, 39, 60, 109, 110]. Wasike [60] determined total aflatoxin levels in randomly sampled maize grains from Bungoma using ELISA method and found 2.51–3.56 ppb of total aflatoxins (based on dry weight) and concluded that there was no significant variation ($p < 0.05$) with site. He also reported lack of awareness among farmers on aflatoxins in the areas where samples were taken from and listed harvesting, drying, storage methods and prevailing rainy weather during harvesting as main factors that influenced the production of aflatoxins [60]. Okech [110] used solvent extraction and LC–MS to analyse branded (milled and packaged by commercial Millers) flour samples taken from supermarkets and unbranded (milled by traditional posho mills, packed in sacks and weighed according to customer needs in open markets) flour samples obtained from various open markets in Nairobi, Thika and Machakos. He found AFB1 in 67% of the unbranded flour samples with mean concentrations ranging from 1.07 to 8.89 ppb. About 33% of the samples from Kiambu showed aflatoxin levels with one sample having 8.89 ppb which was above the KEBS and Codex maximum level limit of 5 ppb, while 16.7% of the samples from Nairobi and Machakos had aflatoxins levels but were lower than the 5 ppb limit [110]. One sample of unbranded maize flour from Machakos contained AFG2 which was detected at a mean concentration of 6.02 ppb which was above the 5 ppb limit [110]. In terms of total aflatoxins, 22.2% of the samples of unbranded maize flour had aflatoxins but were below the 10 ppb KEBS and Codex maximum level limit [110]. There were no aflatoxins (all were below detection limit) in all samples of the branded flour samples which showed that commercial maize milling process in Kenya, which involves removal of unsuitable grains, dehulling, and removal of bran, lowers risks of aflatoxin exposure in human in Kenya [26, 110]. It was concluded that the levels of AFB1 were lower after commercial milling with concentrations in unbranded maize flour being much lower than corresponding dried grains [110]. Nduti et al. [26] analysed dried maize grains and flour samples taken from Western, Eastern and Nairobi regions of Kenya by ELISA and found significant variations ($p < 0.05$) in the three regions, with mean total aflatoxin level in grains ranging from 7.95 ± 1.57 ppb (Nairobi samples) to 22.54 ± 4.94 ppb (eastern samples), which were higher than the 10 ppb KEBS and Codex maximum limit and therefore a major source of concern. No significant difference in aflatoxins levels with site in flour was found, and the total aflatoxins levels were detected but were below the 10 ppb limit. Nduti et al. [26] found maize grains to be contaminated with aflatoxins (including AFB1) in samples from Nairobi and Eastern Kenya detecting aflatoxins in all samples with levels higher than the Codex and KEBS maximum limit of 10 ppb usage. The variations with site were insignificant ($p > 0.005$), and slight differences in mean concentration levels were attributed to differences in weather such as wind, temperature, insect damage of produce and storage and handling [26]. However, in maize flour which is the staple food for most of the population, the mean total level was slightly >5 ppb which was lower than the WHO level. In this study, aflatoxin contamination was confirmed by the presence of AFM1 in urine of the population [26, 35]. Nduti et al. [26] proposed that sorting, cleaning, bran removal and the use of chemical and biological agents to reduce the levels may have influenced lower concentrations in flour than maize grains. The results of Nduti et al. [26] suggested that cooked mixture of maize and beans (traditionally known as *githeri*) as the most likely source of human exposure of AFB1 in humans in the Eastern province of Kenya.

Recently, Orony et al. [59] reported mean total aflatoxins ranging from 0.33 to 1.58 ppb (wet weight) in sun-dried dagaa fish (*Rastrineobola argentea*) obtained from markets located along the Lake Victoria, caused by contamination due to poor handling and storage conditions. They estimated a daily intake of total aflatoxins of 0.0079 μg/kg/day during the rainy season when sun-drying is not effective. The risks involved in consumption of this fish in Kenya were found to be lower when considering the recommended maximum limits [50]. However, aflatoxins are remarkably potent, often causing disease even when ingested in minute quantities. They are accumulative, resistant to degradation and also heat resistant implying that ingestion of minute amounts still poses risks. The generation of aflatoxins in processed dagaa was explained by the fact that the samples were collected from the markets during the rainy season in July, when drying was incomplete; hence, the sun-dried dagaa were packed in plastic sacks when they were not completely dry resulting in the growth of moulds [59]. The samples which were dried on a rack with some aeration were found to have lower levels of aflatoxin [59]. In Kenya, aflatoxin contamination was reported to be less common in foods during dry seasons as the drying process is more efficient during that period [50]. Incomplete drying condition has been associated with production of aflatoxins in previous studies [85]. Studies done in Nigeria by Bukola et al. [111] on smoked-dried fishes sold in the markets revealed that aflatoxins B1 (AFB1) and G1 were present in the samples at concentrations between 1.5–8.1 and 1.8–4.5 μg/kg, respectively. These reported cases of aflatoxin contamination in staple foods such as maize flour and fish in Kenya indicate that a very large proportion of the population in Kenya is potentially exposed to sublethal concentrations of aflatoxins including AFB1 in their diet. Previous studies conducted in Uganda, Swaziland, Thailand and Kenya have shown positive correlations between levels of aflatoxin contamination in market food samples and cooked food samples with incidences of hepatocellular cancer and mortalities [25]. However, research on biomarkers to quantify aflatoxin exposure in individuals have still not yet determined to link aflatoxin exposure with cancer risk in Kenya [4, 59].

There have been reported cases of aflatoxin outbreaks in Kenya which have led to severe poisoning in school children and adults fed on maize products, some of the products being donations by WHO food programmes for the school feeding programme [112, 113, 123]. These outbreaks of aflatoxin prevalence and aflatoxicosis have been blamed on the lack of regulations and control measures including lack of adherence to handling procedures such as drying period, maintaining required moisture levels, removal of damaged grains, lack of optimal ventilation and temperature during storage, prevention of insect damage which encourages moulding, failure by the national grain cereal companies to purchase the grains from farmers on time and failure to perform routine analysis of moisture and aflatoxin presence in the produce before milling [76]. It has been reported that the most critical interval of drying maize in Kenya is from when it starts drying up, down to approximately 20% moisture, and during this interval moulds occur more easily than any other period [26]. This period can be very long, ranging from 28 to 58 days, respectively, when traditional storage methods are adopted [26], during which, grains are subjected to extreme fluctuations in weather such as rainfall. In sub-Saharan Africa, weather is critical in addition to the prevalence of the S-strain of *Aspergillus flavus* which is more toxic as it produces more aflatoxins than any other strain of *A. flavus*. Nontoxic L-strain of *A. flavus* has been used to competitively exclude the producers through propagation during crop infection and thereby limit contamination in some countries such as the USA [76]. These highly competitive atoxigenic strains of *A. flavus* are applied to soil after which they spread to the crop, excluding the toxic strains [76]. There are about eight nontoxin-producing strains of *A. flavus*, which are capable of radically reducing aflatoxin in maize by 99% [76] and have been tried in Nigeria.

In Kenya, researchers at the Kenya Agricultural and Livestock Research Organization developed and manufactured a product called Aflasafe KE01 to fight aflatoxins in 2016 although this product has not yet trickled down significantly to the small-scale farmer. Aflasafe KE01 consists of four friendly strains of *A. flavus* which do not produce aflatoxins as active ingredient with sterilized sorghum and a binder making up 97% of the solid formulation which is applied preharvest by broadcast during plant growth in the field (KALRO website, www.kalro.org). A single application is required in each cropping season to protect maize. The product has achieved between 80 and 99% reduction of aflatoxins in maize and groundnuts at harvest and in storage. Since soil is habitat for aflatoxin-producing fungi, contamination while the crop is still in the field or later during storage and processing is irreversible. Although Aflasafe KE01 reduces contamination in the field, it can only be effective if adopted alongside other safe standard procedures such as proper handling and storage of produce. However, the use of such techniques in Kenya has still not been felt nationally even though training of experts and building capability in Kenya for aflatoxin control have been very effective [76]. It has been recommended that contaminated maize and other grains such as millet be sold to ethanol producing factories since aflatoxins do not appear in the distilled alcohol [114], instead of using them to produce animal feed which makes the situation worse. Such developed country approaches for managing aflatoxin menace which include the use of food additives to make grain safe for farm animals by detoxifying the grain with anhydrous ammonia which reacts with aflatoxin molecules to destroy its toxicity have also not been adopted [76]. Such treatment, which must be done by trained personnel to avoid ammonia smell in the feed, can reduce aflatoxin by 95% [76]. No methods of analysis exist for detecting zero tolerance; therefore, tolerance levels should be based on a risk assessment approach rather than on analytical detection limits, the limits below which no detection is possible by analytical means [76]. This has not yet been achieved, and therefore a 'below detection limit' reported is just a product of instrument sensitivity and preparation losses but does not preclude trace level contamination and human exposure. So far more and more research have been concentrated on determining aflatoxin prevalence and levels in various foods, but research focus needs to shift towards effects and the use of biomarkers as well as epidemiological studies to understand the health impacts in Kenya.

Human exposure from milk has been a major issue of concern [113, 115, 116]. This originates from feeding cows with contaminated feeds or encouraging unhygienic conditions during milking, handling and storage of milk. Dairy production is widely practised in Kenya, and it provides a source of income to farmers, animal feed industry workers and all other stakeholders within the value chain [116]. Dairy farming systems in Kenya have changed over the years from direct use of pastures and hay only to commercial type of animal feeding where cowshed feeding is achieved with grain-based concentrates and silage [103, 105]. This practice was adopted due to increased productivity and high demand for the product. Studies have shown that aflatoxin contamination occurs in commercial feeds in Kenya and that exposure of cattle to mycotoxins generally occurs through consumption of contaminated feeds [103, 105, 109, 117]. AFM1 is usually excreted after 12 h in milk and urine when animal feed contaminated with AFB1/AFB2 is administered to the animals [22]. Aflatoxin is highly toxic to livestock, and feed contamination has been linked to increased mortality in farm animals. When cows consume aflatoxin-contaminated feed, they biotransform approximately 3–6% of AFB1 and AFB2 in their liver by hepatic microsomal mixed-function oxidase enzyme system into hydroxylated metabolites AFM1 and AFM2 [118] which are secreted into milk. AFB1, AFM1 and AFM2 aflatoxins have been detected in cow milk in Kenya [105]. Although AFM1 is 1000 times less toxic compared to AFB1, the AFM1 levels are regulated, and milk containing above 0.5 ppb level of AFM1 is considered unfit for human consumption [117]. Many countries have therefore regulated levels of AFB1 in animal feed, and the EU maximum limit has been set to 5 ppb; and it is recommended that animals should consume less than 40 μg/day of AFB1 in order not to exceed the allowed limit of AFM1.

7. Aflatoxin B1 regulation in Kenya

The World Health Organization, in collaboration with the Food and Agriculture Organization, is responsible for assessing the risks to humans caused by mycotoxins through contamination in food and for recommending adequate maximum levels in food and feed. Risk assessments of mycotoxins in food done by the Joint FAO/WHO Expert Committee on Food Additives are used by governments and by the Codex Alimentarius Commission (the intergovernmental standard-setting body for food) to establish maximum levels in food and provide other risk management advice to control or prevent contamination [11]. The outcome of such health risk assessments can either be a maximum tolerable intake (exposure) level or other guidance to indicate the level of health concern (such as the margin of exposure), including advice on risk management measures to prevent and control contamination and on analytical methods and monitoring and control activities [25]. These tolerable daily intakes are used by governments and international risk managers, such as the Codex Alimentarius Commission, to establish maximum levels for mycotoxins in food [11]. The maximum levels for mycotoxins in food are very low due to their severe toxicity. For example, the maximum levels for total aflatoxins set by the Codex in various nuts, grains, dried figs and milk are in the range of 0.5–10 μg/kg [24]. The WHO encourages national authorities to monitor and ensure that levels of mycotoxins in foodstuff on their market are as low as possible and comply with the both national and international maximum levels, conditions and legislation [25].

Different countries and authorities worldwide have rules and regulations governing aflatoxin B1 in foods which include the maximum permissible levels and recommended levels for certain foods. The Kenya Bureau of Standards (KEBS) has adopted the broad Codex standard limits of 5 ppb (for single metabolite) and 10 ppb for total aflatoxins in food but does not have lower limits for sensitive foods such as milk. The US Food and Drug Administration (FDA) had given an action level (maximum permissible) of total aflatoxin (B1) in combination with B2, G1 and G2 in foods as 20 μg/kg above in which the commodity is withdrawn from the markets [59], except milk which has a maximum level of 0.5 ppb. The Food Standards Agency has set a legal limit of total aflatoxins in foods as 10 μg/kg. Higher levels of 100–300 μg/kg are tolerable for some animal feeds. The EU has set maximum permitted levels for aflatoxin B1 in nuts, dried fruits, cereals and spices ranging from 2 to 12 μg/kg, while the maximum permitted level for aflatoxin B1 in infant foods is set at 0.1 μg/kg [119]. The maximum permitted levels for aflatoxin B1 in animal feeds set by the EU range from 5 to 50 μg/kg, and these levels are much lower than those set in the USA [120]. The Joint FAO/WHO Expert Committee on Food Additives has set the maximum permitted total aflatoxin level of AFB1 in combination with the other aflatoxins (B2, G1 and G2) at 15 μg/kg in raw peanuts and 10 μg/kg in processed peanut, while the tolerance level of aflatoxin B1 alone is 5 μg/kg for dairy cattle feed [121, 124, 125]. Results from previous studies have however shown that it is difficult if not impossible to eradicate AFB1 in cereals once produced [26]. For that matter, consumers are left vulnerable to exposure, yet burning of contaminated cereals, one of the most feasible ways of containing the menace, has caused problem of food insecurity in the past.

8. Conclusions

Aflatoxicosis cases are very common in Kenya, and the major cause is contaminated maize and maize flour. The total aflatoxin and AFB1 levels that have been obtained in maize grains and maize flour are indicating that commercial milling and packaging of maize flour reduce the levels of aflatoxins considerably. However, a large population in the rural and urban areas which still rely on maize flour from open markets, through donation or by traditional posho milling, could be more exposed to aflatoxins as these sources increase and fail to reduce the levels, respectively. More research is needed to identify and determine aflatoxin levels in other produce such as beans, peanuts, groundnuts and their processed products. The current KEBS regulation and maximum allowable limits, in terms of total or single metabolite, are adequate for monitoring and controlling aflatoxicosis menace; however, for export produce and for long-term control of aflatoxicosis in the country, the maximum allowable limits need to be reviewed and lowered. With improvements in analytical techniques which are capable of giving lower detection limits, maximum allowable limits can be lowered to almost zero tolerance to reduce aflatoxicosis and hepatocarcinogenesis in human in Kenya. Although a lot of research in Kenya has gone into identification and determination of aflatoxin levels in various human foods and animal feeds and their detoxification mechanisms, it is still not possible to directly link AFB1 exposure to liver cancer as less epidemiological and biomarker studies have been done in Kenya to confirm such linkage.

Acknowledgements

The authors wish to thank the National Research Fund (NRF), Nairobi, Kenya, through a multidisciplinary TUK/MMUST/Maseno/PCPB research grant.

Author details

Joseph Owuor Lalah[1*], Solomon Omwoma[2] and Dora A.O. Orony[3]

1 Department of Chemical Science and Technology, The Technical University of Kenya, Nairobi, Kenya

2 Jaramogi Oginga Odinga University of Science and Technology, Bondo, Kenya

3 Department of Chemistry, Maseno University, Maseno, Kenya

*Address all correspondence to: lalahjoseph@yahoo.com

References

[1] AOAC. AOAC Official Method: AOAC 993.17 - 1996, Aflatoxins in Corn and Peanuts. Thin Layer Chromatographic Method. Washington, DC: US Food and Drug Administration; 1996

[2] Nabil S. Aflatoxins: Occurrence and Health Risks. 2004. Available from: http://www.ansci.cornell.edu/plants/toxicagents/aflatoxin/aflatoxin.html [Accessed: 08 June 2008]

[3] Reddy SV, Waliyar F. Properties of aflatoxin and its producing fungi. International Crop Research Institute for the Semi-Arid Tropics -ICRISAT. 2000;**10**:95-98

[4] Wogan GN, Kensler TW, Groopman JD. Present and future directions of transitional research and hepatocellular carcinoma. Food Additives & Contaminants: Part A. 2012;**29**(2):249-257

[5] Pavao AC, Neto LAS, Neto JF, Leao MBC. Structure and activity of aflatoxins B and G. Journal of Molecular Structure (THEOCHEM). 1995;**337**:57-60

[6] Borzsonyi M, Lapis K, Day NE, Yamsaki H. editors. Models, mechanisms and tumour promotion. International Agency for Research in Cancer (IARC). Scientific Publication. Lyon, France: World Health Organization; 1984. Vol. 562000

[7] Fink-Gremmels J. Mycotoxins in cattle feeds and carry-over to dairy milk: A review. Food Additives & Contaminants. 2008;**25**:172-180

[8] Mompoint J, McGlone L. Aflatoxins in Food and Their Effects on Health. 2011. Available from: http://docs.google.com/viewer?a=v&q=cache:2X8F-K914ugJ:londellmcglone.com/docs/Aflatoxins%2520in%25 [Accessed: 07 December 2011]

[9] Pizzolitto P, Armando MR, Salvano MA, Dalcero AM, Rosa CA. Evaluation of Saccharomyces cerevisiae as an antiaflatoxicogenic agent in broiler feedstuffs. Poultry Science. 2013;**92**:1655-1663

[10] Sydenham EW, Pieter GT, Walter FOM, Gordon SS, Dirk JVS, Klaus RK. Natural occurrence of some Fusarium mycotoxins in corn from low and high esophageal cancer prevalence areas of the Transkei, Southern Africa. Journal of Agriculture and Food Chemistry. 1990;**38**(10):1900-1903

[11] Bankole SA, Adebanjo A. Mycotoxins in food in West Africa: Current situation and possibilities of controlling it. African Journal of Biotechnology. 2003;**2**(9):254-263

[12] Wagacha JM, Muthomi JW. Mycotoxin problem in Africa: Current status, implications to food safety and health and possible management strategies. International Journal of Food Microbiology. 2008;**124**(1):1-12

[13] Yi J, Pauline J, William E, Jia-sheng W, Timothy P, Jonathan W. Aflatoxin B1 albumin adduct levels and cellular immune status in Ghanaians. International Immunology. 2005;**17**(6):807-814

[14] Satini A, Ritieni A. Aflatoxins: Risk, Exposure and Remediation. Rijeka, Croatia: IntechOpen; 2013. DOI: 10.5772/52866. Chapter 16

[15] Piva FB, Galvano RD, Pietri AP, Piva RD. Detoxification methods of aflatoxins: A review. Nutrition Research. 1995;**15**(5):767-776

[16] Rahama F, Basappa SC, Murthy VS. Destruction of aflatoxin in rice by different cooking methods. Journal of Food Science and Technology. 1979;**16**:11-112

[17] Scott PM. Effects of food processing on mycotoxins. Journal of Food Protection. 1984;**47**(6):489-499

[18] O'Neil MJ, editor. The Merck Index-An Encyclopedia of Chemicals, Drugs, and Biologicals. Whitehouse Station, NJ: Merck and Co., Inc.; 2006. p. 33

[19] Bbosa DS, Kitya D, Odda J, Ogwal-Keng J. Aflatoxins metabolism effects on epigenetic mechanisms and their role in carcinogenesis. Health. 2013;**5**(10A):14-34. DOI: 10.4236/health.2013.510A1003

[20] Filazi A, Sireli UT. Occurrence of Aflatoxins in Food. Rijeka, Croatia: IntechOpen; 2013. pp. 143-170. DOI: 10.5772/5103. Chapter 7

[21] WHO. Food Safety Digest. Department of Food Safety and Zoonoses Aflatoxins (Vol. Ref No. WHO/NHM/FOS/RAM/18.1): World Health Organization. Joint FAO/WHO Expert Committee on Food Additives (JECFA). 2018. Additional information available from: www.who.int/foodsafety/areas_work/chemical-risks/en/

[22] Abbas HK. Introduction to the toxin reviews special issue "*Aspergillus flavus*, aflatoxin, cyclopiazonic acid, and biological control". Toxin Reviews. 2011;**30**(2-3):31-32. DOI: 10.3109/15569543.2011.590624

[23] MdQuadri SH, Niranjan MS, Chaluvaraju KC, Shantaram U, Enamul HS. An overview on chemistry, toxicity, analysis and control of aflatoxins. International Journal of Chemical and Life Sciences. 2013;**2**:1071-1078

[24] Logrieco A, Visconti A. An Overview on Toxigenic Fungi and Mycotoxins in Europe. Dordrecht: Kluwer Academic Publishers; 2014

[25] Warburton ML, Williams WP. Aflatoxin resistance in maize: What have we learned lately? Advances in Botany. 2014;**2014**:10. DOI: 10.1155/2014/352831

[26] Nduti NN, Njeru PN, Mwaniki M, Reid G. Aflatoxin variations in maize flour and grains collected from various regions of Kenya. African Journal of Food Agriculture Nutrition and Development. 2017;**17**(1):11743-11756. DOI: 10.18971/ajfand.77.16875

[27] Wild CP, Turner PC. The toxicology of aflatoxins as a basis for public health decisions. Mutagenesis. 2002;**17**:471-481

[28] Gallagher EP, Wienkers LC, Stapleton PL, Kunze KL, Eaton DL. Role of human microsomal and human complementary DNA-expressed cytochromes P4501A2 and P4503A4 in the bioactivation of Aflatoxin B1. Cancer Research. 1994;**54**:101-108

[29] Jard G, Liboz T, Mathieu F, Guyonvarch A, Lebrihi A. Review of mycotoxin reduction in food and feed: From prevention in the field to detoxification by adsorption or transformation. Food Additives & Contaminants: Part A. 2011;**28**:1590-1609

[30] Prandini A, Tansini G, Sigolo S, Filippi L, Laporta M, Piva G. On the occurrence of aflatoxin M1 in milk and dairy products. Food and Chemical Toxicology. 2009;**47**:984-991

[31] Rustom IYS. Aflatoxin in food and feed: Occurrence, legislation and inactivation by physical methods. Food Chemistry. 1997;**59**:57-67

[32] Park DL, Price WD. Reduction of aflatoxin hazards using ammoniation. Reviews of Environmental Contamination and Toxicology. 2001;**171**:139-175

[33] Cole RJ, Cox RH. Handbook of Toxic Fungal Metabolites. Vol. 5. London: Academic Press; 1981. pp. 390-395

[34] Nduti N, McMillan A, Shannon S, Sumarah M, Njeru P, Mwaniki M, et al.

Investigating probiotic yoghurt to reduce an aflatoxin B1 biomarker among school children in Eastern Kenya: Preliminary study. International Dairy Journal. 2016;**63**:124-129

[35] Nduti NN, Reid G, Sumarah M, Hekmat S, Mwaniki M, Njeru PN. *Weissella cibaria* Nn20 isolated from fermented Kimere shows ability to sequester AFB1 in vitro and ferment milk with good viscosity and phin comparison to yogurt. Food Science & Nutrition Technology. 2018, 2018;**3**(1):000137

[36] Giovati L, Magliani W, Ciociola T, Santinoli C, Conti S, Polonelli L. AFM1 in Milk: Physical, biological, and prophylactic methods to mitigate contamination. Toxins. 2015;7:4330-4349

[37] Jebali R, Abbès S, Salah-Abbès JB, Ben Younes R, Haous Z, Oueslati R. Ability of *Lactobacillus plantarum* MON03 to mitigate aflatoxins (B1 and M1) immunotoxicities in mice. Journal of Immunotoxicology. 2014;**12**:290-299

[38] El-banna AA, Scott PM. Fate of mycotoxins during processing of food stuffs. Journal of Food Protection. 1983;**46**:301-304

[39] Kirui. Assessment of the traditional and improved processing methods in the reduction of aflatoxin levels in maize and maize products [MSc thesis]. Nairobi, Kenya: Jomo Kenyatta University of Agriculture and Technology (JKUAT); 2016

[40] Abrar M, Anjum FM, Butt MS, Pasha I, Randhawa MA. Aflatoxins: Biosynthesis, occurrence, toxicity and remedies. Critical Review of Food Science and Nutrition. 2013;**53**(8):43-57

[41] Singh R, Hsich DP. Aflatoxin biosynthetic pathway: Elucidation by using blocked mutants of *Aspergillus parasiticus*. Archives of Biochemistry and Biophysics. 1977;**178**(1):285-292

[42] Yu J, Whitelaw CA, Nierman WC, Bhatnagar D, Cleveland TE. *Aspergillus flavus* expressed sequence tags for identification of genes with putative roles in aflatoxin contamination of crops. FEMS Microbiology Letters. 2004;**237**(2):333-340

[43] Dewick PM. Medicinal Natural Products: A Biosynthetic Approach. 3rd ed. Sussex, UK: Wiley and Sons Ltd.; 2009. pp. 122-124. ISBN: 978-04707427/92

[44] Zain ME. Impact of mycotoxins on humans and animals. Journal of Saudi Chemical Society. 2011;**15**:129-144

[45] International Agency for Research of Cancer (IARC). Aflatoxins. IARC – Summaries and Evaluations. Lyon, France: International Agency for Research on Cancer,World Health Organization; Vol. 561993. p. 245

[46] Ada JP, Matcha B. Analysis of aflatoxin B1 in contaminated feeds, media, and serum samples of *Cyprinus carpio* L by high performance liquid chromatography. Food Quality and Safety. 2018;**2**(4):199-204. DOI: 1093/fqsafe/fyy013

[47] Lahouar A, Marin S, Crespo-Sempere A, Saïd S, Sanchis V. Effects of temperature, water activity and incubation time on fungal growth and aflatoxin B1 production by toxinogenic *Aspergillus flavus* isolates on sorghum seeds. Revista Argentina De Microbiologia. 2016;**48**:78-85

[48] Nelson DB, Kimbrough R, Landrigan PS, Hayes AW, Yang GC, Benanides J. Aflatoxin and Reye's syndrome: A case control study. Pediatrics. 1980;**66**:865-869

[49] Wacoo AP, Wendiro D, Vuzi PC, Hawumba JF. Methods for detection of aflatoxins in agricultural food crops. Journal of Applied Chemistry. 2014;**2014**:15. DOI: 10.1155/2014/706291

[50] FAO. Worldwide Regulations for Mycotoxins in Food and Feed. Food and Nutrition Paper. Rome, Italy: Food and Agriculture Organization; 2003

[51] Manabe M, Goto T, Masuura S. High performance liquid chromatography of aflatoxin with fluorescence detection. Agricultural and Biological Chemistry. 1978;**42**(11):57-59

[52] AOAC. Official Methods of Analysis of the Association of Official Analytical Chemists: Test Method; AOAC 2003.02. AOAC; Washington, DC: US Food and Drug Administration; 2006

[53] Muscarella M, Iammarino D, Nardeiello D, LoMagro SL, Palermo C, Centonze D, et al. Validation of a confirmatory analytical method for the determination of aflatoxins B1, B2, G1 and G2 in foods and feeds materials by HPLC with online photochemical derivation and fluorescence detection. Food Additives and Contaminants. 2009;**26**(10):1402-1410

[54] Seo JH, Min WK, Kweon DH, Park K, Park YC. Characterization of monoclonal antibody against aflatoxin B1 produced in hybridoma $2C_{12}$ and its single-chain variable fragment expressed in recombinant *Escherichia coli*. Food Chemistry. 2011;**126**:1316-1323

[55] Lamphugh SM, Hendrick RG. Aflatoxin and Kwashiorkor. African Health. 1983;**5**:20-25

[56] Hooper DG, Bolton VE, Guilford FT, Straus DC. Mycotoxin detection in human samples from patients exposed to environmental molds. International Journal of Molecular Sciences. 2009;**10**(4): 1465-1475. ISSN: 2422-0067

[57] Langone JJ, Van Vunakis H. Aflatoxin B specific antibodies and their use in radioimmunoassay. Journal of the National Cancer Institute. 1976;**56**(3):591-595

[58] William H, George WL. Natural Toxins. Official Methods of analysis of AOAC International. 18th ed. Gaithersburg, MD; Washington, DC: US Food and Drug Administration; 2005. pp. 21-22. Chapter 49

[59] Orony DNA, Lalah JO, Jondiko IO. Carcinogenic polycyclic aromatic hydrocarbons (PAHs), Aflatoxins and nitrosamines in processed fish from the Winam Gulf area of Kenya. Polycyclic Aromatic Compounds. 2015. DOI: 10.10801.10406638.2014.980433. Published online on July 30, 2015;**36**(4):295-317

[60] Wasike C. Determination of presence of aflatoxins in sun-dried maize from Kabuchai location—Bungoma county, Kenya [Bachelor of Technology Research Project]. Nairobi: Technical University of Kenya; 2015

[61] Leszczynka J, Maslowska J, OwczarekaA, KucharskaU. Determination of aflatoxin in foods products by the ELISA methods. Czech Journal of Food Science. 2001;**19**:8-12

[62] Kachapulula PW, Akello J, Bandyopadhyay R, Cotty PJ. Aflatoxin contamination of groundnut and maize in Zambia: Observed and potential concentrations. Journal of Applied Microbiology. 2017;**122**(6):1471-1482. DOI: 10.1111/jam.13448

[63] EC Commission Regulation No 1881/2006 of 19th December 2006. Setting maximum levels for certain contaminants in foodstuffs. Official Journal of the European Union. EU, Brussels

[64] Marchese S, Polo A, Ariano A, Velotto S, Costantini S, Severino L. Aflatoxin B1 and M1: Biological properties and their involvement in cancer development. Toxins. 2018;**10**:214. DOI: 10.3390/toxins10060214. Available from: www.mdpi.com/journal/toxins

[65] CDC. Definition of *Aspergillus flavus*/Aspergillosis/Types of Fungal diseases/Fungal diseases. 2017. Available from: www.cdc.gov

[66] Nesheim S, Stack ME. Preparation of mycotoxin standards. Methods in Molecular Biology (Clifton, N.J.). 2001;**157**:31-36

[67] Wild CP et al. Aflatoxin-albumin adducts: A basis for comparative carcinogenesis between animals and humans. Cancer Epidemiology, Biomarkers & Prevention. 1996;**5**:179-189

[68] Maddock J, editor. Public Health, Public Health—Methodology, Environmental and Systems Issues. London, UK: IntechOpen; 2012. ISBN: 978-953-51-0641-8

[69] Brown KA et al. Modified hydra bioassay to evaluate the toxicity of multiple mycotoxins and predict the detoxification efficacy of a clay-based sorbent. Journal of Applied Toxicology. 2014;**34**:40-48

[70] Fouad AM, Ruan D, El-Senousey HK, Chen W, Jiang S, Zheng C. Harmful effects and control strategies of aflatoxin B1 produced by *Aspergillus flavus* and *Aspergillus parasiticus* strains on poultry: Review. Toxins. 2019;**11**:176. DOI: 10.3390/toxins11030176

[71] Kumar P, Mahato DK, Kamle M, Mohanta TK, Kang SG. Aflatoxins: A global concern for food safety, human health and their management (A review). Frontiers in Microbiology. 2017;7:2170

[72] FAO. Food Agriculture Organization of the United Nations, Food and Nutrition Paper No. 81: Worldwide Regulations for Mycotoxins in Food and Feed in 2003. Rome, Italy: Food and Agriculture Organization; 2004. p. 165

[73] AOAC. Official Methods of Analysis of the Association of Official Analytical Chemists: Test Method; AOAC 2003.02. AOAC; Washington, DC: US Food and Drug Administration; 2004

[74] Anitha S, Waliyar F, Reddy AS, Rao R, Rao R, Kumar PL. Development of a simple enzyme-linked immunosorbent assay for quantitative estimation of aflatoxin B1 albumin adduct in humans. Current Science. 2011;**101**(7):844-846. ISSN: 0011 - 3891

[75] EFSA. Opinion of the scientific panel on contaminants in the food chain on a request from the commission related to aflatoxin B1 as undesirable substance in animal feed. EFSA Journal. 2004;**39**:1-27

[76] Moturi WKN. Factors likely to enhance mycotoxin introduction into the human diet through maize in Kenya. African Journal of Food Agriculture Nutrition and Development. 2008;**8**(3):265-277

[77] Battilani P, Toscano P, van de Fels-Klerx HJ, Moretti A, Leggieri CM, Brera C, et al. Aflatoxin B1 contamination in maize in Europe increases due to climate change. Scientific Reports. 2016;**6**:24328

[78] Pitt JI. Toxigenic fungi and mycotoxins. British Medical Bulletin. 2000;**56**:184-192

[79] Diener UL, Cole RJ, Sanders TH, Payne GA, Lee LS, Klich MA. Epidemiology of aflatoxin formation by *Aspergillus flavus*. Annual Review of Phytopathology. 1987;**25**:249-270

[80] Payne G, Brown MP. Genetics and physiology of aflatoxin biosynthesis. Annual Review of Phytopathology. 1998;**36**:329-362

[81] Atherstone C, Grace D, Waliyar F, Lindahl JF, Osiru M. Aflatoxin Literature Synthesis and Risk Mapping: Special Emphasis on Sub-Saharan Africa. Nairobi, Kenya: ILRI; 2014

[82] Hell K, Mutegi C. Aflatoxin control and prevention strategies in key crops of Sub-Saharan Africa. African Journal of Microbiology Research. 2011;**5**(5):459-466

[83] Fountain JC, Scully BT, Ni X, Kemerait RC, Lee RD, Chen Z-Y, et al. Environmental influences on maize-*Aspergillus flavus* interactions and aflatoxin production. Frontiers in Microbiology. 2014;**5**:40. DOI: 10.3389/fmicb.2014.00040

[84] Mutegi CK, Hendricks SL, Jones RB, Okello JJ, Ngugi HK. Paper Presented at the African Crop Science Conference Proceedings. 2007

[85] Obioha IW, Craft AA, Starh MH. Effect of sodium nitrate on aflatoxin production in pork sausages at different temperatures and the effect of nitrite on growth of *Aspergillus parasiticus* in culture. Journal of Agricultural and Food Chemistry. 1983;**31**(5):1039-1042

[86] WHO. International Programme on Chemical Safety, Environment Health Criteria 11: Mycotoxins. Geneva: World Health Organization; 1979. ISBN: 924154071

[87] Heidtmann-BemvenutiR,MendesGL, Scaglioni PT, Badiale-Furlong E, Souza-Soares LA. Biochemistry and metabolism of mycotoxins: A review. African Journal of Food Science. 2011;**5**(16):861-869. Available from: https://www.researchgate.net/publication/265035156_Biochemistry_and_metabolism_of_mycotoxins_A_review [Accessed: 12 July 2019]

[88] Eaton DL, Gallagher EP. Mechanisms of aflatoxin carcinogenesis. Annual Review of Pharmacology and Toxicology. 1994;**34**:135-172

[89] Haddad LM. Clinical Management and Drug Overdose. 2nd ed. Philadelphia, PA: W.B. Saunders Co.; 1990. p. 515

[90] Klaassen CD, editor. Casarett and Doull's Toxicology. The Basic Science of Poisons. 6th ed. New York, NY: McGraw-Hill; 2001. p. 75

[91] Chen C, Wang L, Lu S, Wu M, You S, Zhang Y, et al. Elevated aflatoxin exposure and risk of hepatocellular carcinoma. Hepatology. 1996;**24**:38-42

[92] Neal GE, Eaton DL, Judah DJ, Verma A. Metabolism and toxicity of aflatoxins M1 and B1 in human-derived in vitro systems. Toxicology and Applied Pharmacology. 1998;**151**:152-158

[93] Bhosa GS, Kitya D, Lubega A, Ogwal-Okeng J, Anokbonggo WW, Kyegombe DB. Review of the biological and health effects of aflatoxins on body organs and body systems. In: Razzaghi-Abyaneh M, editor. Aflatoxins—Recent Advances and Future Prospects. Rijeka, Croatia: InTech; 2013. pp. 239-265. ISBN: 978-953-51-0904-4

[94] Verma RJ. Aflatoxin cause DNA damage. International Journal of Human Genetics. 2004;**4**:231-236

[95] Searle CE, editor. Chemical Carcinogens. ACS Monograph 173. Washington, DC: American Chemical Society; 1976. p. 670

[96] Liu Y, Wang W. Aflatoxin B1 impairs mitochondrial functions, activates ROS generation, induces apoptosis and involves Nrf2 signal pathway in primary broiler hepatocytes. Animal Science Journal. 2016;**87**:1490-1500

[97] Li D, Cao Y, He L, Wang NJ, Gu JR. Aberrations of p53 gene in human hepatocellular carcinoma from China. Carcinogenesis. 1993;**14**:169-173

[98] Battista JR, Marnett LJ. Prostaglandin H synthase-dependent epoxidation of aflatoxin B1. Carcinogenesis. 1985;**6**:1227-1229

[99] Weng MW, Lee HW, Choi B, Wang HT, Hu Y, Mehta M, et al. AFB1 hepatocarcinogenesis is via lipid peroxidation that inhibits DNA repair, sensitizes mutation susceptibility and induces aldehyde-DNA adducts at p53 mutational hotspot codon 249. Oncotarget. 2017;**8**:18213-18226

[100] Hussein HS, Brasel JM. Toxicity, metabolism, and impact of mycotoxins on humans and animals. Toxicology. 2001;**167**(2):101-134

[101] Kowalska A, Walkiewicz K, Koziel P, Muc-Wierzgon M. Aflatoxins: Characteristics and impact on human health. Postępy Higieny i Medycyny Doświadczalnej (Online). 2017;**71**:315-327

[102] Nduti NN. Isolation and characterization of *Lactobacillus* in Kimere, a fermented Pearl Millet product in Kenya and screening their ability to retain viability and health benefit in a new developed product [PhD thesis]. Nairobi, Kenya: Technical University of Kenya; 2017

[103] Ngindu A, Johnson BK, Kenje PR, Ngira JA, Ochieng DM, Nandwa H, et al. Outbreak of acute aflatoxicosis caused by aflatoxin poisoning in Kenya. Lancet. 1982;**1**:1346-1348

[104] Burger HM, Lombard MJ, Shephard GS, Rheeder JR, van der Westhuizen L, Gelderblom WC. Dietary fumonisin exposure in a rural population of South Africa. Food and Chemical Toxicology. 2010;**48**(8-9):2103-2108. DOI: 10.1016/j.fct.2010.05.011

[105] Kangethe EK, MIbui GM, Randolph TF, Langat AK. Prevalence of aflatoxin M1 and B1 in milk and animal feeds from urban smallholder dairy production in Dagoretti Division, Nairobi, Kenya. East African Medical Journal. 2007;**84**(11):583-587

[106] Mutiga SK, Were V, Hoffmann V, Harvey JW, Milgroom MG, Nelson RJ. Extent and drivers of mycotoxin contamination: Inferences from a survey of Kenyan maize mills. Phytopathology. 2014;**104**(11):1221-1231. DOI: 10.1094/phyto-01-14-0006-r

[107] Okoth S, Nyongesa B, Ayugi V, Kang'ethe E, Korhonen H, Joutsjoki V. Toxigenic potential of *Aspergillus* species occurring on maize kernels from two agro-ecological zones in Kenya. Toxins (Basel). 2012;**4**(11):991-1007. DOI: 10.3390/toxins4110991

[108] Center for Disease Control Report. Prevention, Effectiveness Analysis of Aflatoxin Screening Program in Rural Eastern Africa. Washington, DC: Center for Disease Control Report, US Department of Health and Human Services; 2012

[109] Nyangaga DN. Traders' awareness and level of aflatoxins in human foods and cattle feed in selected markets and stores in Nairobi County, Kenya [MSc thesis]. Nairobi, Kenya: Kenyatta University; 2014

[110] Edward OO. Determination of aflatoxin in maize flour sold in Nairobi, Machakos and Kiambu counties [BTech Project]. Nairobi, Kenya: Technical University of Kenya; 2019

[111] Bukola CA, Abiodun AO, Ukpe GP. Mycofloral of smoke-dried fishes sold in Uyo Eastern Nigeria. World Journal of Agricultural Sciences. 2008;**4**(3):346-350

[112] Bennett JW, Klich M. Mycotoxins. Clinical Microbiology Reviews. 2003;**16**(3):497-516. DOI: 10.1128/CMR.16.3.497-516.2003

[113] Azziz-Baumgartner E, Lindblade K, Gieseker K, Rogers HS, Kieszak S, et al. Case-control study of an acute aflatoxicosis outbreak, Kenya, 2004. Environmental Health Perspectives. 2005;**113**:1779-1783

[114] Vincelli P, Parker G, Mcneill S. Aflatoxins in Corn. Department of Cooperative Extension Service, College of Agriculture Food and Environment, University of Kentucky; 1995. Publication ID-59

[115] Behfar A, Khorasgani ZN, Alemzadeh Z, Goudarzi M, Ebrahimi R, Tarhani N. Determination of aflatoxin M1 levels in produced pasteurized milk in Ahvaz City by using HPLC. Jundishapur Journal of Natural Pharmaceutical Products. 2012;**7**(2): 80-84. DOI: 10.5812/jjpharma.4707

[116] Armando MR, Dogi CA, Pizzolitto RP, Escobar F, Peirano MS, Salvano MA. et al. *Saccaromyces cerevisiae* strains from animal environmental with aflatoxin B1 detoxification ability and anti pathogenic bacteria influence in vitro. World Mycotoxin Journal. 2011;**4**(1):59-68. ISSN: 1875-0710

[117] Govaris A, Roussi V, Koidis PA, Botsoglou NA. Distribution and stability of aflatoxin during processing, ripening and storage of Telemes cheese. Food Additives and Contaminants. 2001;**18**:437-444

[118] Van Egmond HP. Introduction in Mycotoxins in Dairy Products. London: Elsevier Applied Science; 1989

[119] Wageh SD, Yoshinori I, Shouta MMN, Mayumi I. An overview on mycotoxin contamination of foods in Africa. Journal of Veterinary Medical Science. 2014;**76**(6):789-797

[120] EC Commission Directive 91/126/ EEC of 13th February 1991. Amending the Annexes to Council Directive 74/63/ EEC on undesirable substances and products in animal nutrition. Official Journal of the European Union. EU, Brussels

[121] FAO/WHO. FAO/WHO Standards Programme. Codex Alimentarius Commission, Alinorm 93/12. The Hague, Netherlands: Report of the 24th Session of Codex Commision on Food Additives and Contaminants; 1992

[122] Wacoo AP, Wendiro D, Vuzi PC, Hawumba JF. Methods for detection of aflatoxins in agricultural food crops: A review. Journal of Applied Chemistry. 2014;**2014**:706291. DOI: 10.1155/2014/706291

[123] Mwihia JT, Straetman M, Ibrahim A, Njau J, Muhenje O, Guracha A, et al. Aflatoxin levels in locally grown maize from Makueni District. East African Medical Journal. 2008;**85**:311-317

[124] Park DL, Liang B. Perspectives on aflatoxin control for human food and animal feed. Trends in Food Science and Technology. 1993;**4**:334-342

[125] Park DL, Njapau H. Contamination issues and padding. Journal of the American Oil Chemists' Society. 1989;**66**:1402-1405

Chapter 2

Aflatoxin Occurrence in Dairy Feeds: A Case of Bulawayo, Zimbabwe

Nancy Nleya, Lubanza Ngoma and Mulunda Mwanza

Abstract

Aflatoxin contamination in feeds used by Bulawayo peri-urban farmers for dairy cows was assessed. Semi-intensive farming was the most common farming type practised by the farmers where the animal feeds were supplemented with mixed rations, concentrated feed, grass and brewers' spent grains. Mixed ration was the most commonly used feed supplement. Feed analysis by high-performance liquid chromatography (HPLC) showed the presence of all four naturally occurring aflatoxins: aflatoxins B_1, B_2, G_1 and G_2. Total aflatoxin concentration in the feeds ranged from 0 to 250.9 μg/kg. Mixed ration had the highest average total aflatoxin concentration of 29.0 μg/kg, which is above the European Union (EU) standard adopted by Zimbabwe. AFB_1, the most potent aflatoxin was the predominant aflatoxin across all feeds with an average concentration of 9.0 μg/kg and highest concentration of 149.6 μg/kg in a mixed ration sample which is also above the EU 5.0 μg/kg for lactating cows. Farm personnel responses to the questionnaire showed that most of them were not aware of aflatoxins. These findings call for stringent measures to be put in place with regard to aflatoxin testing in feeds for the dairy sector as well as educating the farmers on the importance of aflatoxin monitoring feed ingredients and livestock feeds.

Keywords: aflatoxins, feeds, dairy, cows, chromatography, farming systems, monitoring

1. Introduction

Animal feed ingredients are at risk of mould contamination with subsequent mycotoxin production during preharvest, harvest and postharvest times [1–3]. The sources of the individual components used in the formulation of dairy feeds are quite diverse ranging from cereals, cereal products, oil seeds as well as hay and forages [3, 4]. Also the high cost of feed has led to the addition of stale bread, kitchen and bakery wastes to the feed. Furthermore scarcity of protein sources for animal feeds has led to the use of alternative protein sources such as brewers' spent grains (BSG) [5]. These waste products are usually tainted with fungus and may be a contributing factor in mycotoxin production in cattle feed. Aflatoxins are the most toxic mycotoxins produced by members of the genus *Aspergillus* [6], and their presence in animal feedstuffs has become a potential health hazard to both animals and humans [7]. Toxic effects of aflatoxins in ruminants include liver damage, diminished growth efficiency, diminished milk production and quality and impaired resistance to infectious diseases [7–9].

In dairy farming, depending on the farming system adopted, the diet consists of the concentrates, alternative protein sources as well as forage; hence the animals are exposed to more than one type of mycotoxins [4]. Although there are more than 20 aflatoxins known, only four of these occur naturally, namely, aflatoxins (AF) B_1, B_2, G_1 and G_2, based on their fluorescence under UV light (blue or green) [10–12]. The most abundant aflatoxin in cow feeds and rations is aflatoxin B_1 and is also the most potent of them all [13, 14].

Animals differ in their sensitivity to mycotoxin toxicity [15] with ruminants being more resistant than the monogastrics [16] mainly because they have microorganisms in their rumen which play significant roles in the deactivation and degradation of the aflatoxins as well as alteration of the binding of the aflatoxins to some essential nutrients [17, 18]. However, aflatoxins are poorly degraded by ruminants as most of the rumen microbiota are inhibited by AFB_1 concentration of 10 μg/ml [16]. The aflatoxins will get to the bioconversion sites of nutrients and xenobiotics like the intestinal epithelium, liver and kidneys unaltered [16]. In the liver, AFB_1 is bio-transformed to AFM_1 which enters the circulatory system or is conjugated to glucuronic acid. The conjugated AFM_1 is excreted through the biliary system, and the one in circulation may be excreted through urine and milk. It has been shown that AFM_1 retains some carcinogenic activity resulting in its reclassification by IARC as a group 1 carcinogen [19–21]. Consumption of AFB_1-contaminated feed by lactating cows results in its metabolism into AFM_1 subsequently secreted into milk thereby making milk a source of aflatoxin contamination in humans. In this study the extent of aflatoxin contamination of feeds used in different feeding systems adopted by dairy farmers was assessed.

2. Methodology

2.1 Data collection

Convenience sampling coupled with snowball sampling methods was used to identify farmers willing to participate in the research. Questionnaires were used to get information from the farmers. The information required from the farmers included the following: plot size in acres, number of cattle owned by the farmer, number of cows that were being milked, age, breed, lactation stage, milking method, volume of milk produced on the farm per day, volume of milk produced by each cow per day, number of milking per day, amount of feed given to each cow per day and also if the farmer had any knowledge on aflatoxins. A total of 14 farmers participated in this study with farm size of 8.5 hectares and above. Most of them were milking cows ranging between 20 and 250, and a few had less than 10 cows. The cows that were being milked were 25 months old and above, and the common breeds were the Jersey, Holstein and crossbreed (Holstein/Jersey) across all milking stages. Majority of the farmers were milking by hand getting a volume of 100 to over 200 litres per farm per day with each cow giving an average of 6–10 litres.

2.2 Sample collection

A total of 96 feed samples which consisted of dairy feed concentrates (CN), mixed ration (MR), brewers spent grain (BSG) and grass (GR) were collected from 13 farms during the dry season (August–October 2016) and the rainy season (January–March 2017). Samples were collected in sterile polythene ziplock bags which were sealed and transported in cooler boxes to the laboratory where they were ground to a fine powder using IKA® M20 universal batch mill (Germany) and stored in the freezer at −20°C until time for analysis [22].

2.3 Sample preparation for HPLC analysis

Aflatoxins from feeds were extracted using the immunoaffinity extraction method [23] using Easi-Extract® aflatoxin immunoaffinity columns (R-Biopharm Rhone Limited, Glasgow G20 OXA, Scotland). Extraction was carried out according to the manufacturer's protocol with some modifications as follows: a portion of 50 g of the sample was mixed with 5 g of sodium chloride (NaCl) in a laboratory blender followed by 100 ml of methanol: water (80:20 v/v) and blended for 5 minutes. The mixture was filtered through a fluted filter paper (Whatman No.1) into a clean vessel. A volume of 2 ml of the filtrate was then diluted with 14 ml phosphate buffer saline (PBS) solution and passed through an immunoaffinity column. The column was washed with 20 ml of PBS and the aflatoxins finally eluted with 1 ml methanol (LiChrosolv®, Merck, Germany) into a glass cuvette and diluted with 1 ml of distilled water and then stored at −20°C prior to analysis. Aflatoxin B_1, B_2, G_1 and G_2 standards (Trilogy Analytical Laboratory, Washington, USA) were diluted using acetonitrile (LiChrosolv®, Merck, Germany) to give the following concentrations: 5×10^{-6}, 5×10^{-5}, 5×10^{-4}, 5×10^{-3} and 5×10^{-2} mg/ml. Aflatoxin detection and quantification were done using HPLC (Shimadzu FCV-20H2) with operation conditions as given in the KOBRA® cell instruction manual as follows: derivatisation using KOBRA ® cell at 100 μA setting, with an analytical column Inertsil ODS-3 V 5 μm, 4.6 × 150 mm equipped with a C18 4 × 3 mm^2 ID security guard cartridge (Phenomenex, Torrance, CA, USA). Mobile phase was modified from the recommended water: methanol (60:40) to a working condition of 55:45 with 119 mg/litre of potassium bromide (KBr) and 1 ml/litre of 65% nitric acid added at a flow rate of 1.0 ml/minute, and fluorescence detector is set at 362 nm for excitation and emission 425 nm (AFB_1 and B_2) and 455 nm (AFG_1 and G_2). Injector was an auto sampler which injected 100 μl of sample, and elution of the aflatoxins was in the order (AF) G_2, G_1, B_2 and B_1.

Calibration curves for each aflatoxin, AF (B_1), B_2, G_1 and G_2, were constructed using standard solutions which were diluted with acetonitrile to give the following concentrations: 0.005, 0.05, 0.5, 5 and 50 μg/kg. The limit of detection for all the standards was 0.005 μg/kg. The linearity of the standard curves was determined using correlation regression (r^2). A curve with good linearity will have an r^2 value close to 1. Aflatoxin concentration of the samples was calculated by measuring the area of the peak and then interpolating from the standard curve.

2.4 Statistical analysis

Descriptive statistics was used to show the distribution of aflatoxins in the different feeds and one-way ANOVA used for significance testing using IBM SPSS Statistics 25.

3. Results

3.1 Farmer survey

Most of the farmers who took part in the study were practising semi-intensive farming followed by extensive and lastly intensive farming as summarised by **Figure 1**.

The cows were mainly fed with concentrates, mixed ration, brewers' spent grain and grass ranging from 6 to 10 kg per animal per day. Only 36% of the farmers had some knowledge on aflatoxins. The most utilised feed was mixed ration as shown by **Figure 2**.

3.2 Analysis of aflatoxins

HPLC analysis of aflatoxins showed the presence of all the major aflatoxins AF (B_1), B_2, G_1 and G_2 in the bulk of the samples indicated by the peaks in the

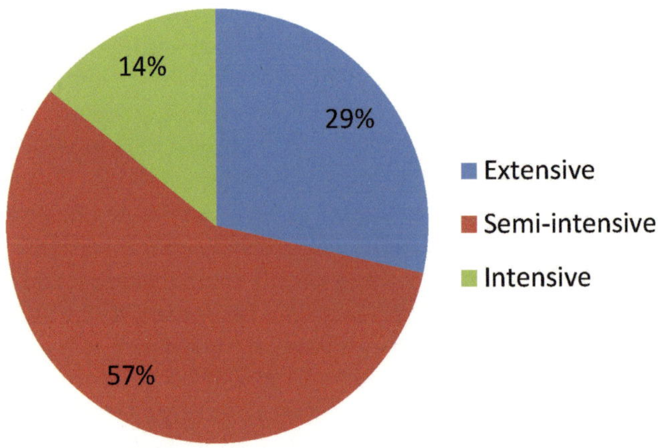

Figure 1.
Farming systems adopted by dairy farmers in Bulawayo peri-urban showing that most the farmers practise semi-intensive farming.

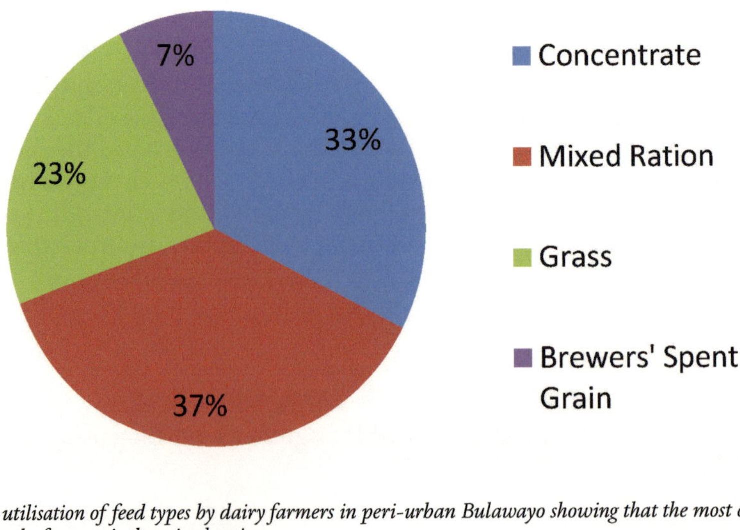

Figure 2.
Percentage utilisation of feed types by dairy farmers in peri-urban Bulawayo showing that the most common feed used by the farmers is the mixed ration.

chromatograms as shown in **Figure 3**. The calibration curves gave good linearity for the different aflatoxins with r^2 values of 1. Total aflatoxin concentration in the feeds ranged from 0 to 250.9 μg/kg.

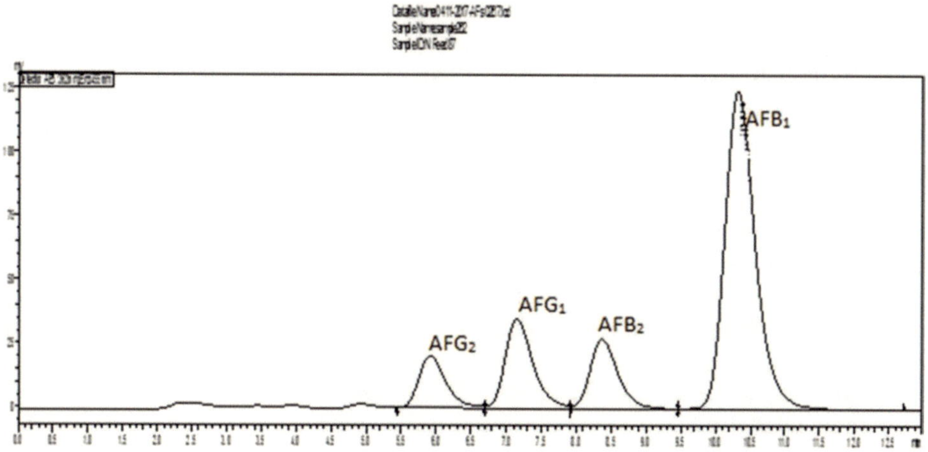

Figure 3.
Representative chromatogram showing four peaks indicating the presence of all major aflatoxins.

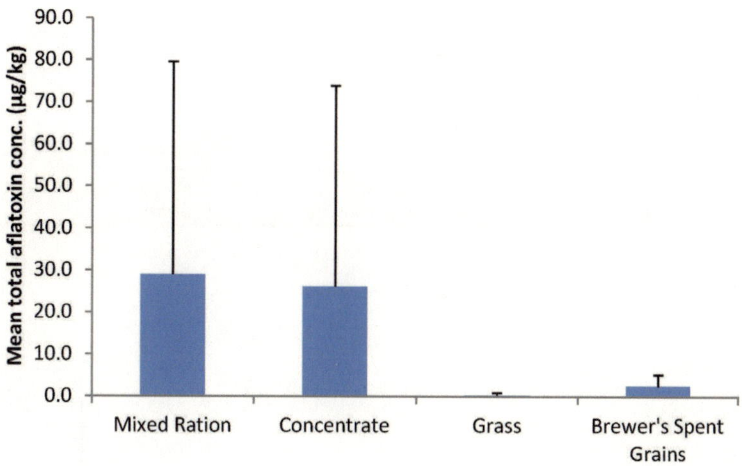

Figure 4.
Average total aflatoxin concentrations in the feeds. A p *value of 0.043 shows that there was significant difference in the aflatoxin concentrations in the different feeds with mixed ration had the highest contamination.*

ANOVA					
Total AF conc (ug/kg)					
	Sum of squares	df	Mean square	F	*p* value
Between groups	14860.674	3	4953.558	2.832	**0.043**
Within groups	159185.082	91	1749.287		
Total	174045.756	94			

A p value <0.05 indicates that there is a significant difference in the levels of aflatoxin in the different types of feeds used for feeding the dairy cows.

Table 1.
One-way ANOVA for all feed types.

3.3 Aflatoxin distribution in feeds

Mixed ration had the highest total AF concentrations with an average concentration of 29.8 μg/kg, and grass had the lowest concentrations as shown in **Figure 4**. The one-way analysis of variance (ANOVA) (**Table 1**) gave a p value of 0.043, meaning that at 95% confidence level ($p < 0.05$) there is enough evidence to conclude that there is a significant difference in the total mean concentration of aflatoxins across the feeds. However, looking at MR and CN (**Table 2**), $p = 0.766$; therefore there was no significant difference in the mean total aflatoxin concentrations.

The distribution of aflatoxins in the feeds showed that AFB_1 was the most common aflatoxin across all feeds as shown by **Figure 5**. However, there was variation with individual feeds as shown in **Figure 6a–d**.

Looking at the distribution of total aflatoxins across the different farming systems, **Figure 7** shows that the semi-intensive system had the highest aflatoxins with an average of 21.6 μg/kg. One-way ANOVA (**Table 3**), however, indicated that there is no significant difference in the mean total aflatoxin concentration in the feeds from semi-intensive and intensive farming systems as $p = 0.937$ which is greater than p value of 0.05 at 95% confidence level.

ANOVA					
Total AF conc (μg/kg)					
	Sum of squares	**df**	**Mean square**	**F**	***p* value**
Between groups	218.928	1	218.928	0.089	**0.766**
Within groups	159133.265	65	2448.204		
Total	159352.193	66			

A p value >0.05 indicates that there is no significant difference in the levels of aflatoxin.

Table 2.
One-way ANOVA between the mixed ration and feed concentrate.

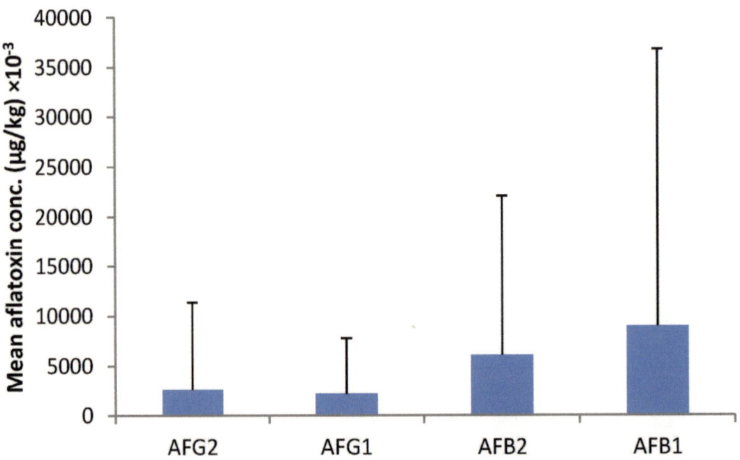

Figure 5.
Distribution of aflatoxins across all feed types. One-way ANOVA analysis gave a p *value of 0.017, indicating a significant difference between the concentrations of the individual aflatoxins with* AFB_1 *being the most dominant aflatoxin.*

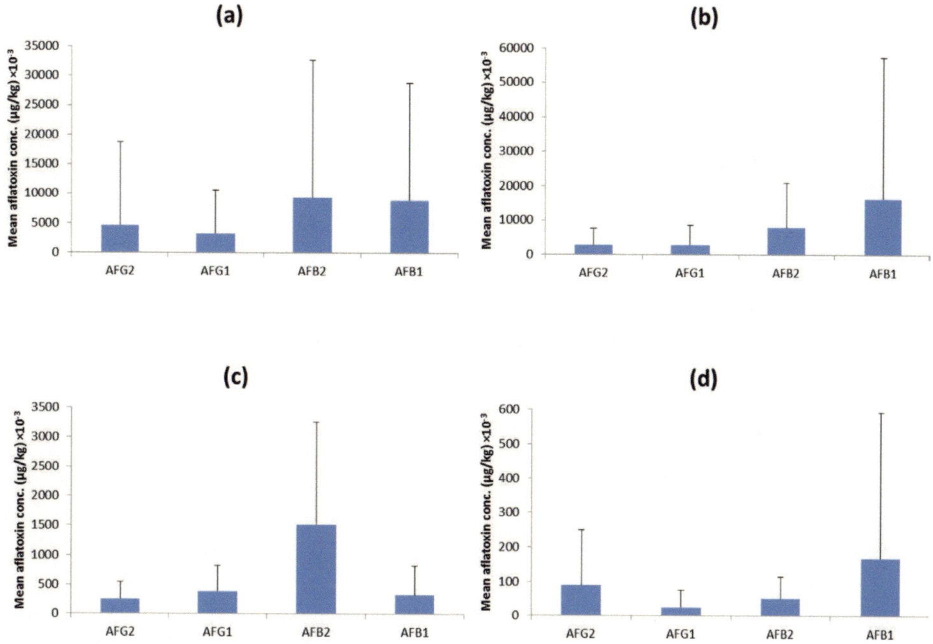

Figure 6.
Distribution of aflatoxins in the feeds, (a) feed concentrates, (b) mixed ration, (c) brewers' spent grains and (d) grass. One-way ANOVA gave a p *value of 0.017, indicating a significant difference in the concentration of individual toxins across all feeds.* AFB_1 *was the dominant aflatoxin in mixed ration and grass, whereas for concentrates and brewers' spent grains,* AFB_2 *was the predominating aflatoxin.*

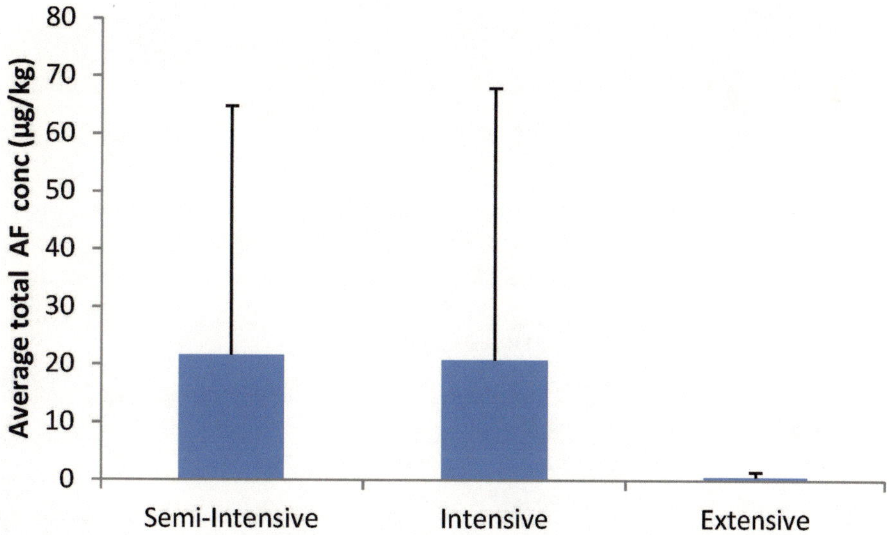

Figure 7.
Distribution of aflatoxins across the three farming systems. Descriptive statistics shows that extensive farming has the lowest aflatoxin concentration and semi-intensive farming has more aflatoxin concentrations in their feeds. However, one-way ANOVA gave $p = 0.470$*, indicating no significant difference among the different farming systems.*

Distribution of AFB_1 in the feeds from the different dry and rainy seasons is shown in **Figure 8**, and ANOVA analysis showed that there is a significant difference in AFB_1 concentrations in the different seasons (**Table 4**).

ANOVA					
Total AF conc (µg/kg)					
	Sum of squares	df	Mean square	F	*p* value
Between groups	12.581	1	12.581	0.006	**0.937**
Within groups	171580.359	87	1972.188		
Total	171592.940	88			

A p value >0.05 indicates that there is no significant difference in the levels of aflatoxin concentration between.

Table 3.
One-way ANOVA results comparing the semi-intensive and intensive farming systems.

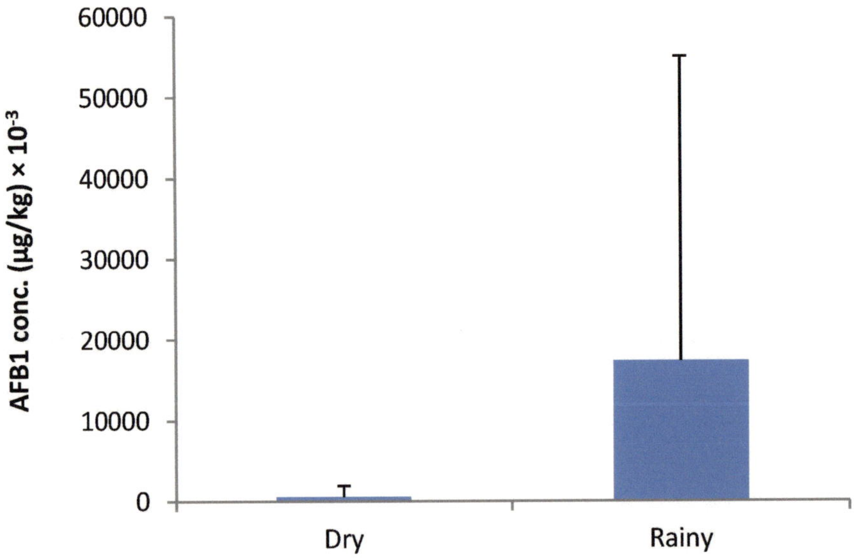

Figure 8.
Seasonal variation in the distribution of AFB_1. There was a significant difference in AFB_1 concentrations (p = 0.003) with samples from the rainy season having more of AFB1 than dry season samples.

ANOVA					
AFB_1 conc (µg/kg) × 10^{-3}					
	Sum of squares	df	Mean square	F	*p* value
Between groups	6747185610.100	1	6747185610.100	9.500	**0.003**
Within groups	66758340020.045	94	710195106.596		
Total	73505525630.144	95			

A p value <0.05 indicates that there is a significant difference in the levels of AFB_1 concentration in feeds in the rainy season.

Table 4.
One-way ANOVA results for dry season and rainy season.

4. Discussion

Feed quality is of great importance in animal husbandry as it affects both animal health and productivity [24]. Consumption of aflatoxin-contaminated feeds by dairy cows may result in the aflatoxins occurring in milk posing health risks to humans [18]. Research has shown that some feedstuffs used in formulating animal feeds can become infected by aflatoxin-producing fungi [25]. Researchers worldwide have been analysing dairy feed for aflatoxin contamination and have reported various findings with most feeds exceeding the regulatory limits [26–29].

This study also showed that 96% of feeds used in feeding dairy cows in peri-urban Bulawayo that were analysed were contaminated with at least one of the naturally occurring aflatoxins. The results also indicate that 21% of the samples analysed had total aflatoxin levels above the regulatory limit set by international governing bodies of 20 μg/kg for animal feeds. This concurs with the findings by Reddy and Salleh [30] who reported that 22.5% of their samples had aflatoxin concentrations above this regulatory limit. Zimbabwe reviewed the AFB_1 regulatory limit to 20 μg/kg in 1990 [31] for food intended for human consumption. However, there are no regulatory limits in terms of animal feeds [32].

The feeds that are used in feeding dairy cows by farmers in peri-urban Bulawayo included feed concentrates, mixed ration, grass and brewer's spent grains. This is in accordance with the requirements of the diets of dairy cows which should consist of a component that provides protein and energy and a component of roughage [33]. In this study, the protein and energy were supplied by the concentrates, mixed ration and the brewer's spent grains, whereas the roughage was provided in the form of hay stored at the farm or fresh grass in the grazing land.

Mixed rations are considered a whole meal for the cow as they contain basically all the nutrients that are found in forages and concentrates. Formulation of a mixed ration involves combining forages, by-products of other processes such as whole cottonseed or cottonseed cake, grains, protein source, minerals and vitamins [34]. Findings of this study showed that mixed ration had the highest total aflatoxin concentrations with an average of 29.0 μg/kg. ANOVA also showed that at 95% confidence level, there was a significant difference in the mean total aflatoxins in the feeds with the mixed rations having the highest total aflatoxin mean. Findings from this study concur with Mozafari et al. [35] who detected the highest aflatoxin concentrations in mixed ration among the other feeds they analysed. The diversity of the components used could have been potential sources of aflatoxigenic fungi which result in contamination of this feed type with aflatoxins. Other researchers [25] also reported high aflatoxin concentration in noug cake, a product of oil processing industry used in feeding dairy cows. Cottonseed was the most utilised feed ingredient for mixed rations by the farmers who participated in this study. However, Chohan et al. [36] reported feed concentrate having the highest aflatoxin concentration followed by mixed ration in their study on aflatoxin contamination of different feeds and feed ingredients used to feed dairy cows in Pakistan.

From this study it was shown that grass samples had the least aflatoxin concentrations with an average total aflatoxin concentration of 2.5 μg/kg and 169×10^{-3} μg/kg of AFB_1. These results are similar to the finding by Gizachew et al. [25] who also had grass as the least contaminated feed. However, they got a minimum AFB_1 concentration 7 μg/kg for their samples, higher than what was established in this study. Sassahara et al. [37] analysed feedstuffs supplied to dairy cows in North of Paraná state, Brazil, and did not detect any aflatoxins in the silage samples. Work done by Driehuis et al. [33] in the Netherlands also showed the absence of aflatoxins in silage samples used to feed dairy cows. These findings suggest that grass in the form of silage or pasture is not really prone to fungal infections which may result in aflatoxin production. In this study most of the aflatoxigenic strains were isolated from the grass, but it was the feed with the least aflatoxin concentration. Gonzalez Pereyra et al. [38] highlighted that the presence of aflatoxigenic fungi on a substrate does not mean that the toxin is present in that particular food/feed matrix, but there is a risk of toxin production if the environmental conditions become favourable for aflatoxin production. Nonetheless, detection of aflatoxins in a sample means the substrate has been contaminated by toxigenic species which could either be present or absent at the time of sampling. This was the case with the feed concentrates which had aflatoxin concentrations higher than the grass samples, but fewer toxigenic strains were isolated.

The most dominant aflatoxin across all feeds was AFB_1 with an average concentration of 9.0 μg/kg and was detected in all the samples that tested positive for aflatoxin contamination. This is above the EU 5 μg/kg set for lactating cows. Udom et al. [39] and Gizachew et al. [25] also reported their samples having AFB_1 concentrations exceeding the EU regulatory limit. The high levels of AFB_1 in most samples could be attributed to the fact that it was the most common and prevalent aflatoxin in most food matrices [40, 41]. Moreover, some authors have indicated that most toxigenic *Aspergillus* strains produce AFB_1 and therefore it occurs more frequently than the other aflatoxins [10, 42, 43]. AFB_1 was predominant in the rainy season (**Figure 8**). These results are in agreement with the findings by Chohan et al. [36] which also showed high concentrations of AFB_1 during the rainy season. For aflatoxin production, high temperatures and high humidity are required, and these conditions prevail during the rainy season.

However, for brewers' spent grains (BSG), AFB_2 was the predominant aflatoxin. The BSG are a product of beer brewing industry [44] and has been found to be of valuable use in the feedstock industry mainly because it is affordable and available throughout the year [45]. BSG used in this study were from the production of opaque beer. The presence of aflatoxins in beer production has been associated with contaminated malt. Malt production involves increasing the moisture content of the grains to allow partial germination of the grain. Aflatoxigenic fungi are known to contaminate cereal grains which are also used in the beer production process [46]. If the malt is not properly dried or stored, fungal growth may be promoted resulting in the production of aflatoxins. Research on the fate of mycotoxins during the beer fermentation process showed that recovery of AFB_2 in BSG is higher than other aflatoxins [47]. Some researchers [48] showed that AFB_2 is able to adsorb onto yeast cells during fermentation. The yeast cells and the grain particles that are removed through filtration are collectively known as brewers' spent grains. This could be the possible reason why AFB_2 levels were higher in BSG samples. Nevertheless, Gonzalez Pereyra et al. [38] were not able to detect any AFB_2 in barley malt and brewers' spent grains from Argentina breweries. AFB_1 has been reported as the most common aflatoxin occurring naturally in feedstuffs, but for this study it was not the case for BSG as the concentration of AFB_2 was higher than that of AFB_1.

This study also showed that aflatoxin contamination of brewers' spent grains, a known source of nitrogen and roughage, and grass were within the regulatory limits making them safer when compared to the concentrates and mixed ration. However, nutritional composition of the grass will not meet the dietary demands of the cows.

5. Conclusion

Detection of aflatoxins in the feed samples used for this study is a cause of concern as this may be indicating the possibility of transfer into the milk by the dairy cows. Although most samples were within the acceptable limit for total aflatoxin, it was noted that concentrations of AFB_1, the most potent of them, were above the regulatory limit. Moreover, research has shown that AFB_1 can be carried over into milk as its hydroxylated metabolite AFM_1 making milk a route through which humans are exposed to aflatoxins. High prevalence of AFB_1 during the rainy season could be an indication of poor storage of the feeds which may result in increased moisture content resulting in proliferation of aflatoxin-producing *Aspergillus*. Therefore, there is a need to educate the farmers and their personnel on the importance of proper feed storage facilities in order to control contamination of the feeds.

Acknowledgements

I would like to thank the farmers who participated in this research; without you I would not have done it. I am also grateful to the farm personnel who assisted in the collection and safe storage of the samples, thank you for your immense support.

I also want to thank the NRF (Grant number 105882)and the NUST Research Board (Grant number RB No. 43/16) for the funds that were made available towards this research.

Conflicts of interest

The authors declare no conflict of interest.

Author details

Nancy Nleya[1,2*], Lubanza Ngoma[1] and Mulunda Mwanza[1]

1 Department of Animal Health, Northwest University, Mafikeng, South Africa

2 Department of Applied Biology and Biochemistry, National University of Science and Technology, Bulawayo, Zimbabwe

*Address all correspondence to: ndangwa@gmail.com; nancy.nleya@nust.ac.zw

References

[1] Bryden WL. Food and feed, mycotoxins and the perpetual pentagram in a changing animal production environment. Animal Production Science. 2012;**52**(7):383-397. DOI: 10.1071/AN12073

[2] Peng WX, Marchal J, van der Poel A. Strategies to prevent and reduce mycotoxins for compound feed manufacturing. Animal Feed Science and Technology. 2018;**237**:129-153. DOI: 10.1016/j.anifeedsci.2018.01.017

[3] Sultana N, Hanif N. Mycotoxin contamination in cattle feed and feed ingredients. Pakistan Veterinary Journal. 2009;**29**(4):211-213

[4] Fink-Gremmels J. Mycotoxins in cattle feeds and carry-over to dairy milk: A review. Food Additives and Contaminants. 2008;**25**(2):172-180. DOI: 10.1080/02652030701823142

[5] Li X, Zhao L, Fan Y, Jia Y, Sun L, Ma S, et al. Occurrence of mycotoxins in feed ingredients and complete feeds obtained from the Beijing region of China. Journal of Animal Science and Biotechnology. 2014;**5**(1):37. DOI: 10.1186/2049-1891-5-37

[6] Kagot V, Okoth S, De Boevre M, De Saeger S. Biocontrol of *Aspergillus* Mycotoxins in Africa: Benefits and limitations. Toxins. 2019;**11**(2):109. DOI: 10.3390/toxins11020109

[7] Danesh Mesgaran M, Mojtahedi M, Vakili SA, Hayati-Ashtiani M. Effect of aflatoxin B_1 on in vitro rumen microbial fermentation responses using batch culture. Annual Review and Research in Biology. 2013;**3**:686-693

[8] Queiroz O, Han J, Staples C, Adesogan A. Effect of adding a mycotoxin-sequestering agent on milk aflatoxin M_1 concentration and the performance and immune response of dairy cattle fed an aflatoxin B_1-contaminated diet. Journal of Dairy Science. 2012;**95**(10):5901-5908. DOI: 10.3168/jds.2011-5287

[9] Bbosa GS, Kitya D, Odda J, Ogwal-Okeng J. Aflatoxins metabolism, effects on epigenetic mechanisms and their role in carcinogenesis. Health. 2013;**5**(10):14-34. DOI: 10.4236/health.2013.510A1003

[10] Baranyi N, Kocsubé S, Vágvölgyi C, Varga J. Current trends in aflatoxin research. Acta Biologica Szegediensis. 2013;**57**(2):95-107

[11] Arapcheska M, Jovanovska V, Jankuloski Z, Musliu Z, Uzunov R. Impact of aflatoxins on animal and human health. The International Journal of Innovative Research in Science, Engineering and Technology. 2015;**2**(2):156-161

[12] Reid CX, Sparks DL, Williams WP, Brown AE. Single corn kernel aflatoxin B1 extraction and analysis method. Natural Resources. 2016;**7**(07):405. DOI: 10.4236/nr.2016.77035

[13] Tajkarimi M, Shojaee MH, Yazdanpanah H, Ibrahim SA. Aflatoxin in agricultural commodities and herbal medicine. In: Aflatoxins-Biochemistry and Molecular Biology. IntechOpen; 2011. Available from: http://www.intechopen.com/books/aflatoxins-biochemistry-and-molecular-biology/aflatoxin-in-agricultural-commodities-and-herbal-medicine

[14] Bräse S, Gläser F, Kramer C, Lindner S, Linsenmeier AM, Masters KS, et al. Progress in the chemistry of organic natural products. The chemistry of mycotoxins. Progress in the Chemistry of Organic Natural Products. 2013;**97**:v

[15] Denli M. Implications of mycotoxins in livestock feeds. AgroLife Scientific Journal. 2015;**4**(1):52-55

[16] Jouany J, Yiannikouris A, Bertin G. Risk assessment of mycotoxins in ruminants and ruminant products. Options Mediterranéennes, A. 2009;**85**:205-224

[17] Gallo A, Giuberti G, Frisvad JC, Bertuzzi T, Nielsen KF. Review on mycotoxin issues in ruminants: Occurrence in forages, effects of mycotoxin ingestion on health status and animal performance and practical strategies to counteract their negative effects. Toxins. 2015;**7**(8):3057-3111. DOI: 10.3390/toxins7083057

[18] Afsah-Hejri L, Jinap S, Hajeb P, Radu S, Shakibazadeh S. A review on mycotoxins in food and feed: Malaysia case study. Comprehensive Reviews in Food Science and Food Safety. 2013;**12**(6):629-651. DOI: 10.1111/1541-4337.12029

[19] Ketney O, Ovidiu T, Tifrea A. Structural diversity and biochemical and microbiological characteristics of aflatoxins. Acta Universitatis Cibiniensis Series E: Food Technology. 2014;**18**(2):3-18. DOI: 10.2478/aucft-2014-0010

[20] Sarica DY, Has O, Tasdelen S, Ezer Ü. Occurrence of aflatoxin M_1 in milk, white cheese and yoghurt from Ankara, Turkey markets. Journal of Biological and Chemical Research. 2015;**2015**:36-49

[21] Janković VV, Vukojević JB, Lakićević BM, Mitrović RR, Vuković DI. Presence of moulds and aflatoxin M_1 in milk. Zbornik Matice srpske za prirodne nauke. 2009;(117):63-68. DOI: 10.2298/ZMSPN0917063J

[22] Beukovic D, Krstovic S, Perisic B, Jajic I, Glamocic D. Presence of aflatoxin in complete feeding mixtures for different categories of pigs in Serbia. 2015:231-236

[23] Mwanza M. A comparative study of fungi and mycotoxin contamination in animal products from selected rural and urban areas of South Africa with particular reference to the impact of this on the health of rural black people [thesis]. University of Johannesburg; 2012

[24] Raju S, Padamadan CJ, Shenpagam NH. Mycotoxin production by fungi isolated from commercially prepared livestock feed in Kerala. International Journal of Advanced Research. 2016;**2**(5):154-159

[25] Gizachew D, Szonyi B, Tegegne A, Hanson J, Grace D. Aflatoxin contamination of milk and dairy feeds in the Greater Addis Ababa milk shed, Ethiopia. Food Control. 2016;**59**:773-779. DOI: 10.1016/j.foodcont.2015.06.060

[26] Sumantri I, Murti T, van der Poel A, Boehm J, Agus A. Carry-over of aflatoxin B1-feed into aflatoxin M_1-milk in dairy cows treated with natural sources of aflatoxin and bentonite. Journal of the Indonesian Tropical Animal Agriculture. 2012;**37**(4):271-277

[27] Ismail A, Riaz M, Akhtar S, Yoo S, Park S, Abid M, et al. Seasonal variation of aflatoxin B_1 content in dairy feed. Journal of Animal and Feed Sciences. 2017;**26**(1):33-37. DOI: 10.22358/jafs/69008/2017

[28] Kang'ethe E, Sirma A, Murithi G, Mburugu-Mosoti C, Ouko E, Korhonen H, et al. Occurrence of mycotoxins in food, feed, and milk in two counties from different agro-ecological zones and with historical outbreak of aflatoxins and fumonisins poisonings in Kenya. Food Quality and Safety. 2017;**1**(3):161-170. DOI: 10.1093/fqsafe/fyx018

[29] Changwa R, Abia W, Msagati T, Nyoni H, Ndleve K, Njobeh P. Multi-mycotoxin occurrence in dairy cattle feeds from the Gauteng Province of South Africa: A pilot study using UHPLC-QTOF-MS/MS. Toxins. 2018;**10**(7):294. DOI: 10.3390/toxins10070294

[30] Reddy K, Salleh B. A preliminary study on the occurrence of *Aspergillus* spp. and aflatoxin B_1. in imported wheat and barley in Penang, Malaysia. Mycotoxin Research. 2010;**26**:267-271

[31] Siwela AH, Nziramasanga N. Regulatory aspects of aflatoxin control in Zimbabwe—A review. Journal of Applied Science in Southern Africa. 1999;**5**(2):141-147

[32] Mazumder PM, Sasmal D. Mycotoxins—Limits and regulations. Ancient Science of Life. 2001;**20**(3):1

[33] Driehuis F, Spanjer M, Scholten J, Te Giffel M. Occurrence of mycotoxins in maize, grass and wheat silage for dairy cattle in the Netherlands. Food Additives and Contaminants. 2008;**1**(1):41-50. DOI: 10.1080/19393210802236927

[34] Amaral-Phillips DM, Bicudo JR, Turner LW. Feeding Your Dairy Cows a Total Mixed Ration: Getting Started. Bulletin ID-141A Cooperative Extension service, College of agriculture, University of Kentucky, Lexington, US Consultado a; 2002;9

[35] Mozafari S, Mohsenzadeh M, Mehrzad J. Seasonally feed-related aflatoxins B_1 and M_1 spread in semiarid industrial dairy herd and its deteriorating impacts on food and immunity. Journal of Food Quality. 2017;**2017**:1-7. DOI: 10.1155/2017/4067989

[36] Chohan KA, Awan F, Ali MM, Iqbal U, Ijaz M. Assessment of aflatoxin in dairy concentrate feeds, total mixed rations, silage and various feed ingredients in Pakistan. Pakistan Journal of Zoology. 2016;**48**(1):277-280

[37] Sassahara M, Netto DP, Yanaka E. Aflatoxin occurrence in foodstuff supplied to dairy cattle and aflatoxin M_1 in raw milk in the North of Parana state. Food and Chemical Toxicology. 2005;**43**(6):981-984. DOI: 10.1016/j.fct.2005.02.003

[38] Gonzalez Pereyra M, Rosa C, Dalcero A, Cavaglieri L. Mycobiota and mycotoxins in malted barley and brewer's spent grain from Argentinean breweries. Letters in Applied Microbiology. 2011;**53**(6):649-655. DOI: 10.1111/j.1472-765X.2011.03157.x

[39] Udom I, Ezekiel C, Fapohunda S, Okoye Z, Kalu C. Incidence of *Aspergillus* Section *Flavi* and concentration of aflatoxin in feed concentrates for Cattle in Jos, Nigeria. Journal of Veterinary Advances. 2012;**2**(1):39-46

[40] Patel SV, Bosamia TC, Bhalani HN, Singh P, Kumar A. Aflatoxins: Causes and effects. Journal of Agricultural and Biological Sciences. 2015;**13**(9):140-141

[41] Wacoo AP, Wendiro D, Vuzi PC, Hawumba JF. Methods for detection of aflatoxins in agricultural food crops. Journal of Applied Chemistry. 2014;**2014**:1-16. DOI: 10.1155/2014/706291

[42] Bellio A, Bianchi DM, Gramaglia M, Loria A, Nucera D, Gallina S, et al. Aflatoxin M_1 in cow's milk: Method validation for milk sampled in northern Italy. Toxins. 2016;**8**(3):57. DOI: 10.3390/toxins8030057

[43] Gherbawy YA, Shebany YM, Hussein MA, Maghraby TA. Molecular detection of mycobiota and aflatoxin contamination of chili. Archives of Biological Sciences. 2015;**67**(1):223-234. DOI: 10.2298/ABS141010028G

[44] Aghabeigi R, Moghaddaszadeh-Ahrabi S, Afrouziyeh M. Effects of brewer's spent grain on performance and protein digestibility in broiler chickens. European Journal of Experimental Biology. 2013;**3**(3):283-286

[45] Mussatto SI. Brewer's spent grain: A valuable feedstock for industrial applications. Journal of the Science of Food and Agriculture. 2014;**94**(7):1264-1275. DOI: 10.1002/jsfa.6486

[46] Tangni E, Larondelle Y, editors. Malts, moulds and mycotoxins. In: Bacteria, Yeasts and Moulds in Malting and Brewing: Proceedings of the Xth Symposium "Chair J de Clerck", Leuven (Belgium); 2002

[47] Inoue T, Nagatomi Y, Uyama A, Mochizuki N. Fate of mycotoxins during beer brewing and fermentation. Bioscience, Biotechnology, and Biochemistry. 2013;**77**(7):1410-1415. DOI: 10.1271/bbb.130027

[48] Deepak M, Jhanvi S, AnuAppaiah K. Aflatoxin binding and detoxification by non-saccharomyces yeast A New Vista for decontamination. International Journal of Current Microbiology and Applied Sciences. 2015;**4**(5):310-317

Chapter 3

α-Amylase Production by Toxigenic Strains of *Aspergillus* and *Penicillium*

Adekunle Odunayo Adejuwon
and Victoria Anatolyivna Tsygankova

Abstract

Aflatoxins are produced by a variety of fungal species and these have contributed to devastating health problems globally. However, apart from the capability of the production of aflatoxins, the productions of enzymes by like fungi have been explored. Aflatoxin B1-producing-toxigenic strains of *Aspergillus flavus* (A_1), *Aspergillus parasiticus* (A_2), *Penicillium citrinum* (P_1) and *Penicillium rubrum* (P_2) isolated from rice were grown on a defined medium with varying carbon and nitrogen sources. They were also grown on rice as sole carbon and nitrogen source for fungal growth. In an attempt to purify, the extracellular α-amylases produced were subjected to ammonium sulfate precipitation (40–90% saturation) followed by dialysis. The aflatoxin B1-producing toxigenic strains of *Aspergillus flavus* (A_1), *Aspergillus parasiticus* (A_2), *Penicillium citrinum* (P_1) and *Penicillium rubrum* (P_2) were able to produce α-amylases in both the growth medium with varying C and N sources of fungal and also in the rice medium. The most active α-amylase activity was produced by toxigenic *A. flavus* (A_1) with a value of 3.25 ± 0.15 Units and this was when ammonium sulfate was nitrogen source with starch as carbon source of fungal growth in the defined growth medium. These toxigenic fungal strains can be explored for the industrial production of α-amylases.

Keywords: α-amylase, toxigenic, fungi, aflatoxin B1

1. Introduction

1.1 *Aspergilli* and pathogenicity

Aspergilli are of the taxonomic Division Eumycota, Subdivision Eumycotina, Class Ascomycetes, Order Eurotiales, Family Trichocomaceae [1]. *Aspergillus* is a filamentous cosmopolitan and ubiquitous fungus commonly isolated from soil, plant debris and indoor air environment [2]. While the teleomorphic state exists for *Aspergillus species*, some are accepted to be mitosporic without any known sexual spore [3]. The genus *Aspergillus* includes over 185 species and about 20 species have so far been reported as causing opportunistic infections in man [4, 5]. Among these species, *Aspergillus fumigatus* is the most commonly isolated species followed by *Aspergillus flavus* and *Aspergillus niger. Aspergillus clavatus*, *Aspergillus glaucus*, *Aspergillus oryzae*, *Aspergillus terreus*, *Aspergillus ustus* and *Aspergillus versicolor* are among the other species less commonly isolated as opportunistic pathogens [6, 7]. Food infected by *Aspergillus flavus* may be carcinogenic to humans and animals [8]. *Aspergillus flavus* is a saprophyte of grains. It produces mycotoxins in infected food [2]. Infection of peanuts (*Arachis hypogaea*) seeds by *Aspergillus flavus* and *Aspergillus parasiticus* is a serious problem that can result in aflatoxin contamination in the seed [9]. *Aspergillus flavus* produces aflatoxins B, G and cyclopiazonic acid CPA [10].

Beta-1,3-Glucanase activity in peanut seed is induced by infection with *Aspergillus flavus* [9]. Maize seeds are susceptible to *Aspergillus flavus* infection [11]. *Aspergillus flavus* causes Ear rot in corn with aflatoxin production. Resistance to aflatoxin production can be controlled by epistasis [12]. *Aspergillus flavus* causes kernel infection in maize, the Southwestern corn borer (SWCB) has been reported to substantially increase aflatoxin levels in such infection [13]. Kernels of corn genotype GT-MAS:gk are resistant to *Aspergillus flavus* [14]. A 14-KDa protein in corn kernel makes it resistant to *Aspergillus flavus* infection [15]. *Aspergillus flavus* found around corn storage cribs and bins are point sources of inoculum/infection with *Aspergillus flavus* in the corn agroecosystem [16]. Ear corn rot caused by *Aspergillus flavus* and *Aspergillus parasiticus* is severe in areas with high temperatures and drought [2]. *Aspergillus flavus* causes the post-harvest disease of *Arachis hypogaea* [3].

According to Norton [17], carotenoids in endosperm may decrease the amount of aflatoxin produced by *Aspergillus flavus. Aspergillus flavus* can be divided into S and L strains on the basis of sclerotial morphology [18]. Atoxigenic *Aspergillus flavus* L strain reduce formation of both sclerotia and aflatoxin when coinoculated with S strain isolate [18]. *Aspergillus flavus* L strain reduce formation of both sclerotia and aflatoxin when coinoculated with S strain isolate [18]. *Aspergillus flavus* produces aflatoxin in cotton seed with the S strain being highly toxigenic [19]. *Aspergillus parasiticus* isolated from soil from a corn field produced aflatoxin B(1) B(2) and G(1) G(2) [20]. *Aspergillus flavus* produces beta-glucuronidase [21]. *Aspergillus flavus* and *Aspergillus parasiticus* can contaminate agricultural crops with the production of toxic fungal metabolite aflatoxins. An endochitinase which is an inhibitory protein with M(r) of 29,000 is capable of inhibiting growth of *Aspergillus flavus* on maize [22]. Onion seeds stalk and flowers are susceptible to infection by *Aspergillus niger* Tiegh [23, 24]. The black-spored *Aspergillus* isolates that have been found to cause the disease fig smut are *Aspergillus niger* var. niger, *Aspergillus niger* var. awamori, *Aspergillus japonicus* and *Aspergillus carbonarius* [25]. Epiphytic fungi found on table grapes include *Epiccocum nigrum*, *Cladosporium herbarum*, *Alternaria alternata*, *Aspergillus niger* [26].

1.2 Penicilli and pathogenicity

Penicilli belongs to the taxonomic Division Eumycota, Subdivision Eumycotina, Class Ascomycetes, Order Eurotiales, Family Trichocomaceae [1]. Grape fruit green mold is caused by *Penicillium digitatum* [27]. *Penicillium* is common on citrus, gelly and preservatives. It is abundant in the soil and on decaying materials [3]. *Penicillium* spores are present in the air [3]. Studies have shown that *Penicillium* is important in the production of antibiotics such as Penicillin and Griseofluvin [5]. *Penicillium digitatum* causes the green mold of citrus fruits. Optimum temperature of their mycelia on such fruits is about 25°C [28]. The food borne pathogen *Listeria monocytogenes* has been observed to grow on apple infected with *Penicillium expansum* but not after 5 days [29]. The blue mold of decayed pear fruit is caused by *Penicillium expansum* [30]. *Penicillium expansum* has been observed to cause gray mold disease in apple and blue mold in pear [31]. *Penicillium* spp. have been isolated from pear stem [32] while *Penicillium italicum* cause citrus blue mold and green mold [33, 34]. Postharvest green mold of oranges is caused by *Penicillium digitatum* [35, 36]. *Penicillium* sp. has been isolated from grapes [26]. *Penicillium expansum* causes the blue mold decay of pear [37]. *Penicillium digitatum* and *Penicillium italicum* cause postharvest green and blue molds of citrus fruits. Sporulation of both molds can be prevented or reduced by gaseous ozone without noticeable ozone phytotoxicity to the fruits [33, 34]. Apple fruits with stem pulls have been reported to be more susceptible to blue mold decay caused by *Penicillium expansum* than fruits with stems [38]. According to Spotts and Holz [39], *Penicillium expansum* can infect and cause disease in grape and plum fruits. Aqueous chlorine has been reported to reduce the viable spores of *Penicillium digitatum*, the causative fungi of the green mold and sour rot of citrus [40]. Sodium bicarbonate has been found to reduce postharvest decay of apple [41]. The level of resistance to decay of apple cultivars, caused by *Penicillium expansum*, varies from cultivar to cultivar [42]. Ziram but not calcium chloride control gray mold and bull's-eye rot, the postharvest decay of pear associated with the pathogen *Penicillium expansum* [43]. *Penicillium digitatum* has been associated with the postharvest green mold of oranges. Soda ash was observed to control this post-harvest disease [35, 36]. According to Smilanick et al. [35, 36], the effectiveness of imazalil for the control of citrus green mold caused by *Penicillium digitatum* improved significantly when the citrus fruits were treated with heated aqueous solutions of the fungicide as compared with the current commercial practice of spraying wax containing imazalil on the fruits. According to Smilanick et al. [44], fungicide applications with thiabendazole (TBZ) and sodium bicarbonate reduce green mold caused by *Penicillium digitatum* of citrus fruits and lemon fruits. It was also observed that pre harvest applications of thiophanate methyl to the fruits controlled postharvest green mold. Blue mold caused by *Penicillium* is an important postharvest disease of apple. *Penicillium expansum* and *Penicillium solitum* have been identified and isolated from rotten apple and pear fruits [45]. According to Sirois et al. [23, 24], onion seeds are affected by species of *Penicillium*.

1.2.1 α-Amylases

Amylases are hydrolytic enzymes that catalyze the degradation of starch molecules and other carbohydrates to yield dextrins and progressively smaller polymers composed of glucose units [46, 47]. Based on their pattern of catalysis and yield of products, amylases can be categorized as: alpha (α) amylase (endoamylase) (α-1,4-glucan-4-glucanohydrolase, EC 3.2.1.1); beta (β) amylase (exoamylase) (1,4-α-D-glucan maltohydrolase, EC 3.2.1.2); glucoamylase (exohydrolase) (Glucan-1,4-α-glucosidase, EC 3.2.1.3); pullulanase (α-dextrin endo-1,6-α-glucosidase, EC 3.2.1.41); isoamylase (EC 3.2.1.68). Pullulanases and isoamylases are termed debranching enzymes [46, 48, 49]. They can be of plant and microbial sources [50–52].

1.2.2 Microbial α-amylases

α-Amylases are produced by bacteria and fungi [53–58]. The two types of amylases commonly encountered in microbial degradation of starch are α and β amylases.

Degradation of substrate is important in enzymatic hydrolysis [59]. Starch is the substrate used in microbial amylase assay [60]. The starch molecules are hydrolyzed into polymers of glucose units [47]. According to Vihinen and Mantsala [61], starch-degrading enzymes are widely distributed among microbes and several activities are required to hydrolyze the starch into glucose units. *Bacillus subtilis* isolated from flour mill wastes produced a thermostable α-amylase in a complex medium containing starch [62]. According to Ajayi and Fagade [63], corn starch can be used as substrate for β-amylase production by *Bacillus macerans*, *Bacillus licheniformis*, *Bacillus circulans*, *Bacillus coagulans*, *Bacillus megaterium*, *Bacillus polymyxa*, *Bacillus cereus* and *Bacillus subtilis*. According to Reiss et al. [64], approximately 80% of potato starch and 40–50% of grain starch were hydrolyzed by alpha amylase of certain microbes. Lactic acid bacteria have been found to ferment starchy foods to recover RNA though digestion with alpha amylase did not improve extraction [65]. *Rhizopus oligosporus*, a prolific amylase producer can degrade cassava tuber containing 65% starch into glucose [66]. *Thermoactinomyces thalpophilus* isolated from flour mill waste has been found to be capable of hydrolyzing 2% soluble starch [62]. A thermostable α-amylase activity from *Bacillus subtilis* isolated from flour mill waste was found to be more strongly expressed with corn starch than soluble starch [62]. Alpha amylase from *Bacillus licheniformis*, an hyperthermostable enzyme, is able to hydrolyze starch to medium-size oligosaccharides [67]. *Fusarium moniliforme* was found to produce alpha amylase in a culture medium containing starch [68].

Certain environmental (physical) factors affect amylase activity [48]. Lactic acid was found to be produced from *Lactobacillus delbrueckii* subsp.delbrueckii and defatted rice bran powder containing starch with coupled saccharification with amylase at 37°C and pH 5.0 [69]. An α-amylase produced by *Bacillus* sp. isolated from soil sample was optimally active at 75–80°C [70]. Alpha-amylase from *Bacillus licheniformis* is able to hydrolyze soluble starch within a temperature range of 60–75°C [71]. A thermophilic, moderately halophilic anaerobic *Halothermothrix orenii* synthesized an amylase similar to *Bacillus megaterium* amylase with optimal activity at 65°C [72]. Thermophilic *Thermus* sp. was reported to produce an extracellular α-amylase able to degrade starch at 70°C [73]. *Bacillus stearothermophilus* was found to produce a thermostable α-amylase active at 43°C [74]. According to Saito [75], *Bacillus licheniformis* produced a thermophilic extracellular α-amylase stable at 25°C but more active at an optimum temperature of 76°C. Manning and Campbell [76] reported that *Bacillus stearothermophilus* synthesized a thermostable α-amylase. *Rhizopus arrhizus* and *Rhizopus oryzae* were found to be capable of hydrolyzing starch at 30°C [77]. *Bacillus halodurans* produced an alkaline active maltohexaose-forming α-amylase active at 60°C. According to Oh et al. [57], *Lactobacillus gasseri* is able to synthesize a maltogenic amylase exhibiting optimum activity for β-CD hydrolysis at 55°C. Based on studies carried out by Najafi and Kembhavi [50], a marine *Vibrio* sp. produced an extracellular α-amylase with maximum activity at 55–60°C. According to Ogasahara et al. [78], *Bacillus stearothermophilus* was able to produce a thermophilic α-amylase with optimum temperature range of 65–73°C.

α-Amylase from *Pyrococcus woesei* has maximal activity at pH 5.6 [79]. A *Bacillus* sp. isolated from piglet cacum produced an extracellular alpha amylase optimally active at pH 7.0 [80]. A microorganism from uncultured soil was observed to produce amylolytic enzyme with optimal pH of 9.0 [81]. A mutant of *Bacillus amyloliquefaciens* has been reported to synthesize alpha amylase with optimal activity at pH 7.0 [82]. An extracellular alpha amylase isolated from cell free broth of *Streptomyces megasporus* grown in glucose, soluble starch and raw starch was stable at a pH range of 5.5–8.5 but with optimum activity at pH 6.0 [83]. Amylases in culture supernatants of an environmentally derived microbial mixed culture selected for its ability to utilize starch-containing plastic films as sole carbon sources produced amylases active at pH 5.5 and 8.0 [84]. Alpha amylase from *Thermoactinomyces vulgaris* had optimum activity at pH 4.8–6.0 [85]. Starch degradation by *Rhizopus oryzae* was favorable at pH 6.0 [77]. Akindahunsi [86] reported that waste water from cassava mash fermented by pure strains of *Saccharomyces cerevisiae*, *Lactobacillus delbrueckii* and *Lactobacillus coryniformis* produced amylase after 3 days with maximal activity at pH 6.0.

According to Mijts and Patel [72], the thermophilic, moderately halophilic anaerobic *Halothermothrix orenii* is able to synthesize alpha amylase active with specific activity of 2232 U mg^{-1} requiring $CaCl_2$ for optimum activity and thermostability. The maltooligosaccharide-forming amylase from *Bacillus circulans* is enhanced by $C0^{2+}$ and Mg^{2+} [87]. Amylase synthesized by *Lipomyces starkeyi* was found to be actively stable in a commercial mouthwash [88]. A salt-tolerant thermostable amylase produced by *Bacillus megaterium* was reported to be stable at 5 M NaCl [89]. A thermophilic *Thermoascus aurantiacus* has been observed to produce amylase with thermostability enhanced by calcium chloride [90]. Amylase production from *Bacillus sphaericus* was reported to be maximum with 3 mM divalent cations Mg^{++} and Ca^{++} incorporated in a growth medium [91]. Cadmium, Cobalt, Copper, Manganese, Nickel and Lead incorporated into Czapek-Dox liquid medium supported growth and production of amylase by soil yeasts *Geotrichum capitatum* and *Geotrichum candidum* [92]. Activity of α-amylase from a marine *Vibrio* sp. was found to be restored by Fe^{2+}, Mn^{2+}, Co^{2+}, Ca^{2+}, Mg^{2+} and Cu^{2+} to nearly 25–55% [50]. A *Bacillus* sp. produced an alkaliphilic amylase which was enhanced by Na^{+} and Co^{2+} [93]. According to Mishra et al. [94], *Bacillus subtilis* produced an α-amylase. Herbizid has been reported to activate amylase production in culture of *Fusarium oxysporum*, *Mucor niemalis* and *Penicillium chrysogenum* [95].

Amylase from *Fusarium verticillioides* has been found to be inhibited by a hydrophobic 19.7-KDa inhibitor from corn kernel [96, 97]. *Fusarium moniliforme*, a mycotoxigenic fungus has been reported to produce an amylase inhibited by a specific amylase inhibitor found in corn [96, 97]. Alpha-amylase inhibitor has been isolated from culture medium of *Streptomyces parvullus* [98]. *Streptomyces aureofaciens* produces a novel polypeptide inhibitor [99]. A strain of *Streptomyces nigrifaciens* has been reported to produce an amylase inhibitor having inhibitory effects on alpha amylase and glucoamylase [100].

Bacillus subtilis isolated from soil produced a starch degrading amylase with molecular weight of 50 KDa and an isoelectric point of 4.9 [101]. *Streptomyces lividans* has been reported to have a molecular weight of 107,054 KDa [102]. Alpha amylases from some *Bacillus* spp. were detected to possess molecular weight of approximately 65,5854 and 49 KDa [103]. Alpha-amylase of *Clostridium thermosulfurogenes* has been reported to have a molecular mass of 75,112 Da [104]. According to Kang et al. [105], *Bacillus stearothermophilus* produces an alpha-amylase which was glycosylated and with molecular weights of approximately 61–75 KDa.

According to Lorentz [106], Protected 4-Nitrophenyl-1,4–1-D-maltoheptaoside can be used in routine amylase assay. A simple and rapid method using Remazol Brilliant Blue-starch as substrate which is non-destructive allows direct visualization and isolation of amylolytic microorganisms from the environment [107].

Alpha amylase can be used in improving anaerobic solid waste treatment [108]. Carbohydrate-hydrolyzing enzymes have long been used by industrial product markers as major catalysts to transform raw materials into end products in such areas as food processing, beverage production, animal nutrition, leather and textiles [109].

With the advent of new frontiers in biotechnology, the spectrum of amylase application has widened in many fields such as clinical, medicinal and fine-chemical industries, as well as a widespread application of starch saccharification in the textile, food, brewing and distilling industries [110].

1.2.3 *Aflatoxin B_1 and α-amylase production*

According to Mellon et al. [111], an aflatoxin B1 producer strain of *Aspergillus flavus* seem to possess the ability to produce numerous extracellular hydrolases (α-amylase inclusive). Aflatoxin B1 have been detected in groundnut and maize contaminated with *Aspergillus flavus* [112]. The removal of lipids from ground substrates significantly reduced the substrate's potential for aflatoxin B1 (AFB1) production by *Aspergillus flavus*. However, maltose, glucose, arginine, glutamic acid, aspartic acid and zinc significantly induced the AFB1 production up to 1.7–26.6 fold [113]. Aflatoxins B_1, B_2, G_1 and G_2 and α-amylase were detected in *Aspergillus oryzae*, *Aspergillus flavus*, *Talaromyces spectabilis*, *Pacilomyces variotii* and *Lichtheimia* sp. isolated from nuruks in several regions of Korea [114]. According to Fakhoury and Woloshuk [115], a mutant strain of *Aspergillus flavus* failed to produce extracellular α-amylase when the Amy1 gene necessary for the production of α-amylase was disrupted in an aflatoxigenic strain (an aflatoxin B1 producing strain) of the fungus. Mycotoxigenic strains (aflatoxin B1 producing strains) of *Fusarium moniliforme* and *Aspergillus flavus* were capable of α-amylase production in a medium composed of 2% ground corn in milky stage corn [116]. In their attempt to increase aflatoxin B1 resistance in maize, Rajasekaran et al. [117] discovered that the α-amylase inhibitor-like protein (AILP) seem to play a role in the inhibition of *Aspergillus flavus* α-amylase and fungal growth. Fountain et al. [118] reviewed the nature of the interaction occurring between aflatoxin production by *Aspergillus flavus*, the environment in which the fungus thrives and its susceptibility to crop host before harvest. They proposed future directions for elucidating future relationship between resistance and susceptibility to the fungus' colonization, abiotic stress and its relationship to oxidative stress in which its aflatoxin B1 production may function as a form of antioxidant protection to the producing fungus. In a known positive transcriptomic database, E-probe Diagnostic for Nucleic acid Analysis (EDNA), a bioinformatic tool, originally developed to detect plant pathogens in mutagenomic databases, is capable of discriminating between production and non-production of aflatoxin B1 by *Aspergillus flavus* [119]. Substrate-induced lipase gene expression might be indirectly related to aflatoxin formation by providing the basic building block "acetate" for aflatoxin B1 synthesis in aflatoxin-producing *Aspergillus flavus* and *Aspergillus parasiticus* [120]. According to Smith et al. [121], silencing of the aflatoxin gene cluster in a certain strain of aflatoxin B1 producing *Aspergillus flavus* is suppressed by ectopic aflR gene (the transcriptional regulator of the aflatoxin biosynthetic gene cluster) expression.

1.2.4 Rice (Oryza sativa)

Rice (*Oryza sativa*) is a monocotyledonous cereal which belongs to the Grass family Gramineae or Poaceae [122]. With over 7000 varieties of rice, its pericarp and embryo contain 70–80% starch, 7% proteins, 1.5% oils, some vitamins (mostly A, B and C) and some essential minerals [3]. According to Sizer and Whitney [123], rice contains fiber and the vitamin folate and provides 80% of the calories consumed by humans worldwide [122]. It contains 12 chromosomes in a haploid set [124]. The domestication of rice formed part of the basis for civilization in the near East, far East and the New World [125]. Feeding more people worldwide than any other crop, rice is the only crop grown exclusively for human consumption [125]. Sedentary irrigated rice production in tropical lowlands can support hundreds of people per square kilometer, explaining the wide spread importance of rice crops in the tropics [126]. The discovery of Gibberellins arose from infected rice [122]. *Oryza sativa* is the main cultivated rice species but over 20 species in the genus are known [125].

This research was designed to examine the production and activity of α-amylases by some toxigenic aflatoxin B1-producing strains of *Aspergillus* and *Penicillium* isolated from deterioration rice. Attempts were made to purify the α-amylases.

1.2.5 Contribution to knowledge

The present research will establish the presence of α-amylases in rice during mycotic spoilage by toxigenic strains of *Aspergillus flavus* (A_1), *Aspergillus parasiticus* (A_2), *Penicillium citrinum* (P_1) and *Penicillium rubrum* (P_2). These fungi, being capable of producing these enzymes can be used in the production of amylases. Rice as substrate can be explored in such production.

Amylases are used in clinical chemistry most especially in diagnosis. Their combination with proteases and lipases are also employed industrially in the bio-remediation of recalcitrants/organic pollutants and the hydrolytic digestion of the peptidoglycan layers of both gram positive and gram negative bacteria in wastewaters before chlorination [109].

2. Materials and methods

2.1 Sources and identification of isolates

The isolates of aflatoxin B1-producing-toxigenic strains of *Aspergillus flavus* (A_1), *Aspergillus parasiticus* (A_2), *Penicillium citrinum* (P_1) and *Penicillium rubrum* (P_2) for this research were from deteriorated rice and identified at the Seed Health Unit of the International Institute for Tropical Agriculture, Ibadan, Nigeria using techniques contained in the illustrated Handbook of fungi [127, 128].The identification was done by observing cultural and morphological characteristics. Each isolate was cultured on Potato Dextrose agar. The nature of growth, rate of growth, colony color and sporulation patterns were carefully observed. Sporulating mature cultures was used in microscopic examination. Fungal samples were taken from advancing margins and centers of the growth regions with the aid of sterile inoculating needle. The samples were smeared on glass slides and stained with lactophenol cotton blue. After placing the cover slips, macroscopic and microscopic morphological characteristics like arrangement and shape of spores, type of sporangia, type of hyphae, presence or absence of septa on hyphae was examined under the high power objective of a compound binocular microscope.

2.2 Culture conditions and preparation of inocula

The isolates were subcultured and maintained on Potato Dextrose agar plates and slants. Each fungus was further subcultured into test tubes of the same medium and incubated at 25°C. A 96-hr-old culture of toxigenic strains of *Aspergillus flavus* (A_1), *Aspergillus parasiticus* (A_2) and *Penicillium rubrum* (P_2) and 120-h-old culture of *Penicillium citrinum* (P_1) was used as inocula. According to the modified method of Olutiola and Ayres [129], cultures was grown in a defined medium of the under-listed composition: $MgSO_4.7H_20$, K_2HPO_4, KH_2PO_4, L-cysteine, biotin, thiamine and $FeSO_4.7H_20$ with added carbon and nitrogen sources (Sigma). Conical flasks (250 ml) containing 100 ml growth medium will be inoculated with 1 ml of an aqueous spore suspension containing approximately 6×10^4 spores per ml of each isolate. Experimental and control flasks was incubated without shaking at 25°C [130].

2.3 Rice as a source of carbon

Rice (Caprice) from Spain was bought at the main market, Bodija, Ibadan, Nigeria. The rice was added to distilled water (1% w/v) and autoclaved at 15Ib/in^2 at

121°C. Experimental Conical flasks (250 ml) containing 100 ml of the rice medium was inoculated with 1 ml of an aqueous spore suspension containing approximately 6×10^4 spores per ml of each isolate. Control flasks contained sterilized rice medium not inoculated with aqueous spore suspension of the isolate. Experimental and control flasks was incubated without shaking at 25°C.

On a daily basis, the contents of each flask was filtered through glass fiber filter paper (Whatman GF/A). The protein content of the filtrates was determined using the method of Lowry et al. [131]. The filtrates were analyzed for amylase activity using the modified methods of Pfueller and Elliott [132] and Xiao et al. [133]. The filtrates were used as crude preparation.

2.4 Ammonium sulfate fractionation

The crude enzymes were treated with ammonium sulfate (analytical grade) within the limits of 40–90% saturation. Precipitation was allowed to continue at 4°C for 24 h. The mixtures were then centrifuged 10,000 g for 30 min at 4°C using a high speed cold centrifuge (Optima LE-80 K Ultracentrifuge, Beckman, USA). The supernatant was discarded. The precipitate was re-dissolved in 0.2 M citrate phosphate buffer, pH 6.0. The protein contents were determined using the Lowry et al. [131] method while amylase activity was determined using the modified methods of Pfueller and Elliott [132] and Xiao et al. [133].

2.5 Dialysis

Using acetylated dialysis tubings (Visking dialysis tubings, Sigma) [134] and a multiple dialyser (Pope Scientific Inc. Model 220, USA), the enzyme preparations were dialysed under several changes of 0.2 M citrate phosphate buffer pH 6.0 at 4°C for 24 h. The protein contents of the dialysed enzymes were determined using the Lowry et al. [131] method while amylase activity was determined using the modified methods of Pfueller and Elliott [132] and Xiao et al. [133].

2.6 Enzyme assay

Both experimental (fungal isolate inoculated) and control (un-inoculated) flasks were assayed for amylase activity.

2.6.1 α-Amylase

α-Amylase activity was determined using the modified methods of Pfueller and Elliott [132] and Xiao et al. [133]. The reaction mixtures consisted 2 ml of 0.1% (w/v) starch (Sigma) in 0.2 M citrate phosphate buffer, pH 6.0 as substrate and 0.5 ml of enzyme. These were the experimentals in the assay procedure. The controls in the assay procedure consisted only 2 ml of the prepared substrate. The contents of both experimental and control tubes were incubated at 35°C for 30 min. The reactions were terminated with 3 ml of 1 N HCl. Enzyme (0.5 ml) was added to the contents of each control. About 2 ml of the mixture from each of the sets of experimentals and controls was transferred into new sets of clean test tubes. About 3 ml of 0.1 N HCl was added into the contents of each test tube after which 0.1 ml of iodine solution was added. Optical density readings were taken spectrophotometrically at 620 nm. Enzyme activity was defined in units and specific activity as enzyme units per mg protein.

One unit of α-amylase activity was defined as the amount of enzyme which produced 0.1% reduction in the intensity of the blue color of starch-iodine complex under conditions of the assay.

3. Results

3.1 Amylase activities of isolates on growth media

Toxigenic strains of *Aspergillus flavus* (A_1), *Aspergillus parasiticus* (A_2), *Penicillium citrinum* (P_1) and *Penicillium rubrum* (P_2) grew and exhibited amylase activities, varyingly, in modified growth medium used for this research.

Using different carbon sources (rice, starch, maltose, sucrose, lactose, glucose and galactose) in the growth medium, amylase activity expressed by each isolate on the tenth day of incubation is shown in **Table 1**.

With different sources of nitrogen (NH_4Cl, urea, KNO_3, ammonium sulfate, glycine, sodium nitrate, tryptone and peptone) in the growth medium, amylase activity expressed varyingly by each isolate on the tenth day of incubation is shown in **Table 2**.

Toxigenic *P. citrinum* (P_1) produced active α-amylase (0.75 ± 0.01 Units) and this was when potassium nitrate was nitrogen source with maltose as carbon source of the defined growth medium. Toxigenic *A. parasiticus* (A_2) also expressed an α-amylase activity value of 0.72 ± 0.04 Units when rice was both carbon and nitrogen source of medium for fungal growth (**Table 1**).

Carbon source	Isolate	Amylase activity (Units)
Rice	*Aspergillus flavus* (A_1)	0.54 ± 0.01
	Aspergillus parasiticus (A_2)	0.72 ± 0.04
	Penicillium citrinum (P_1)	0.43 ± 0.23
	Penicillium rubrum (P_2)	0.62 ± 0.06
Galactose	*Aspergillus flavus* (A_1)	0.06 ± 0.01
	Aspergillus parasiticus (A_2)	0.53 ± 0.13
	Penicillium citrinum (P_1)	0.36 ± 0.05
	Penicillium rubrum (P_2)	0.09 ± 0.04
Glucose	*Aspergillus flavus* (A_1)	0.50 ± 0.04
	Aspergillus parasiticus (A_2)	0.63 ± 0.08
	Penicillium citrinum (P_1)	0.44 ± 0.08
	Penicillium rubrum (P_2)	0.32 ± 0.11
Lactose	*Aspergillus flavus* (A_1)	0.10 ± 0.00
	Aspergillus parasiticus (A_2)	0.66 ± 0.10
	Penicillium citrinum (P_1)	0.40 ± 0.17
	Penicillium rubrum (P_2)	0.37 ± 0.08
Maltose	*Aspergillus flavus* (A_1)	0.52 ± 0.03
	Aspergillus parasiticus (A_2)	0.68 ± 0.04
	Penicillium citrinum (P_1)	0.75 ± 0.01
	Penicillium rubrum (P_2)	0.58 ± 0.12
Starch	*Aspergillus flavus* (A_1)	0.45 ± 0.04
	Aspergillus parasiticus (A_2)	0.57 ± 0.12
	Penicillium citrinum (P_1)	0.68 ± 0.03
	Penicillium rubrum (P_2)	0.60 ± 0.14
Sucrose	*Aspergillus flavus* (A_1)	0.46 ± 0.05
	Aspergillus parasiticus (A_2)	0.69 ± 0.03
	Penicillium citrinum (P_1)	0.59 ± 0.13
	Penicillium rubrum (P_2)	0.39 ± 0.06

Each value represents the mean of three replicates with standard error.

Table 1.
Effect of carbon sources on activity of amylase produced by isolates.

Nitrogen source	Isolate	Amylase activity (Units)
Ammonium sulfate	*Aspergillus flavus* (A_1)	3.25 ± 0.15
	Aspergillus parasiticus (A_2)	0.05 ± 0.00
	Penicillium citrinum (P_1)	0.38 ± 0.13
	Penicillium rubrum (P_2)	0.13 ± 0.03
Glycine	*Aspergillus flavus* (A_1)	0.38 ± 0.13
	Aspergillus parasiticus (A_2)	2.48 ± 0.03
	Penicillium citrinum (P_1)	0.00 ± 0.00
	Penicillium rubrum (P_2)	1.53 ± 0.48
Potassium nitrate	*Aspergillus flavus* (A_1)	0.50 ± 0.00
	Aspergillus parasiticus (A_2)	1.30 ± 0.10
	Penicillium citrinum (P_1)	0.25 ± 0.25
	Penicillium rubrum (P_2)	0.68 ± 0.03
Ammonium chloride	*Aspergillus flavus* (A_1)	3.02 ± 0.18
	Aspergillus parasiticus (A_2)	0.05 ± 0.05
	Penicillium citrinum (P_1)	0.13 ± 0.13
	Penicillium rubrum (P_2)	0.13 ± 0.03
Peptone	*Aspergillus flavus* (A_1)	0.25 ± 0.00
	Aspergillus parasiticus (A_2)	1.50 ± 0.15
	Penicillium citrinum (P_1)	0.13 ± 0.13
	Penicillium rubrum (P_2)	2.48 ± 0.03
Sodium nitrate	*Aspergillus flavus* (A_1)	0.38 ± 0.13
	Aspergillus parasiticus (A_2)	1.48 ± 0.13
	Penicillium citrinum (P_1)	0.25 ± 0.00
	Penicillium rubrum (P_2)	0.93 ± 0.73
Tryptone	*Aspergillus flavus* (A_1)	0.25 ± 0.00
	Aspergillus parasiticus (A_2)	0.20 ± 0.05
	Penicillium citrinum (P_1)	0.38 ± 0.13
	Penicillium rubrum (P_2)	2.40 ± 0.10
Urea	*Aspergillus flavus* (A_1)	0.15 ± 0.00
	Aspergillus parasiticus (A_2)	2.32 ± 0.03
	Penicillium citrinum (P_1)	0.00 ± 0.00
	Penicillium rubrum (P_2)	2.33 ± 0.08

Each value represents the mean of three replicates with standard error.

Table 2.
Effect of nitrogen sources on activity of amylase produced by isolates.

Toxigenic *A. flavus* (A_1) produced the most active α-amylase (3.25 ± 0.15 Units) and this was when ammonium sulfate was nitrogen source with starch as carbon source of the defined growth medium. Toxigenic *A. flavus* (A_1) also expressed an α-amylase activity value of 3.02 ± 0.18 Units when starch was carbon source and ammonium chloride was nitrogen source of the defined fungal growth medium (**Table 2**).

4. Discussion

The results of this investigation show that the toxigenic strains of *A. flavus* (A_1), *A. parasiticus* (A_2), *P. citrinum* (P_1) and *P. rubrum* (P_2) grew in a synthetic medium with varying carbon and nitrogen sources exhibiting α-amylase activities. α-Amylase activities were detected in the extracts of growth medium with rice as carbon source, infected with the toxigenic strains of *A. flavus* (A_1), *A.*

parasiticus (A_2), *P. citrinum* (P_1) and *P. rubrum* (P_2). When the carbon source was varied, potassium nitrate was the nitrogen source. When the nitrogen source was varied, starch was the carbon source for fungal growth. According to Olutiola [135], *Aspergillus chevalieri* from moldy maize produced extracellular amylase when grown in a liquid medium containing starch as carbon source. According to Barnett and Fergus [136], increasing the amount of starch-yeast extract medium increased the extracellular amylase produced by *Humicola lanuginosa*. Studies carried out by Okafor et al. [137] revealed that *Lactobacillus delbrueckii*, *Lactobacillus coryniformis* and *Saccharomyces* sp., isolated from cassava processing environments were high amylase producers. Among a series of starch sources of carbon, wheat and soluble starch were inducers of a thermostable amylase by a yeast strain isolated from starchy soil [138]. According to Bluhm and Woloshuk [139], amylopectin, an important constituent of starch, induces fumonisin B(1) production in *Fusarium verticillioides* during colonization of maize. According to Coleman [140], extracellular α-amylase was secreted by *Bacillus subtilis* in a complex medium containing maltose, starch, glycerol or glucose as carbon source; the general characteristics of secretion indicated a low but definite production of exoenzyme from the moment the cells of the organism started to grow until the end of the logarithmic phase after which, the rate of increase in cell mass decreased, the rate of enzyme secretion increased to a high linear value which was maintained even in the stationary phase.

4.1 Significance of study

Aflatoxin B1-producing-toxigenic strains of *Aspergillus flavus*, *Aspergillus parasiticus*, *Penicillium citrinum* and *Penicillium rubrum* can be explored industrially for α-amylase production using the specific growth medium and the rice medium used in this investigation. Varying the specific C and N source of this growth medium is of upmost significance in such an exploration.

4.2 Limitations

The genetic make-ups of these aflatoxin B1-producing-α-amylase-producing fungal strains are important in their ability to produce the enzyme α-amylase. Specific genes are necessary and important in the production of this enzyme. Mutant strains lacking the specific genes for α-amylase production will not be ideal in the exploration for production of the enzyme. More so, there seems to be a significant relationship between the ability to produce α-amylase and aflatoxin B1 production in mycotoxigenic fungi from literature.

5. Conclusion

The toxigenic strains of *A. flavus* (A_1), *A. parasiticus* (A_2), *P. citrinum* (P_1) and *P. rubrum* (P_2) can be explored in the industrial production of α-amylases.

Acknowledgements

Authors are thankful to the British Mycology Society (BMS), United Kingdom for Grant supports.

A. Appendix

A.1 Acetylation of cellophane tubings [134]

Material
Visking dialysis tubings (Sigma- Aldrich).
Reagents

(i) Aqueous ethanol (50% V/V)

(ii) Absolute ethanol

(iii) Diethyl ether

(iv) A mixture of benzene, acetic anhydride and pyridine in the ratio 5:4:2 (V/V)

(v) 10% KCl (10 g of KCl in 100 ml distilled water)

Procedure
The cellophane tubings were filled with distilled water and soaked in distilled water for 24 hours. The tubings were then soaked in turn, for 30 min each time in 50% ethanol, absolute ethanol and diethyl ether successively. The tubings were thereafter soaked in the mixture of benzene, acetic anhydride, and pyridine, prepared as described above, for 18 hours. Each tubing was then properly rinsed in distilled water and stored in 10% KCl solution at 4°C until required.

A.2 Protein content determination [131]

Reagents

(i) Reagent A—2% Na_2CO_3 in 0.1 N NaOH

(ii) Reagent B—0.5% $CuSO_4.5H_2O$ in 1% Sodium Potassium tartrate

(iii) Reagent C—50 ml of reagent A mixed with 1 ml of reagent B

(iv) Folin-Ciocalteu's phenol reagent (Sigma-Aldrich Chemie GmbH, Fluka Biochemika) diluted with distilled water in the ratio 1:1(V/V). This is labeled reagent D.

Procedure
5 ml of reagent C was added to 1 ml of the test sample. This was thoroughly mixed and left at room temperature for 10 min. Thereafter, 0.5 ml of reagent D was added and allowed to remain at room temperature for 30 min. Absorbance was determined at 620 nm.

Serial dilutions of Bovine serum albumin (Sigma) were treated likewise and used to plot standard graph. The unknown protein value in each test sample is meant to be extrapolated from the standard graph.

A.3 Iodine solution

(0.3% Iodine in 3% KI)

Reagents

(i) Iodine

(ii) Potassium iodide (KI)

Procedure

3 g of KI was dissolved in 100 ml of warm distilled water. 0.3 g of Iodine was thereafter added and allowed to dissolve in the solution by mixing and warming.

Author details

Adekunle Odunayo Adejuwon[1*] and Victoria Anatolyivna Tsygankova[2]

1 School of Health Information Management, University College Hospital, Ibadan, Nigeria

2 Department for Chemistry of Bioactive Nitrogen-Containing Heterocyclic Compounds, Institute of Bioorganic Chemistry and Petrochemistry of the National Academy of Sciences of Ukraine (NAS), Kyiv, Ukraine

*Address all correspondence to: ao_adejuwon@yahoo.ca

References

[1] Alexopoulos CJ. Introductory Mycology. New York/London: John Wiley and Sons Inc.; 1962. pp. 263-273

[2] Streets RB. Diseases of the Cultivated Plants of the Southwest. Tucson, Arizona: The University of Arizona Press; 1969

[3] Dutta AC. Botany for Degree Students. New Delhi: Oxford University Press; 2007. 708pp

[4] Prescott LM, Harley JR, Klein DA. Microbiology. New York: McGraw Hill; 2005. 992pp

[5] Tortora GJ, Funke BR, Case CL. Microbiology: An Introduction. San Francisco, California: Pearson Education Inc.; 2004. 898pp

[6] Brock DT, Madigan MT. Biology of Microorganisms. Prentice-Hall International Inc.; 1991. 900pp

[7] Brock DT, Madigan MT, Martinko JM, Parker J. Biology of Microorganisms. Eaglewood Cliffs, New Jersey: Prentice-Hall, Inc.; 1994. pp. 528-530

[8] Willey JM, Linda MS, Woolverton CJ. Prescott, Harley and Klein's Microbiology. New York: McGraw Hill Companies Inc.; 2008. 1088pp

[9] Liang XQ, Holbrook CC, Lynch RE, Guo BZ. Beta-1,3-glucanase activity in peanut seed (*Arachis hypogaea*) is induced by inoculation with *Aspergillus flavus* and copurifies with a conglutin-like protein. Phytopathology. 2005;**95**:506-511

[10] Novas MV, Cabral D. Association of mycotoxin and sclerotia production with compatibility groups in *Aspergillus flavus* from peanut in Argentina. Plant Disease. 2002;**86**:215-219

[11] Windham GL, Williams WP. *Aspergillus flavus* infection and aflatoxin accumulation in resistant and susceptible maize hybrids. Plant Disease. 1998;**82**:281-284

[12] Walker RD, White DG. Inheritance of resistance to Aspergillus ear rot and aflatoxin producton of corn from C12. Plant Disease. 2001;**85**:322-327

[13] Windham GL, Williams WP, Davis FM. Effects of the southwestern corn borer on *Aspergillus flavus* kernel infection and aflatoxin accumulation in maize hybrids. Plant Disease. 1999;**83**:535-540

[14] Russin JS, Guo BZ, Tubajika KM, Brown RL, Cleveland TE, Widstrom NW. Comparison of kernel wax from corn genotypes resistant or susceptible to *Aspergillus flavus*. Phytopathology. 1997;**87**:529-533

[15] Chen ZY, Brown RL, Lax AR, Guo BZ, Cleveland TE, Russin JS. Resistance to *Aspergillus flavus* in corn kernels is associated with a 14-KDa protein. Phytopathology. 1998;**88**:276-281

[16] Olanya OM, Hoyos GM, Tiffany LH. Waste corn as a point source of inoculum for *Aspergillus flavus* in the corn agroecosystem. Plant Disease. 1997;**81**:576-581

[17] Norton RA. Effect of carotenoids on aflatoxin B(1) synthesis by *Aspergillus flavus*. Phytopathology. 1997;**87**:814-821

[18] Garber RK, Cotty PJ. Formation of sclerotia and aflatoxins in developing cotton balls infected by the S strain of *Aspergillus flavus* and potential for biocontrol with an atoxigenic strain. Phytopathology. 1997;**87**:940-945

[19] Orum TV, Bigelow DM, Cotty PJ, Nelson MR. Using predictions based on geostatics to monitor trends in

Aspergillus flavus strain composition. Phytopathology. 1999;**89**:761-769

[20] McAlpin CE, Wicklow DT, Platis CE. Genotypic diversity of *Aspergillus parasiticus* in an Illinois corn field. Plant Disease. 1998;**82**:1132-1136

[21] Brown RL, Chen Y, Cleveland TE, Russin JS. Advances in the development of host resistance in corn to aflatoxin contamination by *Aspergillus flavus*. Phytopathology. 1999;**89**:113-117

[22] Moore KG, Price MS, Boston RS, Weissinger AK, Payne GA. A chitinase from Tex 6 maize kernels inhibits growth of *Aspergillus flavus*. Phytopathology. 2004;**94**:82-87

[23] Sirois KL, Loparco DP, Lobeer JW. Systemic infection of onion seedlings by *Aspergillus niger* and *Fusarium* sp. Phytopathology. 1999;**89**:S73. Publication No: P-1999-0520-AMA

[24] Sirois KL, Lorbeer JW, Holcomb MA. Onion seed infection levels subsequent to sequential exposure of onion seed stalk and flower parts to *Aspergillus niger*. Phytopathology. 1999;**89**:S73. Publication No.: P-1999-0521-AMA

[25] Doster MA, Michailides TJ, Morgan DP. *Aspergillus species* and mycotoxins in Figs from California orchards. Plant Disease. 1996;**80**:484-489

[26] Thompson JR, Latorre BA. Characterization of *Botrytis cinerea* from table grapes in Chile using RAPD-PCR. Plant Disease. 1999;**83**:1090-1094

[27] Shellie KC, Skaria M. Reduction of green mold on grape fruit after hot force-air quarantine treatment. Plant Disease. 1998;**82**:380-382

[28] Zhang J, Swingle PP. Effects of curing on green mold and stem-end rot of citrus fruit and its potential application under Florida packing system. Plant Disease. 2005;**89**:834-840

[29] Conway WS, Leverentz B, Saftner RA. Survival and growth of *Listeria monocytogenes* on fresh-cut apple slices and *Pencillium expansum*. Plant Disease. 2000;**84**:177-181

[30] Spotts RA, Cervantes LA. Disease incidence-inoculum close relationships for *Botrytis cinerea* and *Penicillium expansum* and decay of pear fruit using dry, air borne conidia. Plant Diesease. 2001;**85**:755-759

[31] Tian S, Fan Q, Xu Y, Liu H. Biocontrol efficacy of antagonist yeasts to gray mold and blue mold on apples and pears in controlled atmospheres. Plant Disease. 2002;**86**:848-853

[32] Meyer UM, Spotts RA. Detection and quantification of *Botrytis cinerea* by ELISA in pear stems during cold storage. Plant Disease. 2000;**84**:1099-1103

[33] Palou L, Smilanick JL, Crisostco CH, Mansour M. Effects of gaseous ozone exposure on the development of green and blue molds on cold stored citrus fruit. Plant Disease. 2001;**85**:632-638

[34] Palou L, Smilanick JL, Usall J, Vinas I. Control of post harvest blue and green molds of oranges by hot water, sodium carbonate and sodium bicarbonate. Plant Disease. 2001;**85**:371-376

[35] Smilanick JL, Mackey BE, Reese R, Usall J, Margosan DA. Influence of concentration of soda ash, temperature and immersion period on the control of post harvest green mold of oranges. Plant Disease. 1997;**81**:379-382

[36] Smilanick JL, Michael IF, Mansour MF, Mackey BE, Margosan DA, Flores D, et al. Improved control of green mold of citrus with imazalil in warm water compared with its use in wax. Plant Disease. 1997;**81**:1299-1304

[37] Sugar D, Spotts RA. Control of postharvest decay in pear by four laboratory-grown yeasts and two registered biocontrol products. Plant Disease. 1999;**83**:155-158

[38] Janisiewicz WJ, Peterson DL. Susceptibility of the stem pull area of mechanically harvested apples to blue mold decay and its control with a biocontrol agent. Plant Disease. 2004;**88**:662-664

[39] Spotts RA, Holz G. Adhesion and removal of conidia of *Botrytis cinerea* and *Penicillium expansum* from grape and plum fruit surfaces. Plant Disease. 1996;**80**:688-691

[40] Smilanick JL, Aiyabei J, Gabler FM, Doctor J, Sorenson D, Mackey B. Quantification of the toxicity of the aqueous chlorine to spores of *Penicillium digitatum* and *Geotrichum citri-aurantii*. Plant Disease. 2002;**86**:509-514

[41] Janisiewicz WJ, Peterson DL, Yoder KS, Miller SS. Experimental bin drenching system for testing biocontrol agents to control post harvest decay of apple. Plant Disease. 2005;**89**:487-490

[42] Spotts RA, Cervantes LA, Mielke EA. Variability in post harvest decay among apple cultivars. Plant Disease. 1999;**83**:1051-1054

[43] Sugar D, Benbow JM, Powers KA, Basile SR. Orchard sprays on post harvest decay of pear. Plant Disease. 2003;**87**:1260-1262

[44] Smilanick JL, Mansour MF, Sorenson D. Pre- and post harvest treatments to control green mold of citrus fruit during ethylene degreening. Plant Disease. 2006;**90**:89-96

[45] Pianzzola MJ, Moscatelli M, Vero S. Characterization of Penicillium isolates associated with blue mold on apple in Uruguay. Plant Disease. 2004;**88**:23-28

[46] Bohinski RC. Modern Concepts in Biochemistry. 4th ed. Boston/London/Sydney/Toronto: Allyn and Bacon Inc.; 1983. 531pp

[47] Reddy NS, Nimmagadda A, Sambasiva Rao KRS. An overview of the microbial α-amylase family. African Journal of Biotechnology. 2003;**2**(12):645-648

[48] Dixon M, Webb EC. Enzymes. London: Longmans; 1971. 950pp

[49] Robyt JF. Enzymes in hydrolysis and synthesis of starch. In: Starch Chemistry and Technology. New York: Academic Press; 1984. pp. 88-90

[50] Najafi MF, Kembhavi A. One step purification and characterization of an extracellular α-amylase from marine *Vibrio* sp. Enzyme and Microbial Technology. 2005;**36**(4):535-539

[51] Rahardjo YSP, Jolink F, Haemers S, Tramper J, Rinzema A. Signficance of bed porosity, bran and specific surface area in solid-state cultivation of *Aspergillus oryzae*. Biomolecular Engineering. 2005;**22**(4):133-139

[52] Wu YB, Ravindran V, Pierce J, Hendriks WH. Influence of three phytase preparations in broiler diets based on wheat or corn: *In vitro* measurement of nutrient release. International Journal of Poultry Science. 2004;**3**(7):450-455

[53] Ajayi AA, Adejuwon AO, Olutiola PO. Extracellular α-amylase production by the yam (*Discorea* spp.) rot organism, *Penicillium sclerotigenum* Yamamoto Science. Focus. 2005;**10**(3):197-203

[54] Douzdijian V, Gugliuzza KK. The impact of midline versus transverse incisions on wound complications and outcome in simultaneous pancreas-kidney transplant: A retrospective analysis. Transplant International. 1996;**9**(1):62-67

[55] Hashim SO, Delgado OD, Martinez MA, Kaul RH, Mulaa FJ, Mattiasson B. Alkaline active maltohexaose-forming α-amylase from *Bacillus halodurans* LBK 34. Enzyme and Microbial Technology. 2005;**36**(1):139-146

[56] Hemker M, Stratmann A, Goeke K, Schroder W, Lentz J, Piepersberg W, et al. Identification, cloning, expression and characterization of the extracellular acarbose-modifying glycosyltransferase, AcbD from *Actinoplanes* sp. strain SE 50. Journal of Bacteriology. 2001;**183**(15):4484-4492

[57] Oh KW, Kim MJ, Kim HY, Kim BY, Baik MY, Auh JH, et al. Enzymatic characterization of a maltogenic amylase from *Lactobacillus gasseri* ATCC 33323 expressed in *Escherichia coli*. FEMS Microbiology Letters. 2005;**252**(1):175-181

[58] Papi RM, Chaitidou SA, Trikka FA, Kyriakids DA. Encapsulated *Escherichia coli* in alginate beads capable of secreting a heterologous pectin lyase. Microbial Cell Factories. 2005;**4**:35

[59] Lehninger AL. Principles of Biochemistry. New York: Worth Publishers, Inc.; 1982. 1011pp

[60] Howling D. Mechanisms of starch enzymolysis. International Biodeterioration. 1989;**25**:15-19

[61] Vihinen M, Mantsala P. Microbial amylolytic enzymes. Critical Reviews in Biochemistry and Molecular Biology. 1989;**24**(4):329-418

[62] Uguru GC, Akinyanju JA, Sani A. The use of sorghum for thermostable amylase production from *Thermoactinomyces thalpophilus*. Letters in Applied Microbiology. 1997;**25**:13-16

[63] Ajayi AO, Fagade OE. Utilization of corn starch as substrate for β-amylase by *Bacillus* spp. African Journal of Biomedical Research. 2003;**6**(1):37-42

[64] Reiss M, Heibges A, Metzger I, Hartmeier W. Determination of BOD-values of starch containing waste water by a BOD-biosensor. Biosensors and Bioelectronics. 1998;**13**(10):1083-1090

[65] Ampe F, Ben Omar N, Guyot JP. Recovery of total microbial RNA from lactic acid fermented foods with a high starch content. Letters in Applied Microbiology. 1998;**27**(5):270-274

[66] Doelle HW. Socio-economic microbial process strategies for a sustainable development using environmentally clean technologies: Sagopalm a renewable resource. Livestock Research for Rural Development. 1998;**10**(1):23-32

[67] Rivera MH, Lopez-Munguia A, Soberon X, Saab-Rincon G. Alpha-amylase from *Bacillus licheniformis* mutants near to the catalytic site: Effects on hydrolytic and transglycosylation activity. Protein Engineering. 2003;**16**(7):505-514

[68] Zangrando FEL, Yoko HE. Culture media for amylase production by toxigenic fungi. Brazilian Archives of Biology and Technology. 2000;**43**(5):461-467

[69] Tanaka T, Hoshina M, Tanabe S, Sakai K, Ohtsubo S, Taniguchi M. Production of d-lactic acid from defatted rice bran by simultaneous saccharification and fermentation. Bioresource Technology. 2005;**97**(2):211-217

[70] Sejedi RH, Naderi-Manesh H, Khajeh K, Ahmadvand R, Ranjbar B, Asoodeh A, et al. A Ca-independent α-amylase that is active and stable at low pH from the *Bacillus* sp. KR-8104. Enzyme and Microbial Technology. 2005;**36**(5-6):666-671

[71] Rodriguez VB, Alamenda EJ, Gellegos JFM, Lopez AIG. Thermal deactivation of a commercial α-amylase from *Bacillus licheniformis* used in detergents. Biochemical Engineering Journal. 2006;**27**(3):299-304

[72] Mijts B, Patel BKC. Cloning, sequencing and expression of an alpha-amylase gene, amy A, from the thermophilic halophile *Halothermothrix orenii* and purification and biochemical characterization of the recombinant enzyme. Microbiology. 2002;**148**:2343-2349

[73] Shaw JF, Lin FP, Chen SC, Chen HC. Purification and properties of an extracellular α-amylase from *Thermus* sp. Botanical Bulletin of Academia Sinica. 1995;**36**:195-200

[74] Yutani K. Molecular weight of thermostable α-amylase from *Bacillus stearothermophilus*. Journal of Biochemistry. 1973;**74**:581-586

[75] Saito N. A thermophilic extracellular α-amylase from *Bacillus licheniformis*. Archives of Biochemistry and Biophysics. 1973;**155**:290-298

[76] Manning GB, Campbell LL. Thermostable α-amylase of *Bacillus stearothermophilus*. I. Crystallization and some general properties. The Journal of Biological Chemistry. 1961;**236**(11):2952-2957

[77] Huang LP, Jin B, Lant P, Zhou J. Simultaneous saccharification and fermentation of potato starch waste water to lactic acid by *Rhizopus oryzae* and *Rhizopus arrhizus*. Biochemical Engineering Journal. 2005;**23**:265-276

[78] Ogashara K, Imanishi A, Isemura T. Studies on thermophilic α-amylase from *Bacillus stearothermophilus*. I. Some general and physico-chemical properties of thermophilic α-amylase. The Journal of Biochemistry. 1970;**74**:581-596

[79] Synowiecki J, Grzybowska B, Zdzieblo A. Sources, properties and suitability of new thermostable enzyme in food processing. Critical Reviews in Food Science and Nutrition. 2006;**46**(3):197-205

[80] Peng P, Wu J, Cheng AC, Gao QY, Zhang SZ. Cloning and expression of the alpha-amylase gene from a *Bacillus* sp. WS06 and characterization of the enzyme. Wei Sheng Wu Xue Bao. 2005;**45**(6):876-880

[81] Yun J, Kang S, Park S, Yoon H, Kim MJ, Heu S, et al. Characterization of a novel amylolytic enzyme encoded by a gene from a soil-derived metagenomic library. Applied and Environmental Microbiology. 2004;**70**(12):7229-7235

[82] Bessler C, Schmitt J, Maurer KH, Schmid RD. Directed evolution of a bacterial alpha-amylase: Towards enhanced pH-performance and higher specific activity. Protein Science. 2003;**12**(10):2141-2149

[83] Dey S, Agarwal SO. Characterization of a thermostable alpha-amylase from a thermophilic *Streptomyces megasporus* strain SD12. Indian Journal of Biochemistry and Biophysics. 1999;**36**(3):150-157

[84] Burgess-Cassler A, Imam SH, Gould JM. High-molecular weight amylase activities from bacteria degrading starch-plastic films. Applied and Environmental Microbiology. 1991;**57**(2):612-614

[85] Heese O, Hansen G, Hohne WE, Korner D. A thermostable alpha amylase from *Thermoactinomyces vulgaris.* Purification and characterization. Biomedica Biochimica Acta. 1991;**50**(3):225-232

[86] Akindahunsi AA. Physico-chemical studies on amylases from fermented cassava waste water. In: Scientific

Preprints Automized List. Trieste, Italy: The Abdus Salam International Centre for Theoretical Physics; 2001

[87] Dey G, Palit S, Banerjee R, Maiti BR. Purification and characterization of malto oligosaccharide-forming amylase from *Bacillus circulans* GRS 313. Journal of Indian Microbiology and Biotechnology. 2002;**28**(4):193-200

[88] Doman K, Ryu SJ, Heo SJ, Kim DW, Kim HS. Characterization of a novel carbohydrase from *Lipomyces starkeyi* KSM 22 for dental application. Journal of Microbiology and Biotechnology. 1999;**9**(3):260-264

[89] Jana M, Chattopadhyay DJ, Patti BR. Thermostable, high salt-tolerant amylase from *Bacillus megaterium* VUMB-109. Acta Microbiologica et Immunologica Hungarica. 1997;**44**(3):281-289

[90] Ohno N, Fukuda H, Wang H, Kasamura M, Shinoyama H, Fuji T. Amylases produced by a thermophilic fungus. *Thermoascus aurantiacus* and some of their properties. Sebutsu-Kogaku Kaishi. 1998;**76**(3):111-117

[91] Shekhar HU, Ali MM, Hossain MA. Extracellular amylase production by locally isolated mosquito-pathogenic *Bacillus sphaericus* N11. Bangladesh Journal of Microbiology. 1997;**14**(1-2):17-23

[92] Falih AM. Effect of heavy-metals on amylolytic activity of the soil yeasts *Geotrichum capitatum* and *Geotrichum candidum*. Bioresource Technology. 1998;**66**(3):213-217

[93] Bernhardsdotter ECMJ, Ng JD, Garriott DK, Pusey ML. Enzymatic properties of an alkaline, chelator-resistant alpha-amylase from an alkaliphilic *Bacillus* sp. isolate L1711. Process Biochemistry. 2005;**40**:2401-2408

[94] Mishra S, Noronha SB, Suraishkumar GK. Increase in enzyme productivity by induced oxidative stress in *Bacillus subtilis* cultures and analysis of its mechanism using microarray data. Process Biochemistry. 2005;**40**(5):1863-1870

[95] El-Said AH, Abdel-Hafez SI, Saleem A. Effect of herbizid and touchdown of some extracellular enzymes. Acta Microbiologica et Immunologica Hungarica. 2005;**52**(1):105-130

[96] Figueira ELZ, Hirooka EY, Mendiola-Olanya E, Blanco-Labra A. Characterization of a hydrophobic amylase inhibitor from corn (*Zea mays*) seeds with activity against amylase from *Fusarium verticilliodies*. Phytopathology. 2002;**93**:917-922

[97] Figueira ELZ, Ono EYZ, Mendiola-Olanya E. New amylase inhibitor present in corn seeds active *in vitro* amylase from *Fusarium verticilliodes*. Plant Disease. 2002;**87**:233-240

[98] Hofmann O, Vertesy L, Braunitzer G. The primary structure of alpha-amylase inhibitor Z-2685 from *Steptomyces parvullus* FH-1641. Sequence homology between inhibitor and alpha-amylase. Biological Chemistry Hoppe-Seyler. 1985;**366**(12):1161-1168

[99] Vertesy L, Tripier D. Isolation and structure elucidation of an alpha-amylase inhibitor, A1-3688, from *Streptomyces aureofaciens*. FEBS Letters. 1985;**185**(1):187-190

[100] Su YC, Chiu RJ, Yu N, Chang WR. The microbial production of amylase inhibitor and its application. I. Isolation and cultivation of *Streptomyces nigrifaciens* NTU-3314. Proceedings of the National Science Council, Republic of China. 1984;**B8**(4):292-301

[101] Lin J, Lu C, Yu IT, Wu JF. Effects of starch sources on the production and activity of amylase from *Bacillus subtilis*. Journal of the

Agricultural Association of China. 1999;**185**:22-31

[102] Yin XH, Gerbaud C, Francou FX, Guerineau M, Virolle MJ. Ami C, another amylolytic gene maps close to the ami B locus in *Streptomyces lividans* TK 24. Gene (Amsterdam). 1998;**215**(1):171-180

[103] Lo HF, Lin LL, Chiang WY, Chie MC, Hsu WH, Chang CT. Deletion analysis of the C-terminal region of the alpha-amylase of *Bacillus* sp. strain TS-23. Archives of Microbiology. 2002;**178**(2):115-123

[104] Bahl H, Burchhardt G, Spreinat A, Haeckel K, Wienecke A, Schmidt B. Alpha-amylase of *Clostridium therosulfurgenes* EMI: Nucleotide sequence of the gene, processing of the enzyme and comparison of alpha amylases. Applied and Environmental Microbiology. 1991;**57**(5):1554-1559

[105] Kang DO, Hwang IK, Kim BY, Ahn SC, Mheen TI, Ahn JS, et al. Secretion of Bacillus alpha-amylase from yeast directed by glucoamylase I signal sequence of *Saccharomyces diastaticus*. Biochemistry and Molecular Biology International. 1996;**39**(1):181-190

[106] Lorentz K. Routine alpha-amylase assay using protected 4-nitrophenyl-1,4-alpha-D-maltoheptaoside and a novel alpha-glucoside. Clinical Chemistry. 2000;**46**:644-649

[107] Akpan I, Bankole M, Adesemowo AM. A rapid plate culture method for screening of amylase producing microorganisms. Biotechnology Techniques. 1999;**13**(6):411-413

[108] Higuchi Y, Ohashi A, Imachi H, Harada H. Hydrolytic activity of alpha-amylase in anaerobic digested sludge. Water Science and Technology. 2005;**52**(1-2):259-266

[109] Uhlig H. Industrial Enzymes and their Applications. New York: Wiley and Sons; 1998. 472pp

[110] Pandey A, Nigman P, Soccol CR, Soccol VT, Singh D, Mohan R. Advances in microbial amylase. Biotechnology and Applied Biochemistry. 2000;**31**(2):135-152

[111] Mellon JE, Cotty PJ, Dowd MK. *Aspergillus flavus* hydrolases: Their roles in pathogenesis and substrate utilization. Applied Environmental Microbiology and Biotechnology. 2007;**77**:497-504

[112] Jallow EAA, Twumasi P, Mills-Robertson FC, Dumevi R. Assessment of aflatoxin-producing fungi strains and contamination levels of aflatoxin B1 in groundnut, maize, beans and rice. Journal of Agricultural Science and Food Technology. 2018;**4**(4):71-79

[113] Liu J, Sun L, Zhang N, Zhang J, Guo J, Li C, et al. Effects of nutrients in substrate of different grains on aflatoxin B1 production by *Aspergillus flavus*. Biomedical Research International. 2016;**2016**:10. Article ID 7232858. http://dx.doi.org/10.1155/2016/7232858

[114] Kim HR, Kim JH, Bai DH, Ahn BH. Identification and characterization of useful fungi with α-amylase activity from Korean traditional nuruk. Microbiology. 2011;**39**(4):278-282

[115] Fakhoury A, Woloshuk CR. Amy1, the α-amylase gene of *Aspergillus flavus*: Involvement in aflatoxin biosynthesis in maize kernels. Phytopathology. 1999;**89**(1):908-914

[116] Figueira ELZ, Hirooka EY. Culture medium for amylase production by toxigenic fungi. Brazilian Archives of Biology and Technology. 2000;**43**(5):461-467

[117] Rajasekaran K, Sayler RJ, Majumdar R, Sickler CM, Cary JW.

Inhibition of *Aspergillus flavus* growth and aflatoxin production in transgenic maize expressing the α-amylase inhibitor from *Lablab purpureus* L. Journal of Visualized Experiments. 2019;**144**:e59169. DOI: 10.3791/59169

[118] Fountain JC, Scully BT, Ni X, Kemerait RC, Lee RD, Chen ZY, et al. Environmental influences on maize-*Aspergillus flavus* interactions and aflatoxin production. Frontiers in Microbiology. 2014;**5**:40. DOI: 10.3389/fmicb.2014.00040

[119] Espindola AS, Schneider W, Cardwell KF, Carrillo Y, Hoyt PR, Marek SM, et al. Inferring the presence of aflatoxin-producing *Aspergillus flavus* strains using RNA sequencing and electronic probes as a transcriptomic screening tool. PLoS One. 16 Oct 2018;**13**(10):e0198575. DOI: 10.1371/journal.pone.0198575

[120] Yu J, Mohawed SM, Bhatnagar D, Cleveland TE. Substrate-induced lipase gene expression and aflatoxin production in *Aspergillus flavus*. Journal of Applied Microbiology. 2003;**95**:1334-1342

[121] Smith CA, Woloshuk CP, Robertson D, Payne GA. Silencing of the aflatoxin gene cluster in a diploid strain of *Aspergillus flavus* is suppressed by ectopic aflR expression. Genetics. 2007;**176**(4):2077-2086

[122] Stern KR, Jansky S, Bidlack JE. Introductory Plant Biology. New York: McGraw Hill Higher Education; 2003. 624pp

[123] Sizer FS, Whitney EN. Nutrition: Concepts and Controversies. London: Wadsworth, Thomson Learning; 2000. 567pp

[124] Mauseth JD. Botany: An Introduction to Plant Biology. London: Saunders College Publishing; 1995. 794pp

[125] Leventin E, McMahon K. Plants and Society. New York: WCB McGraw Hill; 1999. 477pp

[126] Graham LE, Graham JM, Wilcox LW. Plant Biology. Upper Saddle River: Pearson Education, Inc.; 2006. 670pp

[127] Cannon PF, Kirk PM. Fungal Families of the World. Wallingford, Oxfordshire: CAB International Publishing; 2007. 4556pp

[128] Hanlin RT. Illustrated Genera of Ascomycetes. St. Paul, Minnesota: American Phytopathological Society Press; 1990. 263pp

[129] Olutiola PO, Ayres PG. Utilization of carbohydrates by *Rhynchosporium secalis*.I. Growth and sporulation on glucose, galactose and galacturonic acid. Physiologia Plantarum. 1973;**29**:92-96

[130] Olutiola PO, Nwaogwugwu RI. Growth, sporulation and production of maltase and proteolytic enzymes in *Aspergillus aculeatus*. Transactions of the British Mycological Society. 1982;**78**(1):105-113

[131] Lowry OH, Rosebrough NJ, Farr AL, Randall RJ. Protein measurement with the folin phenol reagent. Journal of Biological Chemistry. 1951;**193**:265-275

[132] Pfueller SL, Elliott WH. The extracellular α-amylase of *Bacillus stearothemophilus*. Journal of Biological Chemistry. 1969;**244**:48-54

[133] Xiao Z, Storms R, Tsang A. A quantitative starch-iodine method for measuring alpha-amylase and glucoamylase activities. Analytical Biochemistry. 2006;**351**(1):146-148

[134] Whitaker DR, Hanson KR, Datta PK. Improved procedure for purification and characterization of Myrothecium cellulase. Canadian Journal of Microbiology and Physiology. 1963;**41**:671-696

[135] Olutiola PO. α-Amylase activity of *Aspergillus chevalieri* from mouldy maize. Indian Phytopathology. 1982;**35**(3):428-433

[136] Barnett EA, Fergus CL. The regulation of extracellular amylase mycelium and time, in some thermophilic and mesophilic *Humicola* species. Mycopathologia et Mycologia Applicata. 1971;**44**(2):131-141

[137] Okafor N, Umeh C, Ibenugbu C. Amelioration of garri, a cassava based fermented food by the inoculation of microorganisms secreting amylase, lysine and linamarase into cassava mash. World Jounal of Microbiology and Biotechnology. 1998;**14**(6):835-838

[138] Fossi BT, Tavea F, Ndjouenkeu R. Production and partial characterization of a thermostable amylase from ascomycetes yeast strain isolated from starchy soils. African Journal of Biotechnology. 2005;**4**(1):14-18

[139] Bluhm BH, Woloshuk CP. Amylopectin induces fumonisin B(1) production by *Fusarium verticilliodes* during colonization of maize kernels. Molecular Plant-Microbe Interactions. 2005;**18**:1333-1339

[140] Coleman G. Studies on the regulation of extracellular enzyme formation by *Bacillus subtilis*. Journal of General Microbiology. 1967;**49**:421-431

Chapter 4

Prevention by Essential Oils of the Occurrence and Growth of *Aspergillus flavus* and Aflatoxin B1 Production in Food Systems: Review

Yamina Ben Miri, Azem Belasli, Djamel Djenane and Agustín Ariño

Abstract

Aspergillus flavus has been reported to be one of the most common fungal species in foods. Under conditions of high humidity and moderate temperature, this fungus may synthetize the mycotoxin Aflatoxin B1 (AFB1), which is reported to be hepatotoxic, teratogenic, mutagenic and immunosuppressive to human beings and livestock and it is classified as carcinogenic to humans (Group 1 by IARC). AFB1 affects cereals, oilseeds, nuts, spices, legumes, and dried fruits, while Aflatoxin M1 is a metabolite of AFB1 that can occur in milk and milk products. Current control is aimed at controlling fungal growth and AFB1 production in food by eco-friendly, biodegradable and safer alternatives, in contrast to synthetic chemicals that can be toxic to humans and cause adverse environmental effects. Recently, considerable attention has been directed towards natural compounds, such as essential oils (EOs) as a promising approach for controlling AFB1 production in food. The main reason for supporting the application of natural products is the consumer's preference for natural methods to preserve foods. The aim of the present review is to summarize knowledge of EOs and AFB1 production from the literature.

Keywords: *Aspergillus flavus*, aflatoxin B1 (AFB1), essential oils, food system

1. Introduction

Molds are ubiquitous micro-organisms with a high capacity to colonize different types of substrates and to proliferate under extreme environmental conditions [1]. They alter various types of foods namely cereals, nuts, oil seeds, legumes, spices, vegetables, fruits, etc. and some species produce mycotoxins. Of all mycotoxins, Aflatoxin B1 (AFB1) produced primarily by *Aspergillus flavus* and *A. parasiticus* is the most toxic form (hepatotoxic, teratogenic, mutagenic and carcinogenic) for humans and animals [2–5]. The health impact of this compound has justified the introduction of a consumer protection measure by the establishment of maximum levels in certain food categories. However, the existence of these standards also has significant economic repercussions restricting trade from certain areas where the contamination is frequent and strongly decreasing the economic value of some productions in case of contamination. These losses are estimated by FAO (Food and Agriculture Organization of The United Nations) at about 1 billion tons a year. Therefore, it seems imperative to develop ways of combating contamination of food with these toxic compounds and/or to limit their harmful effects.

Pesticides and fungicides have been widely used to prevent the development of fungal agents. However, because of their own toxicity, their use is subjected to certain restrictions. Biological control is also a possible option. Thus, antiaflatoxigenic bacterial and fungal strains were found effective in reducing the development of toxic strains of *A. flavus*. However, none of these strategies seems to be able to solve the problem of contamination of raw materials by aflatoxins, as evidenced by the numerous researches that show high levels of contamination, particularly in areas where the climate is favorable for the development of the toxigenic fungal species. At present, there is growing interest in identifying natural compounds able to limit the growth and/or the production of mycotoxins. Thus, the use of essential oils (EOs) of plants or spices could show their ability to limit food contamination. The aim of this review is to summarize the results from the literature on the effects of EOs against *A. flavus* growth and AFB1 production.

2. Aflatoxins

Aflatoxins are produced primarily by the common fungus *Aspergillus flavus* and the closely related species *A. parasiticus*, and they can be found in feedstuffs and foodstuffs throughout the world. These mycotoxins are a family of several molecules of which the most important are AFB1, B2, G1 and G2 (**Figure 1**). The letters refer to the fluorescence blue (B) or green (G) under UV and the numbers (1 or 2) refer to their relative chromatographic mobility. They are molecules with a polycyclic structure belonging to the furanocoumarin class.

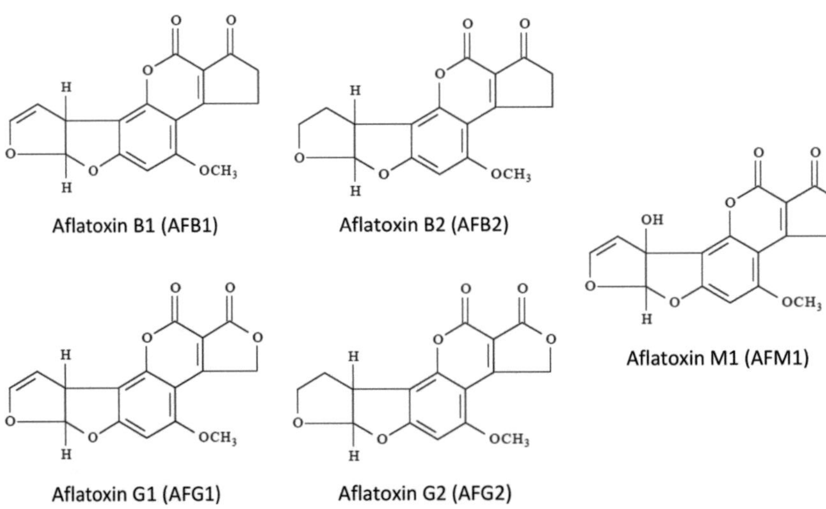

Figure 1.
Chemical structures of AFB1, B2, M1, G1 and G2.

There are also other aflatoxins; there are in total more than a dozen (M_1, P_1, Q_1, B_2a, G_2a, etc.). The most are products resulting from the metabolic metabolism of the four molecules produced by mold in food [6]. For example, after ingestion of contaminated feed, AFB1 is transformed into the liver of mammals by cytochrome P450 into several metabolites, mainly AFM1 excreted in milk, which is produced by hydroxylation of the tertiary carbon of the difuranocoumarin cycle. The hydroxyl group formed makes AFM1 more soluble in water and therefore rapidly excreted in mammalian milk, urine, bile and feces. The AFM1 owes its name to its presence in Milk [7]. Aflatoxins are stable molecules and very resistant to the various processes of food processing such as roasting, extrusion and cooking [8]. Indeed, the decomposition of aflatoxins takes place at very high temperatures which are difficult to comply with the manufacturing or processing processes of food. *A. flavus* and *A. parasiticus* are the main aflatoxin producers; *A. flavus* is responsible for the production of type B aflatoxins, while *A. parasiticus* produces both type B and G [9]. Aflatoxins can contaminate cereals, oil seeds, nuts, spices, legumes, dried fruits, milk and milk products, posing a high risk to public health [10–13]. Maize, peanuts and tree nuts (i.e. pistachios) are susceptible to aflatoxin contamination in the field, while other cereals, oilseeds and dried fruits are mostly contaminated at postharvest and during storage [14–16].

3. Methods of aflatoxin decontamination

Foodstuffs should not be hazardous to consumer health; as consequence, elimination of mycotoxin from products is a challenge for the food industry. Concerns have been directed towards aflatoxins because of their global threat and toxicity. Most of the factors obtained from studies on aflatoxins can be applied to other mycotoxins. Although prevention is the most effective intervention, chemical, physical and biological methods have been investigated to eliminate aflatoxins or reduce them (**Figure 2**). However, these techniques are not completely safe, are expensive and not well preferred by consumers.

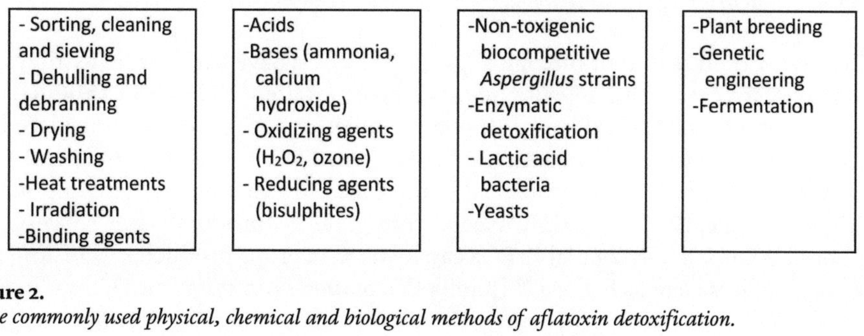

Figure 2.
Some commonly used physical, chemical and biological methods of aflatoxin detoxification.

4. Essential oils: an alternative strategy for control against aflatoxin contamination

The frequency of contamination of world crops by aflatoxins shows that the strategies currently used are insufficient to guarantee the security of the foods and that it is necessary to develop others, as a complement or substitution of those already existing. In this context, strategies based on the use of compounds naturally recognized as not harmful to the environment and to health, seem interesting. Indeed, plants produce different secondary metabolites (terpenoids, phenolic compounds, etc.) for their protection against external agents (mechanical, biological or climatic). These compounds could possibly be used as a means of combating fungal contamination and/or mycotoxins [17].

4.1 Essential oils

4.1.1 Overview

EOs are a mixture of volatile compounds (secondary metabolites) isolated from plants mainly by hydro-distillation. They are mostly consisting of mono- and sesquiterpenes but may also contain non-terpenoid hydrocarbons, phenylpropanoids, esters, lactones, phthalides, nitrogen or sulfurized structures and isothiocyanates. They are lipophilic compounds which are distinguished by their aromatic properties, hence their use as flavorings or perfumes [18]. In addition, certain compounds are also used for their many biological activities: bactericide, fungicide and antioxidant [19].

4.1.2 Mechanism of cellular action of essential oils

The mode of action of EOs has not been completely understood yet [20, 21]. In general, EOs actions are described in three phases. Firstly, EOs spreading on the cell wall of fungi changes the membrane permeability resulting in the loss of cellular components. Secondly, an acidification inside the cell that blocks the production of cellular energy (ATP) due to ion loss, the collapse of proton pumps, the reduction of membrane potential, and destruction of genetic materials that leads to the death of fungus. Furthermore, some reports have indicated that EOs can also coagulate the cytoplasm and damage lipids, proteins, cell walls and membranes that can lead to the leakage of macromolecules and the lysis [22–27].

Phenolic compounds are known to affect microbial cell permeability, allowing the loss of macromolecules from the interior. They could also interact with membrane proteins, causing a deformation in their structure and functionality [28].

4.1.3 Use of essential oils as antifungal and antiaflatoxigenic agents

In view of their different biological properties, EOs have been tested as alternative strategy for combating mycotoxins, especially aflatoxins [29–34] (**Table 1**). EOs are molecules of natural origin, biodegradable, and are therefore considered as a possible alternative to synthetic pesticides [35]. Their use as food additives or flavorings has recently been authorized in the USA [36]. As their active components are highly volatile, they are mainly used as fumigants for products after harvest. A number of commercially available EOs can be used in crops produced according to the specifications such as E-Rase™ (jojoba EO, *Simmondsia californica*), Sporan™ (rosemary EO, *Rosmarinus officinalis*), Promax™ (thyme EO, *Thymus vulgaris*) [37],

Plant scientific name	Plant common name	Applied concentrations in culture medium	Inhibition of *A. flavus* growth	Inhibition of AFB1 production	Reference
Ageratum conyzoides	Mentrasto	0.10 μg/mL 0.04 μg/ mL	49.00% 30.00%	100.00% 65.00%	[1]
Pimpinella anisum	Anise	0.50 μg/g	100.00%	100.00%	[31]
Ocimum sanctum	Holy basil	0.10 μg/ mL 0.20 μg/ mL	72.50% 90.10%	88.40% 100.00%	[63]
Ocimum sanctum	Holy basil	0.10 μL/ mL 0.40 μL/ mL	72.25% 100.00%	82.43% 100.00%	[44]
Piper betle	Betel	0.40 μL/ mL 0.60 μL/ mL	26.70% 77.80%	74.50% 100.00%	[3]
Callistemon lanceolatus	Callistemon	0.546 mg/ mL 0.819 mg/ mL	79.60% 100.00%	100.00% 100.00%	[53]
Cinnamomum jensenianum	Cinnamon	4.00 μL/ mL 6.00 μL/ mL	63.00% 84.00%	84.00% 100.00%	[34]
Amomum subulatum	Cardamom	0.25 mg/ mL 0.50 mg/ mL	25.00% 74.00%	69.00% 100.00%	[64]
Cicuta virosa	Water hemlock	1.00 μL/ mL 4.00 μL/ mL	60.00% 65.70%	31.90% 100.00%	[51]
Cymbopogon citratus	Lemongrass	0.20 mg/ mL	3.00%	100.00%	[32]
Coriandrum sativum	Coriander	0.75 μL/ mL	66.50%	25.00%	[50]
Cuminum cyminum	Cumin	0.40 μL/ mL 0.50 μL/ mL	52.00% 91.00%	67.00% 100.00%	[31]
Curcuma longa	Turmeric	0.50% (v/v)	nd	99.00%	[59]
Foeniculum vulgare	Fennel	0.75 μL/ mL	54.40%	23.00%	[52]
Mentha spicata	Mint	0.60 μL/ mL 0.90 μl/ mL	66.40% 84.90%	50.20% 100.00%	[65]
Cymbopogon martini	Palmarosa-Indian geranium	0.30 μL/ mL 0.40 μL/ mL	50.00% 95.00%	80.00% 100.00%	[66]
Citrus sinensis	Orange	250.00 ppm 1000.00 ppm	18.20% 100.00%	68.32% 100.00%	[49]
Citrus maxima	Pomelo	250.00 ppm 1000.00 ppm	23.40% 100.00%	67.21% 100.00%	
Rosmarinus officinalis	Rosemary	0.45% (v/v)	0.00%	100.00%	[33]
Thymus vulgaris	Thyme	0.30 μL/ mL 0.70 μL/ mL	46.90% 100.00%	75.60% 100.00%	[67]
Thymus daenensis	Thyme	62.50 mg/L 500.00 mg/L	6.45% 100.00%	17.83% 100.00%	
Satureja khozistanica	Sater	62.50 mg/L 500.00 mg/L	12.38% 100%	18.53% 100.00%	[68]
Satureja macrosiphonia	Sater	62.50 mg/L 500.00 mg/L	3.07% 65.22%	10.22% 73.96%	
Lippia rugosa	Verbenacea	600.00 μg/mL 1000.00 μg/mL	5.00% 5.00%	61.00% 100.00%	[48]

Table 1.
Inhibition effect of some EOs on the growth of A. flavus and the production of AFB1.

Cinnamite™ and Valero™ (cinnamon EO, *Cinnamomum verum*) [19], Talent® (based on carvone, EO of cumin or dill) and eugenol-Tween® [38].

The antifungal activity of EOs of *T. vulgaris* and camphor (*Eucalyptus rostrata* L.) was tested on *A. flavus*. They completely inhibited mycelial growth of the fungus at 1000 and 2000 ppm (mg/kg), and aflatoxin production at 500 and 1000 ppm, respectively [39].

The EO of *Satureja hortensis* was assessed for antifungal activity against *A. flavus in vitro* on solid and liquid culture, and under storage conditions. The EO showed strong antifungal activity based on the inhibition zone and minimal inhibitory concentration (MIC) values on solid culture. The very low concentrations of EOs also reduced wet and dry mycelium weight of *A. flavus* in liquid culture [40]. The antifungal potential of EOs of leaves and seeds of *Aframomum daniellii*, *Aframomum melegueta* and *Aframomum latifolium* and those of husk of *A. latifolium* was evaluated against *A. flavus*. Results showed that the inhibition of tested EOs were between 28.06 and 100%, respectively for EOs of seeds of *A. melegueta* and EO of the husk of *A. latifolium* at 500 ppm. EO of leaves of *A. melegueta* and husk of *A. latifolium* exhibited the most effective inhibition [41]. EOs extracted from *Mentha arvensis* (0.5 mg/mL) caused total inhibition of *A. flavus* growth and of AFB1 production [42]. *Cymbopogon martinii*, *Foeniculum vulgare* and *Trachyspermum ammi* EOs were tested against *A. flavus*. The MIC was recorded at 1 μL/mL for *T. ammi* EO and 4 μL/mL for *C. martinii* and *F. vulgare*. At these concentrations, the EOs completely inhibited the growth of *A. flavus* [43].

Ageratum conyzoides EO inhibited *A. flavus* growth and reduced AFB1 production at 0.10 μg/mL. The ultra-structural changes in *A. flavus* cell under transmission electron microscopy (TEM) were observed on the endomembrane system, mainly the mitochondria. The plasma membrane cells lost its linear aspect. The fibrillar layers lost their building and failed to deposit on the cell wall. The mitochondria in treated cells suffered a disruption of the internal structure [1]. *Ocimum sanctum* EO was evaluated to inhibit *A. flavus* growth and AFB1 production. The MIC of *O. sanctum* against *A. flavus* was found at 0.3 μL/mL while AFB1 production was recorded at 0.2 μL/mL [44]. The efficacy of boldo (*Peumus boldus* Mol.), poleo (*Lippia turbinata* var. integrifolia (Griseb.), clove (*Syzygium aromaticum* L.), anise (*Pimpinella anisum*), and thyme (*T. vulgaris*) EOs was tested against *A. flavus* and *A. parasiticus* growth and AFB1 at different water activity (a_W) levels (0.98, 0.95, 0.93). Inhibition was estimated at 75, 83, and 100% at 0.98, 0.95, and 0.93 a_W, respectively [45].

The effects of EOs of *Ocimum gratissimum* and *Plectranthus glandulosus* leaves on growth and AFB1 production by *A. flavus* were assessed at five levels (200, 400, 600, 800 and 1000 mg/L). Growth of *A. flavus* was completely inhibited by 800 mg/L of *O. gratissimum* EO and by 1000 mg/L of *P. glandulosus* EO. The AFB1 production was inhibited by 1000 mg/L of both EOs of *O. gratissimum* and *P. glandulous* [46]. *Cinnamomum camphora* and *Alpinia galanga* EOs inhibited *A. flavus* at 1000 ppm and the AFB1 production at 500 ppm for *A. galanga* and 750 ppm for *C. camphora*. The combination of the two EOs was more effective than the individual ones. The mixture showed total inhibition of the mycelium growth at 750 ppm and AFB1 production starting from 250 ppm [47]. *Lippia rugosa* EO was effective against fungal growth and production of AFB1 from *A. flavus* was totally inhibited at 1000 mg/L. The inhibition was attributed to the presence of geraniol [48].

Both *A. flavus* growth and AFB1 production were inhibited by EOs of *Citrus maxima* Burm, *Citrus sinensis* (L.) Osbeck, and their combination. DL-Limonene inhibited AFB1 productionat a concentration of 250 ppm that is lower than the individual EOs and the combination. It has been suggested that remaining constituents in the EO would mask the efficacy of DL-limonene and they may act in negatively.

Furthermore, the authors declared that there was no synergism between the EO constituents when the two EOs were mixed at the same concentration, attaining aflatoxin inhibition at 500 ppm [49].

Similar types of results were also found in the case of *Piper betle* var. magahi EO, where eugenol was more effective as inhibitor of fungal growth and aflatoxin production than the whole EO. It was suggested that the components of the EO acted synergistically in negative direction and diminished the activity of eugenol [3]. The effect of basil, fennel, coriander, caraway, peppermint and rosemary EOs on *A. flavus* growth and AFB1 production at 500, 750 and 1000 ppm was also studied. The complete inhibition of *A. flavus* growth was observed at 1000 ppm concentrations of basil, coriander, caraway and rosemary EOs. While, EOs of basil and coriander showed interesting inhibition of AFB1 at all concentrations [50].

Cicuta virosa L. EO inhibited the growth of *A. flavus* and AFB1 production at 4 μL/mL of EO. The AFB1 was reduced to about half compared to the control at 2 μL/mL [51]. Similar type of results was found with *Cinnamomum jensenianum* EO, which reduced AFB1 to about half compared to the control at 2 μL/mL. At this concentration of the EO, the plasma membrane of *A. flavus* became rough with continuous folding into the cytoplasm and festooned with small lomasomes. A decreased cytoplasmic matrix was also observed. They showed that some mitochondria suffered extensive disruption of the internal structure with a decrease in mitochondrial cristae. The cell ultrastructure damage was aggravated when the EO concentration was doubled. Major alterations were observed, including massive vacuolation of cytoplasm with vacuole fusion, appearance of numerous lomasomes with folding, and detachment of plasma membrane from the cell wall. The fibrillar layers gradually lost their integrity, becoming thinner, and eventually failing to deposit on the cell wall. The plasma membrane was also folded at many sites. The cytoplasmic matrix and some cytoplasmic organelles were absent. Moreover, the mitochondria suffered a severe disruption of the internal structure with complete lysis. The antifungal mode of action of EO was evaluated by quantification of the ergosterol production in cells. At concentration of 2 μL/mL, the ergosterol content in the plasma membrane of *A. flavus* was significantly reduced by the different concentrations of EO. A dose dependent decrease in ergosterol production was observed when isolates were grown in the presence of the EO. Therefore, this EO exerts its effect directly on the plasma membrane without any obvious damage to the cell wall. This emphasizes that the antimicrobial components of the EOs cross the cell membrane, interact with the enzymes and proteins of the membrane, thus producing a flux of protons towards the cell exterior which induces disruption to the fungal cell organization and, ultimately, their death [34].

The EO of *Anethum graveolens* was evaluated on *A. flavus*. Morphological changes in the cells of *A. flavus* and a reduction in the ergosterol quantity was caused by *A. graveolens* EO. An augmentation of mitochondrial membrane potential (MMP), and the suppression of the glucose-induced decrease in external pH were observed at concentration of 4 mL/mL. A decrease of the activities of ATPase and dehydrogenase in *A. flavus* cells were also observed. The authors attributed the dysfunctions of the mitochondria to the reactive oxygen species (ROS) accumulation in *A. flavus*. The addition of L-cysteine caused a reduction in cell viability, which indicates that ROS is an interesting mediator of the antifungal activity of *A. graveolens* EO [52].

The *Callistemon lanceolatus* (Sm.) Sweet EO inhibited AFB1 production at concentrations lower than its fungitoxic concentration [53]. As well, the EO of *Lantana indica* showed *in vitro* antifungal and antiaflatoxigenic activities against *A. flavus*. The antifungal activity of the *L. indica* EO, tested by disk diffusion test and by SMKY liquid culture, completely inhibited mycelia growth and AFB1 production at 1.5 and 0.75 μg/mL, respectively [54]. The antifungal and antiaflatoxigenic activities of *Litsea cubeba* EO were tested on *A. flavus*. The EO showed a high activity against three toxigenic isolates of *A. flavus*. Under the scanning electron microscopy (SEM), the EO showed alterations of the hyphae and conidiophores structures. The results exhibited that *L. cubeba* EO could inhibit fungal growth and AFB1 production [55]. *Caesulia axillaris* Roxb EO showed complete inhibition of the fungal growth at 1.0 μL/mL and AFB1 at 0.8 μL/mL. Thus, the EO showed antiaflatoxigenic effects at concentration lower than their fungitoxic concentrations indicating two different mode of action for inhibition of fungal growth and AFB1 production [56]. Jamrosa EO (*Cymbopogon khasans*) showed antifungal activity and inhibition of AFB1 production at 0.4 μL/mL. The authors indicated that inhibition of AFB1 production was secondary to inhibition of fungal growth [57]. The capacity of 14 EO components and their combinations to inhibit fungal growth and AFB1 production revealed that thymol, eugenol, menthol, and their combinations were more effective for inhibition of fungal growth and AFB1 was completely inhibited at 1.0 μL/mL. Geranyl acetate, linalool, β-asarone, 1, 8-cineol, and E-citral were moderately antifungal between 1.0 and 5.0 μL/mL [58].

The inhibition of AFB1 production by *A. flavus* was observed at 1.0 and 42.7 μL/mL, respectively, for the samples treated with the EO of *Curcuma longa* L. and curcumin at a concentration of 0.5%. The authors suggested that the antiaflatoxigenic activity might be attributed to phenolic compounds that inhibit lipid peroxidation. Thus, the antioxidant activity of *C. longa* could be important for the inhibition of AFB1 production [59]. The *Boswellia carterii* Birdw EO inhibited *A. flavus* growth and AFB1 production at 1.75 and 1.25 μL/mL, respectively. The EO caused reduction in ergosterol content of plasma membrane of *A. flavus* [60]. This observation showed that plasma membrane is an interesting site for the mechanism of EO supporting the findings of other authors [51]. The *Cuminum cyminum* L. EO was tested on *A. flavus* growth and AFB1 production. The EO inhibited the fungal growth and AFB1 production at 0.6 and 0.5 μL/mL, respectively. The EO totally reduced the ergosterol content at 0.6 μL/mL [31]. *T. vulgaris* L. EO was tested against *A. flavus* growth and AFB1 production. Total inhibition of fungal growth was observed at 250 μg/mL. The *T. vulgaris* EO reduced ergosterol production by *A. flavus*. The morphological structure of *A. flavus* was analyzed by SEM, alterations in conidiophore characteristics were observed. Conidial head size varied between 71.3 and 20.5 μm at concentrations between 50 and 500 μg/mL. A decrease of cytoplasmic content and modifications of membrane integrity were observed. The results were proportional to ergosterol production, which decreased with each EO concentration. Such modifications induced by the EO might be related to the interference caused by its constituents in cell wall synthesis, which affects *A. flavus* growth and morphology. Complete inhibition of AFB1 production was recorded at 150 μg/mL. *T. vulgaris* EO exhibited antiaflatoxigenic activity, as AFB1 biosynthesis inhibition occurred at lower concentration (50 μg/mL) than that required for inhibition of ergosterol production (100 μg/mL) and for morphological alterations of hyphae, conidiophores and conidia (100 μg/mL) [61].

On the other hand, cinnamaldehyde was assessed on AFB1 production of *A. flavus*. The results demonstrated that with cinnamaldehyde treatment, ROS formation reduction was associated with AFB1 production inhibition, which indicate that AFB1 inhibition induced by cinnamaldehyde is related to ROS reduction. Lipid peroxidation is the consequence of ROS formation and has been shown to be involved in AFB1 biosynthesis [62].

Ben Miri et al. [74] reported that *Citrus limon* EO at 1.75 mg/mL and *Citrus sinensis* at 2 mg/mL could totally inhibit fungal growth as well as AFB1 production.

Additionally, the EOs showed notable antioxidant activity and were non phytotoxic to wheat seeds.

5. *In vivo* assays of essential oils

Although *in vitro* assays of EOs is an important first step in determination of the strong activity of plants, *in vivo* confirmation of activity is important because food models may interact with the bioactive compounds, decreasing their efficacy. Generally, to obtain the same effect in food items as those found *in vitro* experiences, higher concentrations of EOs must be applied. Thyme, summer savory and clove EOs was tested in tomato paste and all inhibited the mycelia growth of *A. flavus*. The thyme and summer savory EOs, exhibited the strongest inhibition at concentrations of 350 and 500 ppm, respectively. Taste panel evaluations were carried out in a tomato ketchup base, and the percent of inhibition of each EO in tomato paste was lower than in culture medium. Panelists accepted the results of taste panel with concentration of 500 ppm of thyme EO [69]. Under storage conditions, lemon fruits were completely prevented of *A. flavus* by *S. hortensis* at concentrations of 25, 12.5 and 6.25 μL/mL [40].

The effect of hemlock (*Cicuta virosa* L. var. *latisecta* Celak) EO on inhibition of decay development in cherry tomatoes was assessed by exposing them to EO vapor at 200 μL/mL. Results showed that the *C. virosa* var. latisecta EO has potential to control food spoilage [51]. *Mentha viridis* EO can reduce *A. flavus* and aflatoxin production in stored corn. The authors showed that this of 300 μL of the EO in 100 g of corn is enough to control the fungal growth and the aflatoxin synthesis [70].

EOs of *Origanum majorana* L., *Coriandrum sativum* L., *Hedychium spicatum* Ham. ex Smith, *Commiphora myrrha* (Nees) Engl., and *Cananga odorata* Hook.f. and Thomson, were tested *in vivo* at different concentration against *A. flavus* in chickpea seed. During the investigations in food system all EOs exhibited above 50% protection of chickpea seed from *A. flavus* contamination [71]. The holy basil *O. sanctum* EO reduced the number of *A. flavus* up to 62.94, 67.87 and 74.01% when fumigated at concentrations of 0.3, 0.5 and 1.0 μL/mL, respectively, on *Rauvolfia serpentina* medicinal plant during storage [44]. *Boswellia carterii* Birdw EO showed protection of the fumigated black pepper fruits up to 65.38% from *A. flavus* contamination after 6 months of storage [60]. The efficacy of the combined application of chitosan (CH) and Locust Bean Gum (LBG) in combination with bergamot and bitter orange EOs was evaluated to inhibit *A. flavus* on artificially infected dates. In fruit decay assays coatings based on CH incorporating *Citrus,* EOs were capable to reduce fungal decay between 52 and 62%. Furthermore, the complete absence of off-flavors and off-odors demonstrated the potential of CH coatings carrying bergamot and bitter orange EOs at sub-inhibitory concentrations to control postharvest growth of *A. flavus* in dates [72].

6. Limitations of the use of EOs in food systems

In spite of the great potential of EOs against fungal growth and mycotoxin production, their large scale utilization is limited because of volatile nature, organoleptic effect in food systems and susceptibility to oxidation under light, heat, oxygen and moisture. To develop stability, control the release and enhance the efficacy of EOs in food systems, it is necessary for the current research to develop some structural barriers to enclose these bioactive compounds. In this regards, encapsulation of EOs by different physical, physico-chemical and mechanical methods with the assistance of carrier matrices is a trending area of research.

Thus, although the use of EOs can be an interesting strategy, it faces several constraints:

Phytotoxicity: The alteration of the integrity of the cell membrane following exposure to EO (responsible for their anti-fungal effect) could also affect plants and induce phytotoxicity at slightly higher than those used to control fungi [19]. It should also be noted that the most effective EOs are generally the most phytotoxic [21].

Toxicity to mammals: exposure to EOs or their components may be toxic to mammals. For instance, EO with a high content of furanocoumarins may cause dermal irritation and burns during exposure to light due to photosensitization. The linalool, present in the EO of thyme and lavender is also toxic to human dermal cells [73].

Rapid volatilization: Compounds of EO are highly volatile and may also be oxidatively degraded following exposure to light or temperature rise. This loss of activity would therefore require their reintroduction continuously to maintain the protective effect [35].

Alteration of organoleptic qualities: EOs consists of substances aromatic and are often used in cosmetics industry for their pleasant scent. Their application to foods could change their organoleptic qualities altering the taste [54]. To mitigate this effect, strategies such as encapsulation of EOs have been designed to strengthen the prospective use of EOs in the food industry.

The present review has focused on the antifungal and antiaflatoxigenic activity of essential oils. Additionally, other plant extracts possess potential antifungal activities against *A. flavus* and AFB1 production, but they are generally similar to those observed with the EOs. However, it would seem interesting to further explore the potential of these extracts and their bioactive compounds as they may have several advantages over EOs, such as less sensorial impact on the food.

7. Conclusion

In view of the potential of EOs as inhibitory of *A. flavus* growth and AFB1 production and their efficacy in food system in controlling fungal contamination, the EOs may be recommended for the formulation of plant based preservatives for enhancement of shelf life and safety of foodstuffs during post-harvest processing because consumers are looking for food with natural characteristics.

Acknowledgements

Thanks to the Government of Aragón and FEDER 2014-2020 (Grant Grupo de Investigación A06_17R) and the Ministry of Higher Education and Scientific Research of Algeria (Project number: PRFU/D00L01UN150120180002) for financial support.

Conflict of interest

The authors declare that there are no conflicts of interest.

Author details

Yamina Ben Miri[1]*, Azem Belasli[1], Djamel Djenane[1] and Agustín Ariño[2]

1 Laboratory of Food Quality and Food Safety, University Mouloud MAMMERI, Tizi-Ouzou, Algeria

2 Veterinary Faculty, Instituto Agroalimentario de Aragón-IA2, Universidad de Zaragoza-CITA, Zaragoza, Spain

*Address all correspondence to: sys_yamina@yahoo.com

References

[1] Nogueira JHC, Gonçalez E, Galleti SR, Facanali R, Marques MOM, Felício JD. *Ageratum conyzoides* essential oil as aflatoxin suppressor of *Aspergillus flavus*. International Journal of Food Microbiology. 2010;**137**:55-60

[2] Frisvad CJ, Skouboe P, Samson AR. Taxonomic comparison of three different groups of aflatoxin producers and new efficient producer of aflatoxin B_1, sterigmatocystine and 3-Omethylsterigmatocystine *Aspergillus rumbelli* sp. nov. Systematic and Applied Microbiology. 2005;**28**:442-453

[3] Prakash B, Shukla R, Singh P, Kumar A, Mishra PK, Dubey NK. Efficacy of chemically characterized *Piper betle L*. essential oil against fungal and aflatoxin contamination of some edible commodities and its antioxidant activity. International Journal of Food Microbiology. 2010;**142**:114-119

[4] Prakash B, Shukla R, Singh P, Mishra PK, Dubey NK, Kharwar RN. Efficacy of chemically characterized *Ocimum gratissimum* L. essential oil as an antioxidant and a safe plant based antimicrobial against fungal and aflatoxin B_1 contamination of spices. Food Research International. 2011;**44**:385-390

[5] Reddy KRN, Raghavender CR, Salleh B, Reddy CS, Reddy BN. Potential of aflatoxin B_1 production by *Aspergillus flavus* strains on commercially important food grains. International Journal of Food Science and Technology. 2011;**46**:161-165

[6] IARC Monograph. Some traditional herbal medicines, some mycotoxins, naphthalene and styrene. International Agency for Research on Cancer. 2002;**82**:1-556

[7] Becker-Algeri TA, Castagnaro D, de Bortoli K, de Souza C, Drunkler DA, Badiale-Furlong E. Mycotoxins in bovine milk and dairy products: A review. Journal of Food Science. 2016;**81**(3):R544-R552

[8] Marin S, Ramos AJ, Cano-Sancho G, Sanchis V. Mycotoxins: Occurrence, toxicology, and exposure assessment. Food and Chemical Toxicology. 2013;**60**:218-237

[9] Varga J, Baranyi N, Chandrasekaran M, Vágvölgyi C. Mycotoxin producers in the *Aspergillus* genus: An update. Acta Biologica Szegediensis. 2015;**59**:151-167

[10] Yassin MA, El-Samawaty AMA, Moslem M, Bahkali A, Abd-Elsalam K. Fungal biota and occurrence of Aflatoxigenic *Aspergillus* in postharvest corn grains. Fresenius Environmental Bulletin. 2011;**20**:903, 1018-909, 4619

[11] Moghadam MM, Hokmabadi H. Study on the effect of pistachio testa on the reduction of *Aspergillus flavus* growth and aflatoxin B-1 production in kernels of different pistachio cultivars. Australian Journal of Crop Science. 2010;**4**:744, 1835-749, 2693

[12] Liang XQ, Wang T, Zhang EH, Chen XP, Li L. Identification of seed proteins associated with resistance to pre-harvested aflatoxin contamination in peanut (*Arachis hypogaea* L). BMC Plant Biology. 2010;**10**:1471-2229

[13] Cornea CP, Ciuca M, Voaides C, Gagiu V, Pop A. Incidence of fungal contamination in a Romanian bakery: A molecular approach. Romanian Biotechnological Letters. 2011;**16**:5863, 1224-5871, 5984

[14] Sanchez-Hervas M, Gil JV, Bisbal F, Ramon D, Martinez-Culebras PV. Mycobiota and mycotoxin producing fungi from cocoa beans. International Journal of Food Microbiology. 2008;**125**:336, 0168-340, 1605

[15] Bankole SA, Adenusi AA, Lawal OS, Adesanya OO. Occurrence of aflatoxin B1 in food products derivable from 'egusi' melon seeds consumed in southwestern Nigeria. Food Control. 2010;**21**:974, 0956-976, 7135

[16] Rustom IYS. Aflatoxin in food and feed: Occurrence, legislation and inactivation by physical methods. Food Chemistry. 1997;**59**:57, 0308-67, 8146

[17] Isman MB, Machial CM. Chapter 2 pesticides based on plant essential oils: From traditional practice to commercialization. Advances in Phytomedicine. 2006;**3**:29-44

[18] Chizzola R. Regular monoterpenes and sesquiterpenes (essential oils). In: Ramawat KG, Mérillon JM, editors. Natural Products: Phytochemistry, Botany and Metabolism of Alkaloids, Phenolics and Terpenes. Heidelberg: Springer; 2013:2973-3008

[19] Isman MB. Plant essential oils for pest and disease management. Crop Protection. 2000;**19**:603-608

[20] Burt S. Essential oils: Their antibacterial properties and potential applications in foods: A review. International Journal of Food Microbiology. 2004;**94**:223-253

[21] Carson CF, Mee BJ, Riley TV. Mechanism of action of *Melaleuca alternifolia* (tea tree) oil on *Staphylococcus aureus* determined by time-kill, lysis, leakage, and salt tolerance assays and electron microscopy. Antimicrobial Agents and Chemotherapy. 2002;**46**:1914-1920

[22] Gustafson JE, Liew YC, Chew S, et al. Effects of tea tree oil on *Escherichia coli*. Letters in Applied Microbiology. 1998;**26**:194-198

[23] Cox SD, Mann CM, Markham JL, et al. The mode of antimicrobial action of essential oil of *Melaleuca alternifola* (tea tree oil). Journal of Applied Microbiology. 2000;**88**:170-175

[24] Lambert RJW, Skandamis PN, Coote P, Nychas GJE. A study of the minimum inhibitory concentration and mode of action of oregano essential oil, thymol and carvacrol. Journal of Applied Microbiology. 2001;**91**:453-462

[25] Saad NY, Muller CD, Lobstein A. Major bioactivities and mechanism of action of essential oils and their components. Flavour and Fragrance Journal. 2013;**28**:269-279

[26] Turgis M, Han J, Caillet S, Lacroix M. Antimicrobial activity of mustard essential oil against *Escherichia coli* O157:H7 and *Salmonella typhi*. Food Control. 2009;**20**:1073-1079

[27] Di Pasqua R, Hoskins N, Betts G, Mauriello G. Changes in membrane fatty acids composition of microbial cells induced by addiction of thymol, carvacrol, limonene, cinnamaldehyde, and eugenol in the growing media. Journal of Agricultural and Food Chemistry. 2006;**54**:2745-2749

[28] Fung DYC, Taylor S, Kahan J. Effects of butylated hydroxyanisole (BHA) and butylated hydroxitoluene (BHT) on growth and aflatoxin production of *Aspergillus flavus*. Journal of Food Safety. 1977;**1**:39-51

[29] Abd El-Aziz ARM, Mahmoud MA, Al-Othman MR, Al-Gahtani MF. Use of selected essential oils to control aflatoxin contaminated stored cashew and detection of aflatoxin biosynthesis gene. The Scientific World Journal. 2015;**2015**:958192

[30] Bluma R, Amaiden MR, Daghero J, Etcheverry M. Control of *Aspergillus* section *Flavi* growth and aflatoxin accumulation by plant essential oils. Journal of Applied Microbiology. 2008;**105**:203-214

[31] Kedia A, Prakash B, Mishra PK, Dubey NK. Antifungal and antiaflatoxigenic properties of *Cuminum cyminum (L.)* seed essential oil and its efficacy as a preservative in stored commodities. International Journal of Food Microbiology. 2014;**168-169**:1-7

[32] Paranagama PA, Abeysekera KHT, Abeywickrama K, Nugaliyadde L. Fungicidal and anti-aflatoxigenic effects of the essential oil of *Cymbopogon citratus* (*DC.*) Stapf. (lemongrass) against *Aspergillus flavus* link. Isolated from stored rice. Letters in Applied Microbiology. 2003;**37**:86-90

[33] Rasooli I, Fakoor MH, Yadegarinia D, Gachkar L, Allameh A, Rezaei MB. Antimycotoxigenic characteristics of *Rosmarinus officinalis* and *Trachyspermum copticum L.* essential oils. International Journal of Food Microbiology. 2008;**122**:135-139

[34] Tian J, Huang B, Luo X, Zeng H, Ban X, He J, et al. The control of *Aspergillus flavus* with *Cinnamomum jensenianum Hand.-Mazz* essential oil and its potential use as a foodpreservative. Food Chemistry. 2012;**130**:520-527

[35] Kedia A, Jha DK, Dubey NK. Plant essential oils as natural fungicides against stored product fungi. In: Mendez-Vilas A editor. The Battle Against Microbial Pathogens: Basic Science, Technological Advances and Educational Programs. Badajoz: Formatex Research Center; 2015:208-214

[36] Food and Drug Administration. US Code of Federal Regulations. 2013; Title 21, Part 182, Section 182.20, 129-130

[37] Dayan FE, Cantrell CL, Duke SO. Natural products in crop protection. Bioorganic and Medicinal Chemistry. 2009;**17**:4022-4034

[38] Prakash B, Kedia A, Mishra PK, Dubey NK. Plant essential oils as food preservatives to control moulds, mycotoxin contamination and oxidative deterioration of agri-food commodities–potentials and challenges. Food Control. 2015;**47**:381-391

[39] Salem EA, Shalaby K. Effect of plant essential oils and gamma irradiation on growth and aflatoxin production by *Aspergillus flavus* isolated from wheat grains. Arab Journal of Nuclear Science and Applications. 2016;**94**(1):123-130

[40] Dikbas N, Kotan R, Dadasoglu F, Sahin F. Control of *Aspergillus flavus* with essential oil and methanol extract of *Satureja hortensis*. International Journal of Food Microbiology. 2008;**124**:179-182

[41] Kwazou LN, Dongmo JMP, Ngoune TL, Sameza LM, Dongmo NB, Zollo AHP, et al. Propriétés antifongiques des huiles essentielles de quelques plantes du genre *Aframomoum* du Cameroun contre *Aspergilus flavus*. Cameroon Journal of Experimental Biology. 2009;**5**(1):44-51

[42] Kumar R, Dubey NK, Tiwari OP, Tripathi YB, Sinha KK. Evaluation of some essential oils as botanical fungitoxicants for the protection of stored food commodities from fungal infestation. Journal of Scientific and Food Agriculture. 2007;**87**:1737-1742

[43] Gemeda N, Woldeamanuel Y, Asrat D, Debella A. Effect of essential oils on *Aspergillus*spore germination, growth and mycotoxin production: A potential source of botanical food preservative. Asian Pacific Journal of Tropical Biomedicine. 2014;**4**(1):S373-S381

[44] Kumar A, Dubey NK, Srivastava S. Antifungal evaluation of *Ocimum sanctum* essential oil against fungal deterioration of raw materials of *Rauvolfia serpentina* during storage. Industrial Crops and Products. 2013;**45**:30-35

[45] Passone MA, Girardi NS, Ferrand CA, Etcheverry M. *In vitro* evaluation

of five essential oils as botanical fungitoxicants for the protection of stored peanuts from *Aspergillus flavus* and *A. parasiticus* contamination. International Biodeterioration and Biodegradation. 2012;**70**:82-88

[46] Tatsadjieu NL, Etoa FX Mbofung CMF, Ngassoum MB. Effect of *Plectranthus glandulosus* and *Ocimum gratissimum* essential oils on growth of *Aspergillus flavus* and aflatoxin B1production. Tropicultura. 2008;**26**(2):78-83

[47] Srivastava B, Singh P, Shukla R, Dubey NK. A novel combination of the essential oils of *Cinnamomum camphora* and *Alpinia galanga* in checking aflatoxin B1 production by a toxigenic strain of *Aspergillus flavus*. World Journal of Microbiology and Biotechnology. 2008;**24**:693-697

[48] Tatsadjieu NL, Dongmo PMJ, Ngassoum MB, Etoa FX, Mbofung CMF. Investigations on the essential oil of *Lippia rugosa* from Cameroon for its potential use as antifungal agent against *Aspergillus flavus* link ex. fries. Food Control. 2009;**20**:161-166

[49] Singh P, Shukla R, Prakash B, Kumar A, Singh S, Mishra KP, et al. Chemical profile, antifungal, antiaflatoxigenic and antioxidant activity of *Citrus maxima* Burm. And *Citrus sinensis* (L.) Osbeck essential oils and their cyclic monoterpene, DL-limonene. Food and Chemical Toxicology. 2010;**48**:1734-1740

[50] Deabes MM, Neveen H, El-Soud A, Lamia T, El-Kassem A. *In Vitro* inhibition of growth and Aflatoxin B1 production of *Aspergillus flavus* strain (ATCC 16872) by various medicinal plant essential oils. Macedonian Journal of Medical Sciences. 2011;**4**(4):345-350

[51] Tian J, Ban X, Zeng H, He J, Huang B, Wang Y. Chemical composition and antifungal activity of essential oil from *Cicuta virosa* L. var. latisecta Celak. International Journal of Food Microbiology. 2011;**145**:464-470

[52] Tian J, Ban X, Zeng H, He J, Chen Y, Wang Y. The mechanism of antifungal action of essential oil from dill (*Anethum graveolens* L.) on *Aspergillus flavus*. PLoS One. 2012;7(1):e30147

[53] Shukla R, Singh P, Prakash B, Dubey NK. Antifungal, aflatoxin inhibition and antioxidant activity of *Callistemon lanceolatus* (Sm.) sweet essential oil and its major component 1,8-cineole against fungal isolates from chickpea seeds. Food Control. 2012;**25**:27-33

[54] Kumar A, Shukla R, Singh P, Anuradha, Dubey NK. Efficacy of extract and essential oil of *Lantana indica* Roxb. Against food contaminating moulds and aflatoxin B1 production. International Journal of Food Science and Technology. 2010;**45**:179-185

[55] Li Y, Kong W, Li M, Liu H, Zhao X, Yang S, et al. Litsea cubeba essential oil as the potential natural fumigant: Inhibitionof *Aspergillus flavus* and AFB1 production in licorice. Industrial Crops and Products. 2016;**80**:186-193

[56] Mishra PK, Shukla R, Singh P, Prakash B, Dubey NK. Antifungal and antiaflatoxigenic efficacy of *Caesulia axillaris* Roxb. Essential oil against fungi deteriorating some herbal raw materials, and its antioxidant activity. Industrial Crops and Products. 2012;**36**:74-80

[57] Mishra PK, Shukla R, Singh P, Prakash B, Kedia A, Dubey NK. Antifungal, anti-aflatoxigenic, and antioxidant efficacy of Jamrosa essential oil for preservation of herbal raw materials. International Biodeterioration and Biodegradation. 2012;**74**:11-16

[58] Mishra PK, Singh P, Prakash B, Kedia A, Dubey NK. Assessing essential oil components as plant-based

preservatives against fungi that deteriorate herbal raw materials. International Biodeterioration and Biodegradation. 2013;**80**:16-21

[59] Ferreira FD, Kemmelmeier C, Arrotéia CC, da Costa LC, Mallmann CA, Janeiro V, et al. Inhibitory effect of the essential oil of *Curcuma longa* L. and curcumin on aflatoxin production by *Aspergillus flavus* link. Food Chemistry. 2013;**136**:789-793

[60] Prakash B, Mishra PK, Kedia A, Dubey NK. Antifungal, antiaflatoxin and antioxidant potential of chemically characterized *Boswellia carterii* Birdw essential oil and its *in vivo* practical applicability in preservation of *Piper nigrum* L. fruits. Food Science and Technology. 2014;**56**:240

[61] Kohiyama CY, Ribeiro MMY, Mossini SAG, Bando E, Bomfim NDS, Nerilo SB, et al. Antifungal properties and inhibitory effects upon aflatoxin production of *Thymus vulgaris* L. by *Aspergillus flavus* link. Food Chemistry. 2015;**173**:1006-1010

[62] Sun Q, Wang L, Lu Z, Liu Y. *In vitro* anti-aflatoxigenic effect and mode of action of cinnamaldehyde against aflatoxin B1. International Biodeterioration and Biodegradation. 2015;**104**:419-425

[63] Kumar A, Shukla R, Singh P, Dubey NK. Chemical composition, antifungal and antiaflatoxigenic activities of *Ocimum sanctum L.* essential oil and its safety assessment as plant based antimicrobial. Food and Chemical Toxicology. 2010;**48**:539-543

[64] Singh P, Srivastava B, Kumar A, Kumar R, Dubey NK, Gupta R. Assessment of *Pelargonium graveolens* oil as plant-based antimicrobial and aflatoxin suppressor in food preservation. Journal of the Science of Food and Agriculture. 2008;**88**:2421-2425

[65] Kedia A, Prakash B, Mishra PK, Chanotiya CS, Dubey NK. Antifungal, antiaflatoxigenic, and insecticidal efficacy of spearmint (*Mentha spicata L.*) essential oil. International Biodeterioration and Biodegradation. 2014;**89**:29-36

[66] Mishra PK, Kedia A, Dubey NK. Chemically characterized *Cymbopogon martinii* (Roxb.) Wats. Essential oil for shelf life enhancer of herbal raw materials based on antifungal, antiaflatoxigenic, antioxidant activity, and favorable safety profile. Plant Biosystems. 2015;**3504**:1-10

[67] Kumar A, Shukla R, Singh P, Prasad CS, Dubey NK. Assessment of *Thymus vulgaris L.* essential oil as a safe botanical preservative against post harvest fungal infestation of food commodities. Innovative Food Science and Emerging Technologies. 2008;**9**:575-580

[68] Gorran A, Farzaneh M, Shivazad M, Rezaeian M, Ghassempour A. Aflatoxin B_1-reduction of *Aspergillus flavus* by three medicinal plants (Lamiaceae). Food Control. 2013;**31**:218-223

[69] Omidbeygi M, Barzegar M, Hamidi Z, Naghdibadi H. Antifungal activity of thyme, summer savory and clove essential oils against *Aspergillus flavus* in liquid medium and tomato paste. Food Control. 2007;**18**:1518-1523

[70] Gibriel YAY, Hamza AS, Gibriel AY, Mohsen SM. *In vivo* effect of mint (*Mentha viridis*) essential oil on growth and aflatoxin production by *Aspergillus flavus* isolated from stored corn. Journal of Food Safety. 2011;**3**:445-451

[71] Prakash B, Singh P, Kedia A, Dubey NK. Assessment of some essential oils as food preservatives based on antifungal, antiaflatoxin, antioxidant activities and *in vivo* efficacy in food system. Food Research International. 2012;**49**:201-208

[72] Aloui H, Khwaldia K, Licciardello F, Mazzaglia A, Muratore G, Hamdi M, et al. Efficacy of the combined application of chitosan and locust bean gum with different citrus essential oils to control postharvest spoilage caused by *Aspergillus flavus* in dates. International Journal of Food Microbiology. 2014;**170**:21-28

[73] Prashar A, Locke IC, Evans CS. Cytotoxicity of lavender oil and its major components to human skin cells. Cell Proliferation. 2004;**37**:221-229

[74] Ben Miri Y, Ariño A, Djenane D. Study of antifungal, anti-aflatoxigenic, antioxidant activity and phytotoxicity of Algerian *Citrus limon* var. Eureka and *Citrus sinensis* var. Valencia essential oils. Journal of Essential Oil-Bearing Plants. 2018;**21**(2):345-361

Section 2

Aflatoxin B1 Detection

Chapter 5

A New Approach for Detection of Aflatoxin B1

Xing-Zhi-Zi Wang

Abstract

Aflatoxin B_1 (AFB_1) is harmful to human health, mainly resulting from its toxic effects on the liver. AFB_1 can lead to liver cell necrosis, hemorrhage, fibrosis, cirrhosis, etc. Acute AFB_1 exposure at high levels can lead to hepatitis, whereas chronic exposure can result in liver cancer. In the past decades, a series of methods and techniques for detecting AFB_1, including enzyme-linked immunosorbent assay (ELISA), high-performance liquid chromatography (HPLC), and thin-layer chromatography (TLC), have been developed. This study reviewed the detection methods of AFB_1 and the corresponding utilization and summarizes all methods for evaluating the toxification of AFB_1.

Keywords: aflatoxin B_1, purification, detection, aptasensor, biosensor, reduced graphene nanosheets

1. Introduction

Aflatoxin B_1 (AFB_1) is mainly a metabolite produced by *Aspergillus flavus*. AFB_1 poses a threat to human health due to its three huge toxicities [1]. The toxic effects are as follows [2]. First, it is genetically toxic and can cause DNA damage. Second, aflatoxin shows strong hepatophilic properties when it enters the human body and can cause liver cell necrosis, hemorrhage, fibrosis, and cirrhosis. Finally, aflatoxin has high toxicity and strong carcinogenicity. The data show that its toxicity is 10 times that of potassium cyanide and 68 times that of arsenic. The carcinogenic force is 70 times that of the known carcinogen dimethyl nitrosamines and 900 times that of butter yellow (methyl azobenzene) [3]. The carcinogenic pathway is mainly activated by cytochrome p450 (CYP) monooxygenase system, and AFB_1 is metabolized by CYP1A2 and CYP3A4 to produce epoxy compounds, including active epoxy resins (aflatoxin-8,9-epoxy, AFBO), which generate mutagenic aflatoxin-n7-guanine adduct (AFB1-N7-gua) through interaction with DNA and cause DNA damage to varying degrees [4]. Since AFB_1 is toxic to the human body, it is necessary to monitor the content of AFB_1 in food. However, AFB_1 pollution still exists in a small number of remote areas due to poor living standards and quality. Considering the feasibility and economic feasibility of AFB_1 detection technology, the government needs to add feasible, fast, and accurate new technical schemes for supervision [5]. Therefore, it is of great significance to study the new progress in the detection of AFB_1 in food.

Detection of AFB_1 is divided into two processes, including purification of AFB_1 and quantitative analysis of AFB_1. Purification methods of AFB_1 mainly include liquid–liquid extraction, dispersive liquid–liquid microextraction, solid-phase extraction, molecularly imprinted polymer, immunoaffinity column, etc. [6]. The quantitative analysis methods of AFB_1 mainly include enzyme-linked immunosorbent assay (ELISA), high-performance liquid chromatography (HPLC), thin-layer chromatography (TLC), etc. These methods are tedious, time-consuming, and expensive; moreover, the sample processing is complex and requires professional operation, which is not suitable for the rapid and effective detection and analysis of AFB_1. Therefore finding a fast and sensitive method has important application value.

With the rapid development of science and technology, scientists have been concerned about inventing a fast and sensitive method to detect AFB_1. AFB1 detection based on aptamer AFB_1 sensor is the most widely used detection technology. The aptamer is a single-stranded nucleic acid or peptide molecule; it has a unique secondary structure and can specifically bind to the target, like proteins, drugs, and other biomolecules [7]. Aptamer-based biosensors (aptasensors) have been widely used owing to high sensitivity, selectivity, accuracy, fast response, and low cost [8–10]. Fluorescent-based optical biosensors are the most commonly used method. Combining fluorescent pigment molecules with fluorescent aptasensors leads to the generation of light in the process of biological recognition interaction, so as to achieve the detection of target molecules [11]. In addition, nanomaterials have been widely used in biomolecular detection, such as graphitic carbon nitride nanosheets (g-C3N4 NSs) [12] and reduced graphene nanosheets (rGO) [13].

2. Purification of aflatoxins

The purification is the key step in the detection of the level of AFB_1; traditional methods of AFB_1 mainly include liquid–liquid extraction (LEE), dispersive liquid–liquid microextraction, solid-phase extraction (SPE), molecularly imprinted polymer, immunoaffinity column, etc.; most of these are time-consuming and expensive [14]. Encouragingly, Xie J et al. [6] provide the first report of a broad-spectrum specific mAb-modified reduced graphene nanosheets (rGO) film that can be designed to extract and purify AFB_1, AFB_2, AFG_1, AFG_2, AFM_1, and AFM_2 in rabbit serum. This method is suitable for analysis of different types of analyses from different samples. Compared with the traditional method, this method has the advantages of high selectivity, simplicity, low sample consumption, and the use of a small amount of organic solvent, especially extraction of ultra-trace levels of AFs.

However, in the process of extracting AFB_1, the complexity of food components, especially fat, causes some interference to AFB_1. In addition, AFB_1 is lipophilic; it is difficult to extract AFB_1 from soybean and vegetable oil [14, 15]. The purification is not strong enough, the AFB_1 in vegetable oil cannot be completely removed, and lower lever of AFB_1 will also lead to human liver damage [1, 16]. Xi Yua et al. analyzed trace amounts of AFB_1 in vegetable oils by combining LTC and immuno-magnetic solid-phase extraction (IMSPE) with fluorescence spectroscopy (FL) detection. This process removed fat interference in vegetable oil samples. Subsequently, IMSPE enhances the selectivity and efficiency of extraction through specific antibody–antigen binding. The advantage of this method is that the combined application of traditional LTC and modern IMSPE improves the sensitivity and selectivity of extraction process and meanwhile reduces the time and cost.

3. Application of aptamer

Nucleic acid aptamers are single-stranded oligonucleotides screened in vitro by systematic evolution of ligands by exponential enrichment (SELEX), which are widely concerned as a new biometrics. SELEX technology can be used to screen the combination of the target molecule specific adaptor and target specific [17]. Thus the aptamer has the characteristics of simple preparation, strong specificity, good stability, and a very wide range of target substances, including analysis and detection, biochemistry, food safety [18], clinical medicine [19], and other fields [20]. According to the design principles in different fields, adaptors can be converted into different signals. The commonly used ligand biosensors include fluorescence adaptor sensor, colorimetric adaptor sensor, electrochemical adaptor sensor, etc. In recent years, the aptamer has been applied to the detection of AFB_1, which has greatly improved the detection efficiency and sensitivity of AFB_1 in the field of aflatoxin sensor construction; according to various researches at home and abroad, electrochemical biosensors have been constructed with antibody, enzyme and nucleic acid aptamer as recognition elements; and enzyme catalysis technology, DNA self-assembly technology, ionic liquid, nano materials, conductive polymer have been used to metal compounds, etc. for the detection of aflatoxin [21–23].

4. Fluorometric aptamer

Ye et al. [24] developed a low-cost, high-sensitivity fluorescence polarization (FP) assay by using GO-based fitness biosensors to detect AFB_1. Fluorescein amidite (FAM) labeled the aptamers fitness combines with the surface of GO to form the aptamer/GO macromolecular complex. In the presence of AFB_1, the opposite dissociates from the GO surface and binds to AFB_1 specifically to form the aptamer/AFB_1 complex. As a result, large changes in the molecular weight of the aptamer were observed before and after the combination, leading to significant changes in the fluorescence polarization (FP) value. The lowest detection limit (LOD) of this method was 0.05 nM.

Li et al. [25] use a fluorometric aptamer-based method to detect the level of aflatoxin B1 (AFB_1). Their assay aims to develop a simple and sensitive label-free fluorescence aptasensor to monitor and control AFB_1 in foodstuffs quickly and accurately. In their experiment, the AFB_1 aptamer with the fluorescent dye thioflavin T (ThT) forms a AFB_1 aptamer/ThT G-quadruplex complex in the absence of AFB_1, increasing the fluorescence intensity of ThT. While the AFB_1 aptamer with AFB_1 forms a AFB_1 aptamer/AFB_1 complex in the presence of AFB_1, causing the fluorescence intensity to decrease, the levels of AFB_1 were directly correlated to fluorescence intensity. The general experimental procedures are as follows: first of all, the samples were preprocessed; then, the experimental conditions were optimized, including the optimum ratio of AFB_1 aptamer: ThT, the concentration of KCL and the reaction time (20 min); lastly, using a LUMINA Fluorescence Spectrometer, the fluorescence intensity at excitation/emission wavelengths of 440 nm/487 nm was tested. In this case, the results were in good agreement with those obtained from commercial ELISA kits; the advantages of this method are simpler and more convenient—no label, low cost, and higher efficiency and specificity. The more evidence [8] has proven that this fluorometric aptamer-based method has great practical applications in food industry; not only does it detect AFB_1 and ochratoxin A, but it is more likely to spread to other toxins.

Xia et al. [26] designed a dual-terminal proximity structured aptamer probe; the main purpose of this design is to construct an enzyme-free, ultrafast, single-tube, homogeneous AFB 1 analysis method. This aptamer probe can quickly respond to AFB_1, and the detection process can be completed within 1 min, which is one of the fastest detection methods for AFB_1. Aptamer probe is the design to dual-terminal proximity structures, which allows the binding of one molecule to illuminate the fluorophores of two molecules and achieve enzyme-free amplification and significantly improve the signal-to-background ratio and sensitivity of AFB_1 detection.

Lu et al. [27] discovered another interesting fluorescence method. Their experiments reported a target-driven switch-on fluorescence aptasensor for monitoring AFB_1 determination by employing the fluorescence resonance energy transfer (FRET) between the CdZnTe quantum dots (QDs) and Au nanoparticle (AuNP) pair. AuNPs is considered to be one of the most widely used metal NPs. It can promote electron transfer and act as a tiny conduction center. The crucial design of this switch is that the AuNP acceptors were bioconjugated with the thiol group-modified complementary DNA (cDNA) of aptamer. In this case, as the CdZnTe QDs (energy donor) approaches AuNPs(energy acceptor), FRET is produced, leading to the subsequent fluorescence disappearance of CdZnTe QDs, while AFB1 specifically binds to the aptamer, and aptamer breaks away from AuNPs. Thus, CdZnTe QDs separates from AuNPs, leading to the subsequent fluorescence recovery of CdZnTe QDs. This aptasensor is simple in design and has the advantages of wide linear range, low LOD, high sensitivity, and selectivity.

Wang et al. [28] synthesized a novel fluorescent nitrogen-doped carbon quantum dot (N, C-dots) and combined it with the aptamer/AuNP complex for detection of AFB_1. Initially, they synthesized a positively charged fluorescent N, C-dots by hydrothermal treatment of trypsin, synthesized AuNP by a typical citrate reduction method, and attached a thiol-labeled oligonucleotide (AFB_1 aptamer) to AuNP. N, C-dots/aptamer/AuNP nanocomposite is formed on the surface. N, C-dots are mainly used as a quencher for the construction of aptamer sensors. When AFB_1 is absent, N, C-dots bind to aptamer/AuNPs by electrostatic interaction, and the fluorescence of N, C-dots is quenched by AuNPs. When AFB_1 is present, the aptamer binds to AFB_1, N, C-dots are released, and its fluorescent signal is restored. Therefore, by measuring the fluorescent signal of N, C-dots, the concentration of AFB_1 can be obtained. The detection system is extremely sensitive with a detection limit of 5 pg/mL (16 pM).

Beheshti-Marnani et al. [13] developed aptasensor assembled with assisting reduced graphene oxide nanosheets as the signal amplifier was fabricated and applied for detecting ultralow levels of AFB_1 through a nanobiology interaction system. The detection principle and procedures are different from fluorescence method; the steps are as follows: (1) synthesis of reduced graphene nanosheets (rGO), (2) fabrication of the AFB_1 aptasensor, (3) immobilizing AFB_1 binding ssDNA aptamer on the surface of electrode, and (4) cyclic voltammetry (CV) and electrochemical impedance spectroscopy (EIS) characterized by the modified glassy carbon electrodes. Differential pulse voltammetry (DPV) was used to quantitatively analyze aflatoxin B_1 in practical samples. This new technology is characterized by its simplicity, low cost, and sensitive label-free, in particular, the ability to detect very small quantities of aflatoxin B_1 with a considerable low limit of detection (LOD = 0.07 nM) and good repeatability (RSD = 2.9) and stability.

Wang et al. [29] report a versatile ratiometric fluorescence platform for multiple detection of various targets based on the conjugation of single-stranded DNA (ssDNA) with protonated graphitic carbon nitride nanosheets (Pg-C3N4NSs). This method is also feasible for AFB_1; the principle is that Pg-C3N4NSs promotes oxidation of substrate o-phenylenediamine (OPD) by binding to ssDNA in the presence of H_2O_2. Subsequently, the fluorescence signal at 564 nm of the oxidation product 2,3-diaminophenazine (DAP) was collected and concurrently quenches the intrinsic fluorescence of conjugates ssDNA/Pg-C3N4 NSs at 443 nm upon excitation at 370 nm. Lastly, the transformation of fluorescence was used for ratiometric fluorescence-based analytical. This method applies to for multiplex detection of various targets.

5. Electrochemical aptamer

Wu et al. [30] proposed a simple electrochemical body sensor, and they take advantage of host-guest identification between ferrocene and β-cyclodextrin (β-CD) to detect AFB_1. Despite the long-time consumption and complexity involved in the preparation process of the pβ-CD/AuNPs/GC electrode and AFB1-sensitive dsDNA, they demonstrated the selectivity, stability, and reproducibility of the electrochemical aptasensor in the detection of AFB_1; there is no significant difference in stability between 1 day and 15 days, that is to say, electrochemical aptasensor has good stability.

Abnous et al. [31] built an electrochemical biosensor for accurate detection of AFB_1. AFB_1 is based on aptamer to form a π-shape complementary strand of aptamer (CSs) complex on the surface of electrode and exonuclease I (Exo I). The purpose of π-shape design is to greatly increase the sensitivity of aptamer. In the absence of AFB_1, the PI configuration of the gold electrode surface remains intact, and a double potential barrier is formed on the electrode surface, limiting the contact of $[Fe(CN)_6]^{3-/4-}$ with the electrode surface, and only weak electrochemical signals are measured. When AFB_1 exists,π-shape structure was removed, and a strong current was recorded after the addition of Exo I. Under the optimum conditions, the concentration range of AFB_1 can be detected in the range of 7–500 pg/mL and a limit of detection (LOD) of 2 pg/mL.

Xia et al. [32] designed a new split-type photoelectrochemical (PEC) immunosensing platform for sensitive detection of AFB_1, combined with the etching reaction triggered by the enzymatic hydrolysis of cobalt oxyhydroxide (CoOOH) at the functional interface of cadmium sulfide (CdS) nanoparticles. The concentration of CdS nanoparticles has a great influence on the analytical properties of PEC biosensor. Excessive CdS may induce high background signal, while low concentration produces weak photocurrent response. In their experiment, the optimum concentration of CdS nanoparticles was 0.8 mg/mL^{-1}, and the entire time of the method is within 1.5 h for each sample. Under optimal conditions, the detection limit of this method is 2.6 pg/mL^{-1}, and the accuracy of this method (expressed in RSD) is ±8.6%.

6. Aptamers with chemiluminescence immunoassay

Li et al. [33] developed an aptamer structure switch experiment with horseradish peroxidase (HRP) labeling for sensitive absorbance and chemiluminescence detection of small molecules. Differently from competitive enzyme-linked immunosorbent assay (ELISA), they fixed the cDNA of the aptamer to the surface of the microporous plate.

7. Others

Zhao et al. [34] developed a novel nano-antibody and magnetic beads-based directed competitive ELISA (MB-dcELISA) based on both recombinant antibody and its mimotope for AFB1 detection. The 50% inhibition concentration and detection limit of MB-dcELISA were 0.75 and 0.13 ng/mL, respectively, and the linear range was 0.24–2.21 ng/mL.

Zhang et al. [35] discovered a novel anti-AFB_1 monoclonal antibody in order to establish a sensitive immunoassay for AFB_1, and a novel CdTe/CdS/ZnS quantum dot fluorescence probe was synthesized by binding to the surface of CdTe/CdS/ZnS quantum dots. CdTe/CdS/ZnS quantum dot is a kind of semiconductor nanomaterial, which has strong photostability and fluorescence efficiency and has longer fluorescence time. Compared with the traditional ELISA method, fluorescence immunoassays (FLISA) can be used to measure AFB_1 in grain samples in a wide range of linearity. In addition, CdTe/CdS/ZnS quantum dot fluorescence assay has lower toxicity, high stability, and excellent fluorescence properties.

Based on the competitive response of AFB1 and cy5 modified DNA complementary strands to aptamers, Shim et al. [36] first developed a dipstick assay for AFB1 sensing. This sensor has a minimum detection limit of about 0.1 ng/mL for AFB_1, indicating good potential for practical applications. The whole determination process can be completed in 30 min. Moreover, the dipstick assay is consistent with the ELISA assay results.

8. Discussion

We mainly report on the new detection techniques of aflatoxin in recent years. It mainly includes fluorescence detection, electrochemical detection, immunological detection, and so on. Fluorescence detection method is more and more popular in the industry because of its high sensitivity and high specificity. Electrochemical detection is a powerful analytical technology. Due to its simple operation and low price, it has been widely used in environmental monitoring and food safety [30]. According to the different detection principles, it can be divided into electrochemical enzyme sensor, electrochemical immunosensor, and electrochemical aptamer sensor in the determination of aflatoxin in food. ELISA has been widely used in the determination of AFB_1 in recent years. The method has high sensitivity and selectivity, but the reaction time is long and the operation process is complex. In addition, antibodies and enzymes are easily denatured during storage, which severely limits their practical application.

More and more scholars are committed to the research and development of highly sensitive AFB_1 sensor [37], and biosensors with antibodies, enzymes, and nucleic acid aptamers as recognition elements were constructed. In addition, a large number of new materials have been used for the detection of AFB_1 at home and abroad.

As the research frontier of modern science and technology, nanotechnology has been widely used in the detection of AFB_1 abbreviation in foods in combination with electrophysiology, biology, and immunology and has become a development trend in the field of food safety research. The fabrication of Au nanostructures/graphene nanosheets modified ITO substrate has been reported; it is then used as a high sensitivity and AFB_1 sensor to detect very low concentrations of AFB_1 early by using Raman spectroscopy and electrochemical techniques [38]. Carbon dots (C-dots), as a new type of fluorescent nanomaterials, have attracted great attention in recent years due to their excellent light stability, good biocompatibility, low toxicity, and good water solubility. In order to expand the field of application, many researchers have studied the surface modification of C-dots with various functions [28]. Compared to traditional fluorescent sensors, C-dots-based aptasensors have greater potential because of their chemical inertness, ease of functionalization, and resistance to photobleaching. Based on the highly efficient fluorescence quenching properties of AuNP, a DNA sensor for detecting mRNA in living cells was developed. The results show that the fluorescence sensor based on AuNPs leads to high signal and sensitivity. CdTe quantum dots have the advantages of high fluorescence yield, strong photostability, long fluorescence lifetime, good biocompatibility, and wide excitation wavelength range. It is widely used in biomedical fields such as biochips, protein and DNA detection, and targeted tracing [39–42].

However, nanotechnology itself has its drawbacks. The preparation of CdS nanoparticles and CoOOH nanosheets takes a long time, and it is necessary to verify whether the synthesis is successful. In addition, the concentration of CdS nanoparticles directly affects PEC immunosensor; excessive CdS may lead to high background signal, whereas a low concentration produces a weak photocurrent response.

As an important medium, aptamer combines AFB_1 with nanomaterials and detects it by fluorescence and electrophysiological detection, which greatly shortens the time of detection and reduces the cost, and its accuracy and reliability. There is no change in sex, and the specificity and sensitivity are increased. However, since the AFB_1 aptamer preparation technique may still need improvement, as described above, the AFB_1 aptamer is an oligonucleotide, and the length of the small molecule nucleotide affects the binding to AFB_1. Aptamer Structure Switch coupled with horseradish peroxidase labeling on microplate for sensitive detection of small molecules. It is affected by the concentration of aptamer and AFB_1, and the results of Ye [24] show that when only 10 nM aptamer is used, the change in FP and AFB_1 concentrations has a good linear relationship between 0.05 and 5 nM of AFB_1. Coupled with the time required for preparation, combined with the complex and diverse detection methods, there is no standardized operation in life. However, based on the fluorescence and electrochemical detection of the AFB_1 aptamer, it is most promising for the detection of AFB_1.

Author details

Xing-Zhi-Zi Wang[1,2]

1 Department of Pathology, The Affiliated Hospital of Youjiang Medical University for Nationalities, Baise, China

2 The Centre of Pathology Diagnosis and Research, Youjiang Medial University for Nationalities, Baise, China

*Address all correspondence to: stpwxzz@163.com

References

[1] Kumar P, Mahato DK, Kamle M, et al. Aflatoxins: A global concern for food safety, human health and their management. Frontiers in Microbiology. 2016;**7**:2170. DOI: 10.3389/fmicb.2016.02170

[2] Weng MW, Lee HW, Choi B, et al. AFB_1 hepatocarcinogenesis is via lipid peroxidation that inhibits DNA repair, sensitizes mutation susceptibility and induces aldehyde-DNA adducts at p53 mutational hotspot codon 249. Oncotarget. 2017;**8**(11):18213-18226. DOI: 10.18632/oncotarget.15313

[3] Tao F, Yao H, Hruska Z, et al. Use of visible-near-infrared (Vis–NIR) spectroscopy to detect Aflatoxin B_1 on peanut kernels. Applied Spectroscopy. 2019;**73**(4):415-423. DOI: 10.1177/0003702819829725

[4] Rushing BR, Selim MI. Aflatoxin B_1: A review on metabolism, toxicity, occurrence in food, occupational exposure, and detoxification methods. Food and Chemical Toxicology. 2019;**124**:81-100. DOI: 10.1016/j.fct.2018.11.047

[5] Qi N, Yu H, Yang C, et al. Aflatoxin B_1 in peanut oil from Western Guangdong, China, during 2016-2017. Food Additives & Contaminants: Part B. 2019;**12**(1):45-51. DOI: 10.1080/19393210.2018.1544173

[6] Xie J, Fang X, Dai X, et al. Antibody-functionalized reduced graphene oxide films for highly selective capture and purification of aflatoxins. Microchimica Acta. 2019;**186**(3):193. DOI: 10.1007/s00604-019-3255-6

[7] Famulok M, Mayer G. Aptamer modules as sensors and detectors. Accounts of Chemical Research. 2011;**44**(12):1349-1358. DOI: 10.1021/ar2000293

[8] Wu K, Ma C, Zhao H, et al. Sensitive aptamer-based fluorescence assay for ochratoxin a based on RNase H signal amplification. Food Chemistry. 2019;**277**:273-278. DOI: 10.1016/j.foodchem.2018.10.130

[9] Guo L, Zhao Q. Thrombin-linked aptamer assay for detection of platelet derived growth factor BB on magnetic beads in a sandwich format. Talanta. 2016;**158**:159-164. DOI: 10.1016/j.talanta.2016.05.037

[10] Tong P, Zhao WW, Zhang L, et al. Double-probe signal enhancing strategy for toxin aptasensing based on rolling circle amplification. Biosensors and Bioelectronics. 2012;**33**(1):146-151. DOI: 10.1016/j.bios.2011.12.042

[11] Razmi N, Baradaran B, Hejazi M, et al. Recent advances on aptamer-based biosensors to detection of platelet-derived growth factor. Biosensors and Bioelectronics. 2018;**113**:58-71. DOI: 10.1016/j.bios.2018.04.048

[12] Liu JW, Luo Y, Wang YM, et al. Graphitic carbon nitride nanosheets-based ratiometric fluorescent probe for highly sensitive detection of H_2O_2 and glucose. ACS Applied Materials & Interfaces. 2016;**8**(49):33439-33445. DOI: 10.1021/acsami.6b11207

[13] Beheshti-Marnani A, Hatefi-Mehrjardi A, Es'haghi Z. A sensitive biosensing method for detecting of ultra-trace amounts of AFB1 based on "aptamer/reduced graphene oxide" nano-bio interaction. Colloids and Surfaces B: Biointerfaces. 2019;**175**:98-105. DOI: 10.1016/j.colsurfb.2018.11.087

[14] Yu X, Li Z, Zhao M, et al. Quantification of aflatoxin B_1 in vegetable oils using low temperature clean-up followed by immuno-magnetic solid phase extraction. Food Chemistry.

2019;**275**:390-396. DOI: 10.1016/j.foodchem.2018.09.132

[15] Wang D, Zhang Z, Li P, et al. Europium nanospheres-based time-resolved fluorescence for rapid and ultrasensitive determination of total aflatoxin in feed. Journal of Agricultural and Food Chemistry. 2015;**63**(47):10313-10318. DOI: 10.1021/acs.jafc.5b03746

[16] Rapisarda V, Loreto C, Malaguarnera M, et al. Hepatocellular carcinoma and the risk of occupational exposure. World Journal of Hepatology. 2016;**8**(13):573-590. DOI: 10.4254/wjh.v8.i13.573

[17] Takahashi M. Aptamers targeting cell surface proteins. Biochimie. 2018;**145**:63-72. DOI: 10.1016/j.biochi.2017.11.019

[18] Liu X, Zhang X. Aptamer-based technology for food analysis. Applied Biochemistry and Biotechnology. 2015;**175**(1):603-624. DOI: 10.1007/s12010-014-1289-0

[19] Nimjee SM, White RR, Becker RC, et al. Aptamers as therapeutics. Annual Review of Pharmacology and Toxicology. 2017;**57**:61-79. DOI: 10.1146/annurev-pharmtox-010716-104558

[20] Lauridsen LH, Doessing HB, Long KS, et al. A capture-SELEX strategy for multiplexed selection of RNA aptamers against small molecules. Methods in Molecular Biology. 2018;**1671**:291-306. DOI: 10.1007/978-1-4939-7295-1_18

[21] Chen J, Wen J, Zhuang L, et al. An enzyme-free catalytic DNA circuit for amplified detection of aflatoxin B1 using gold nanoparticles as colorimetric indicators. Nanoscale. 2016;**8**(18):9791-9797. DOI: 10.1039/c6nr01381c

[22] Yang M, Liu G, Mehedi HM, et al. A universal SERS aptasensor based on DTNB labeled GNTs/Ag core-shell nanotriangle and CS-Fe_3O_4 magnetic-bead trace detection of Aflatoxin B_1. Analytica Chimica Acta. 2017;**986**:122-130. DOI: 10.1016/j.aca.2017.07.016

[23] Li Z, Xue N, Ma H, et al. An ultrasensitive and switch-on platform for aflatoxin B1 detection in peanut based on the fluorescence quenching of graphene oxide-gold nanocomposites. Talanta. 2018;**181**:346-351. DOI: 10.1016/j.aca.2017.07.016

[24] Ye H, Lu Q, Duan N, et al. GO-amplified fluorescence polarization assay for high-sensitivity detection of aflatoxin B1 with low dosage aptamer probe. Analytical and Bioanalytical Chemistry. 2019;**411**(5):1107-1115. DOI: 10.1007/s00216-018-1540-6

[25] Li Y, Wang J, Zhang B, et al. A rapid fluorometric method for determination of aflatoxin B_1 in plant-derived food by using a thioflavin T-based aptasensor. Mikrochimica Acta. 2019;**186**(4):214. DOI: 10.1007/s00604-019-3325-9

[26] Xia X, Wang Y, Yang H, et al. Enzyme-free amplified and ultrafast detection of aflatoxin B1 using dual-terminal proximity aptamer probes. Food Chemistry. 2019;**283**:32-38. DOI: 10.1016/j.foodchem.2018.12.117

[27] Lu X, Wang C, Qian J, et al. Target-driven switch-on fluorescence aptasensor for trace aflatoxin B1 determination based on highly fluorescent ternary CdZnTe quantum dots. Analytica Chimica Acta. 2019;**1047**:163-171. DOI: 10.1016/j.aca.2018.10.002

[28] Wang B, Chen Y, Wu Y, et al. Aptamer induced assembly of fluorescent nitrogen-doped carbon dots on gold nanoparticles for sensitive detection of AFB1. Biosensors and Bioelectronics. 2016;**78**:23-30. DOI: 10.1016/j.bios.2015.11.015

[29] Wang L, Zhu F, Liao S, et al. Single-stranded DNA modified protonated graphitic carbon nitride nanosheets: A versatile ratiometric fluorescence platform for multiplex detection of various targets. Talanta. 2019;**197**:422-430. DOI: 10.1016/j.talanta.2019.01.066

[30] Wu SS, Wei M, Wei W, et al. Electrochemical aptasensor for aflatoxin B1 based on smart host-guest recognition of beta-cyclodextrin polymer. Biosensors and Bioelectronics. 2019;**129**:58-63. DOI: 10.1016/j.bios.2019.01.022

[31] Abnous K, Danesh NM, Alibolandi M, et al. A new amplified pi-shape electrochemical aptasensor for ultrasensitive detection of aflatoxin B1. Biosensors and Bioelectronics. 2017;**94**:374-379. DOI: 10.1016/j.bios.2017.03.028

[32] Su L, Song Y, Fu C, et al. Etching reaction-based photoelectrochemical immunoassay of aflatoxin B1 in foodstuff using cobalt oxyhydroxide nanosheets-coating cadmium sulfide nanoparticles as the signal tags. Analytica Chimica Acta. 2019;**1052**:49-56. DOI: 10.1016/j.aca.2018.11.059

[33] Li Y, Sun L, Zhao Q. Aptamer-structure switch coupled with horseradish peroxidase labeling on a microplate for the sensitive detection of small molecules. Analytical Chemistry. 2019;**91**(4):2615-2619. DOI: 10.1021/acs.analchem.8b05606

[34] Zhao F, Tian Y, Shen Q, et al. A novel nanobody and mimotope based immunoassay for rapid analysis of aflatoxin B1. Talanta. 2019;**195**:55-61. DOI: 10.1016/j.talanta.2018.11.013

[35] Zhang F, Liu B, Zhang Y, et al. Application of CdTe/CdS/ZnS quantum dot in immunoassay for aflatoxin B1 and molecular modeling of antibody recognition. Analytica Chimica Acta. 2019;**1047**:139-149. DOI: 10.1016/j.aca.2018.09.058

[36] Shim WB, Kim MJ, Mun H, et al. An aptamer-based dipstick assay for the rapid and simple detection of aflatoxin B1. Biosensors and Bioelectronics. 2014;**62**:288-294. DOI: 10.1016/j.bios.2014.06.059

[37] Wu L, Ding F, Yin W, et al. From electrochemistry to electroluminescence: Development and application in a ratiometric aptasensor for aflatoxin B1. Analytical Chemistry. 2017;**89**(14):7578-7585. DOI: 10.1021/acs.analchem.7b01399

[38] Althagafi II, Ahmed SA, El-Said WA. Fabrication of gold/graphene nanostructures modified ITO electrode as highly sensitive electrochemical detection of Aflatoxin B1. PLoS One. 2019;**14**(1):e0210652. DOI: 10.1371/journal.pone.0210652

[39] Wang K, Zhang R, Sun N, et al. Near-infrared light-driven photoelectrochemical aptasensor based on the upconversion nanoparticles and TiO_2/CdTe heterostructure for detection of cancer cells. ACS Applied Materials & Interfaces. 2016;**8**(39):25834-25839. DOI: 10.1021/acsami.6b09614

[40] Istif E, Kagkoura A, Hernandez-Ferrer J, et al. Self-assembled core-shell CdTe/poly(3-hexylthiophene) nanoensembles as novel donor-acceptor light-harvesting systems. ACS Applied Materials & Interfaces. 2017;**9**(51):44695-44703. DOI: 10.1021/acsami.7b13506

[41] Pan D, Chen K, Zhou Q, et al. Engineering of CdTe/SiO_2 nanocomposites: Enhanced signal amplification and biocompatibility for electrochemiluminescent immunoassay of alpha-fetoprotein. Biosensors and Bioelectronics. 2019;**131**:178-184. DOI: 10.1016/j.bios.2019.02.022

[42] Xiang X, Gao T, Zhang BR, et al. Surface functional groups affect CdTe QDs behavior at mitochondrial level. Toxicology Research. 2018;7(6):1071-1080. DOI: 10.1039/c8tx00160j

Chapter 6

The Blood AFB1-DNA Adduct Acting as a Biomarker for Predicting the Risk and Prognosis of Primary Hepatocellular Carcinoma

Qin-Qin Long, Xiao-Qin Wu and Jin-Guang Yao

Abstract

Aflatoxin B1 (AFB1) is an important carcinogen for primary hepatocellular carcinoma (PHCC). However, the values of blood AFB1-DNA adducts predicting HCC risk and prognosis have not still been clear. We conducted a hospital-based case-control study, consisting of 380 patients with pathologically diagnosed PHCC and 588 controls without any evidence of liver diseases, to elucidate the associations between the amount of AFB1-DNA adducts in the peripheral blood and the risk and outcome of HCC. All subjects had not the history of hepatitis B and C virus infection. AFB1-DNA adducts were tested using enzyme-linked immunosorbent assay. Cases with PHCC featured an increasing blood amount of AFB1-DNA adducts compared with controls (2.01 ± 0.71 vs. 0.98 ± 0.63 μmol/DNA). Increasing adduct amount significantly grew the risk of PHCC [risk values, 1.82 (1.34–2.48) and 3.82 (2.71–5.40) for medium and high adduct level, respectively]. Furthermore, compared with patients with low adduct level, these with medium or high adduct level faced a higher death and tumor-recurrence risk. These results suggest that the blood AFB1-DNA adducts may act as a potential biomarker for predicting the risk and prognosis of PHCC.

Keywords: AFB1, DNA adduct, primary hepatocellular carcinoma, biomarker, risk, prognosis

1. Introduction

Aflatoxin B1 (AFB1) is a knowledge I-type chemical carcinogen for primary hepatocellular carcinoma (PHCC) [1–3]. This carcinogen is mainly produced by *Aspergillus parasiticus* and *Aspergillus flavus* and often found in crops and food (including maize, nuts, and beans), which are raised in the areas with humid and hot environment [1, 4, 5]. Once these AFB1-contaminated crops and food are ingested by human bodies, AFB1 will be metabolized through two stage reactions consisting of detoxification stage (such as reduction, oxidation, and hydrolytic reaction) and covalent stage (such as binding reaction and conjugating reaction) [2, 3]. During the process of AFB1's metabolism, AFB1-DNA adducts, including AFB1-formamidopyrimidine adduct (AFB1-FAPa) and AFB1's 8,9-dihydro-8-(N^7-guanyl)-9-hydroxy–adduct (AFB1-GA), are frequently formed [2, 3]. Growing evidence has shown that AFB1-DNA adducts are usually tested in the tissue samples (such as liver and placenta tissues) of these individuals from high AFB1 exposure areas [6–10]. Recent studies have displayed that they are also found in the peripheral blood white cells of peoples who are from high AFB1 exposure areas and are associated with the time of AFB1 exposure [11–17]. However, the potential of blood AFB1-DNA adducts predicting PHCC risk and prognosis is not clear. Here, we specifically conduced a hospital-based case-control study to investigate whether blood AFB1-DNA adducts were related to the risk and outcome of PHCC.

2. Materials and methods

2.1 Study population

A total of 380 patients were recruited from the affiliated hospitals of Youjiang Medical University for Nationalities and Guangxi Medical University (two main medical universities in the AFB1-exposure areas in China) between 2011 and 2013. All cases were newly diagnosed as patients using histopathological method and they had no history of radiation or chemotherapy treatment before enrollment. A total of 588 controls, who were randomly recruited from a pool of healthy individuals in the same hospitals during the same time, were all volunteers without any evidence with liver diseases. To control the effects of confounder factors such as age, gender, and race, controls were individually matched with the cases on these factors. In this study, all cases and controls had no history of hepatitis B virus (HBV) and/hepatitis C virus (HCV) infection, whereas these subjects with positive status of serum anti-HCV and/or hepatitis B surface antigen (HBsAg) were excluded. They all agreed to participate in this investigation and did not drop out. With informed consent, all clinicopathological data, including age, gender, race, hepatitis virus B and C infection information, survival follow-up information, were collected using healthy examination or medical records. Additionally, 10 ml of peripheral blood samples for all subjects were also collected for AFB1-DNA adduct analysis. In this study, the last following-up date was set on January 31, 2019. Overall survival (OS) and tumor recurrence-free survival (RFS) status were defined according to the previously described methods [11, 14, 18]. The study protocol was approved by the ethics committees of Youjiang Medical University for Nationalities and Guangxi Medical University.

2.2 AFB1-DNA adducts data

The amount of AFB1-DNA adducts in the peripheral blood were tested using the previously published methods [8, 17]. Briefly, DNA samples were first extracted from the peripheral blood samples and adducts were next quantitated by the comparative enzyme-linked immunosorbent assay (ELISA). To investigate the association between different levels of AFB1-DNA adducts and the risk and prognosis of PHCC patients, the levels of AFB1-DNA adducts were divided into three subgroups according to the mean adduct amounts of cases and controls: low AFB1-DNA adduct level (LAL, <1.00 μmol/DNA), medium AFB1-DNA adduct level (MAL, 1.00–2.00 μmol/DNA), and high AFB1-DNA adduct level (HAL, >2.00 μmol/DNA).

2.3 Statistical analysis

All statistical analyses were accomplished with SPSS statistical package (Version 18, SPSS Institute, Chicago, IL, USA). Test for the distribution of age, gender, and race between patients with PHCC and controls was accomplished using chi-square test. The effects of blood AFB1-DNA adducts on PHCC risk were evaluated using odds ratio (OR) and 95% confidence interval (CI) in the conditional logistic regression model. For survival analyses, Kaplan-Meier survival model with *Log-Rank* test and Cox regression model (the selection of significant variates based on forward-step method with likelihood ratio test) was used to analyze the association between blood AFB1-DNA adducts and PHCC outcomes. Cumulative hazard value for the effects of adducts on the prognosis of patients with PHCC and corresponding 95% CI was calculated using hazard ratio (HR) from significant multivariate Cox regression model (including all significant variates). In this study, the P value <0.05 was defined as statistical significance.

3. Results

3.1 The features of study population

A total of 380 cases with PHCC and 588 controls were included in our final analyses. Baseline characteristics of all cases with PHCC and controls were summarized in **Table 1**, and results showed there were no significant distributions of age, gender, and race between cases and controls.

	Controls		PHCCs		*P*
	n	%	n	%	
Total	588	100.0	380	100.0	—
Gender					0.70
Male	426	72.4	271	71.3	
Female	162	27.6	109	28.7	
Age (years)					0.78
≤35	81	13.8	53	13.9	
36–40	62	10.5	38	10.0	
41–45	90	15.3	55	14.5	
46–50	83	14.1	43	11.3	
51–55	94	16.0	56	14.7	
56–60	56	9.5	42	11.1	
61–65	69	11.7	49	12.9	
≥66	53	9.0	44	11.6	
Race					0.88
Han	339	57.7	221	58.2	
Zhuang	249	42.3	159	41.8	

PHCCs, patients with primary hepatocellular carcinoma.

Table 1.
The characteristics of subjects.

AFB1-DNA adduct levels	Controls		PHCCs		OR (95% CI)[a]	*P*
	n	%	n	%		
Low	316	53.7	122	32.1	1	—
Medium	186	31.6	131	34.5	1.82 (1.34–2.48)	1.20×10^{-4}
High	86	14.6	127	33.4	3.82 (2.71–5.40)	2.35×10^{-14}

[a]*OR conditional on matched set.*
AFB1, aflatoxin B1; PHCC, primary hepatocellular carcinoma.

Table 2.
Associations between AFB1-DNA adduct levels and PHCC risk.

3.2 Blood AFB1-DNA adducts correlating with PHCC risk

The amount of AFB1-DNA adducts in the peripheral white blood cells were calculated using ELISA technique. Compared to controls, patients with PHCC featured a higher level of blood AFB1-DNA adducts (0.98 ± 0.63 vs. 2.01 ± 0.71 μmol/DNA), suggesting blood AFB1-DNA adducts may play an important role in the PHCC carcinogenesis. To investigate possible correlation between AFB1-DNA adducts and PHCC risk, the levels of blood AFB1-DNA adducts were divided into three groups. Results from multivariable logistic regression analyses showed that these individuals with medium AFB1-DNA adduct level (MAL) had an increasing risk of PHCC compared to those with low AFB1-DNA adduct level (LAL) (OR = 1.82 and 95% CI = 1.34–2.48), whereas risk value for high AFB1-DNA adduct level (HAL) was 3.82 (2.71–5.40) (**Table 2**). Altogether, these data were indicative of important potential risk role of blood AFB1-DNA adducts in the carcinogenesis of PHCC.

3.3 Blood AFB1-DNA adducts correlating with PHCC outcome

To explore the effects of blood AFB1-DNA adducts on the prognosis of patients with PHCC, we accomplished two survival model analyses. Kaplan-Meier's

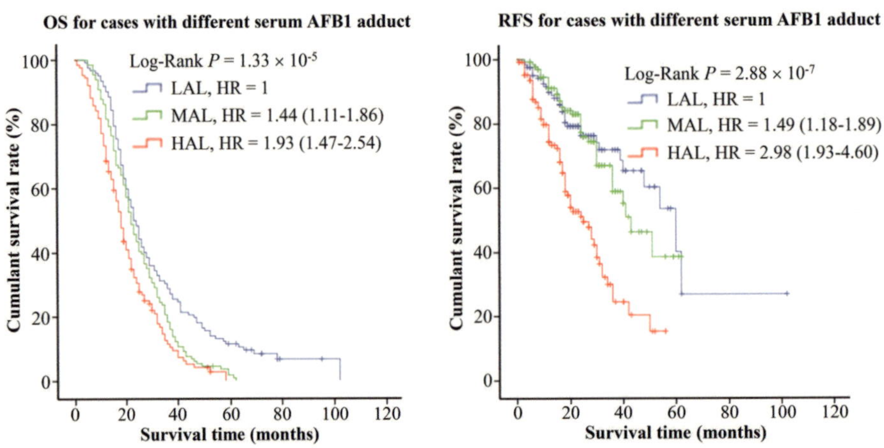

Figure 1.
The aflatoxin B1 (AFB1)-DNA adducts in peripheral blood white cells significantly correlating with the overall survival (OS) and tumor recurrence-free survival (RFS) of primary hepatocellular carcinoma (PHCC). Cumulative hazard function was plotted by Kaplan-Meier's methodology, and P value was calculated with two-sided log-rank tests. The relative hazard ratio (HR) values for genotypes were calculated using multivariable cox regression models (with all significant variables) based on forward-step method with likelihood ratio test. LAL, low AFB1-DNA adduct level; MAL, medium low AFB1-DNA adduct level; HAL, high low AFB1-DNA adduct level.

survival analyses first tested the association between blood AFB1-DNA adducts and patients' OS and results displayed that increasing level of adducts significantly shorten the OS time of patients ($P = 1.33 \times 10^{-5}$) (**Figure 1**, left). Similar effects were also found in the RFS analyses ($P = 2.88 \times 10^{-7}$) (**Figure 1**, right). Results from multivariate Cox's regression models further exhibited that these cases with an increasing level of blood AFB1-DNA adducts faced an increasing risk of death [HRs (95% CIs) = 1.44 (1.11–1.86) for MAL and 1.93 (1.47–2.54) for HAL, respectively] (**Figure 1**, left). For RFS, the corresponding tumor-recurrence risk was 1.49 (1.18–1.89) for MAL and 2.98 (1.93–4.60) for HAL, respectively (**Figure 1**, right).

4. Discussion

In this study, we explored the relationship between the blood AFB1-DNA adducts and the risk and prognosis of PPHCC. We found that individuals with an increasing level of AFB1-DNA adducts in peripheral blood white cells would feature higher PHCC risk (OR = 1.82 for MAL and 3.82 for HAL, respectively). Furthermore, the blood AFB1-DNA adduct levels were significantly associated with poor OS and RFS of patients with PHCC.

AFB1 acts as a major cause of PHCC in the southeast areas of China and is taken into human bodies through its contaminating staple foods [2]. AFB1 is transferred into AFB1-DNA adducts and displays its genic toxicity and hepato carcinogenicity [3, 19]. Mechanically, PHCC induced by AFB1 is mainly concerned with DNA damage (including DNA single-/double-strand breaks, base damage, adduct formation, genic mutation), the dysregulation of DNA repair, the activation of cancer genes (such as ras and myc), the inactivation of cancer suppressor genes (such as TP53, BP1, H2AX, bcl2, p21, and p27), inheritance alterations, and/or abnormal immunoreaction [1, 20–25]. Among these knowledge mechanisms and pathways, AFB1-DNA adducts and mutations at codon 249 of TP53 gene (also termed as hot-spot mutation induced by AFB1) have been especially concerned in the past decades [26–29]. This is mainly because AFB1-DNA adducts are the key central forms in the metabolism of AFB1 in human bodies [19, 26, 30], whereas spot mutations at codon 249 of TP53 gene are highly frequent in HCC patients with AFB1 exposure [31–36]. Evidence from clinical epidemiology and experimental animal models has exhibited that they are constantly tested in biopsy samples, such as liver tissues, tumor tissues, placenta tissues, and blood cells, of individuals from AFB1 exposure areas [6, 8, 11, 12, 15–17].

For example, Hsieh and Hsieh [8] examined the amounts of AFB1-DNA adducts in the 120 placenta tissue samples from women in Taipei, a high AFB1 exposure area, and observed that 57.5% (69/120) of samples were positive AFB1-DNA adducts with the range of 0.6 and 6.3 μmol/mol DNA. Furthermore, they found higher amount of AFB1-DNA adducts in samples collected in the summer than in the winter. Shirabe et al. [37] investigated the association between AFB1-DNA adducts in hepatocyte nuclei and TP53 mutation in PHCC among Japanese population. They found that 6% (118/279) patients with PHCC and 16% (13/83) patients with HBV- and HCV-negative PHCC were positive for AFB1-DNA adducts. Higher hot-spot mutations in the TP53 gene were also found in these with positive AFB1-DNA adduct status [37]. A relatively large-size sample clinical study, including 501 PHCC cases with different AFB1 exposure, also shows that positive status of AFB1-DNA adducts in the tumor tissues significantly increases the risk of TP53 mutations (OR = 3.38 and 95% CI = 2.23–5.11) [7].

Following epidemiological studies on based clinical samples further prove that the amount of AFB1-DNA adducts is higher in the tumor tissues than in the peri-tumor tissues [6]. This increasing tissular AFB1-DNA adducts are significantly associated with poor OS and RFS of patients with PHCC [6].

In this study, we designed and finished a hospital-based case-control study in the southwestern of Guangxi, a knowledge-high AFB1 exposure area. Our data exhibited that increasing the amount of AFB1-DNA adducts in peripheral white blood cells not only increased PHCC risk, but also modified the OS and RFS of patients with PHCC. Supporting our findings through several studies from high AFB1 exposure areas, the amount of blood AFB1-DNA adducts can reflect the levels of AFB1 exposure information and may be related to PHCC risk and prognosis [11, 12, 14, 15, 17, 38]. Taken together, these results suggest that AFB1-DNA adducts in the blood as well as in the tumor tissues may be potential biomarkers for PHCC risk and outcome.

This study has several strengthens. We accomplished the predictive value analyses using these individuals only with AFB1 exposure but without HBV or HCV. This is done mainly because both HBV and HCV infection will alter effects of AFB1-DNA adducts predicting the risk and outcome of PHCC. Additionally, to control potential confounders such as age, gender, and race, the individually matched design was finished in this study. Therefore, our study may represent a relatively more actual predictive role of blood AFB1-DNA adducts.

To conclude, this study explored the association between blood AFB1-DNA adducts and the risk and prognosis of PHCC using a retrospective clinic-sample research approach and displayed that blood AFB1-DNA adduct may be a potential biomarker for HCC risk and outcome. Several limitations should be focused for our study. First, relatively small-size samples may underestimate the effects of blood AFB1-DNA adducts on PHCC risk and outcome. Second, selective bias may happen because of this hospital-based retrospective investigative design. Finally, the mechanical analyses for AFB1-DNA adducts predicting PHCC risk and prognosis were not finished. Thus, the blood AFB1-DNA adducts may be valuable biomarkers for predicting the risk and prognosis of PHCC once the present findings were proved by larger clinic samples and functional analyses.

Acknowledgements

We thank Dr Yuan-Feng Zhou for sample collection and management.

Conflict of interests and source of funding

The authors declare no competing financial interests. This study was supported in part by the National Natural Science Foundation of China (Nos. 81860489, 81760502, 81572353, and 81660495), the Natural Science Foundation of Guangxi (Nos. 2018GXNSFAA281043, 2017GXNSFAA198002, and 2017GXNSFGA198002), Research Program of Guangxi "Zhouyue Scholar" (No. 2017-38), Research Program of Guangxi Specially invited Expert (No. 2017-6th), the "12th Five" Planning Program of Guangxi Education Science (No. 2015C397), the Innovative Program of Guangxi Graduate Education (No. JGY2015139), Research Program of Guangxi Clinic Research Center of Hepatobiliary Diseases (No. AD17129025), and Open Research Program from Molecular Immunity Study Room Involving in Acute and Severe Diseases in Guangxi Colleges and Universities (Nos. kfkt20160062 and kfkt20160063).

Abbreviations

AFB1	Aflatoxin B1
AFB1-FAPa	AFB1-formamidopyrimidine adduct
AFB1-GA	AFB1's 8,9-dihydro-8-(N^7-guanyl)-9-hydroxy–adduct
HAL	high AFB1-DNA adduct level
HBV	hepatitis B virus
HBsAg	hepatitis B surface antigen
HCV	hepatitis C virus
CI	confidence interval
HR	hazard ratio
LAL	low AFB1-DNA adduct level
MAL	medium AFB1-DNA adduct level
OR	odds ratio
PHCC	primary hepatocellular carcinoma
OS	overall survival
RFS	tumor recurrence-free survival

Author details

Qin-Qin Long[†], Xiao-Qin Wu[†] and Jin-Guang Yao*
Department of Pathology, The Affiliated Hospital of Youjiang Medical University for Nationalities, Baise, China

*Address all correspondence to: yyyaojg001@163.com

† These authors contributed equally to this work.

References

[1] Long XD, Deng Y, Huang XY, Yao JG, Su QY, Wu XM, et al. Molecular mechanisms of hepatocellular carcinoma related to aflatoxins: An update. In: Rodrigo L, editor. Liver Research and Clinical Management. Vol. 1.1. Rijeka: InTech; 2018. pp. 113-136. DOI: 10.5772/intechopen.72883

[2] Kew MC. Aflatoxins as a cause of hepatocellular carcinoma. Journal of Gastrointestinal and Liver Diseases. 2013;**22**:305-310. DOI: PMID.24078988

[3] Kensler TW, Roebuck BD, Wogan GN, Groopman JD. Aflatoxin: A 50-year odyssey of mechanistic and translational toxicology. Toxicological Sciences. 2011;**120**(Suppl 1):S28-S48. DOI: 10.1093/toxsci/kfq283

[4] Wu XM, Xi ZF, Lu J, Wang XZ, Zhang TQ, Huang XY, et al. Genetic single nucleotide polymorphisms (GSNPs) in the DNA repair genes and hepatocellular carcinoma related to aflatoxin B1 among Guangxiese population. In: Parine NR, editor. Genetic Polymorphisms. Vol. 1. Rijeka: InTech; 2017. pp. 97-119. DOI: 10.5772/intechopen.69530

[5] Long XD, Yao JD, Yang Q, Huang CH, Liao P, Nong LG, et al. Polymorphisms of DNA repair genes and toxicological effects of aflatoxin B1 exposure. In: Faulkner AG, editor. Aflatoxins: Food Sources, Occurrence and Toxicological Effects. 1st ed. Nova Science Publishers: New York; 2014. pp. 125-156. DOI: 978-1-63117-298-4

[6] Liu YX, Long XD, Xi ZF, Ma Y, Huang XY, Yao JG, et al. MicroRNA-24 modulates aflatoxin B1-related hepatocellular carcinoma prognosis and tumorigenesis. BioMed Research International. 2014;**2014**:482926. DOI: 10.1155/2014/482926

[7] Long XD, Ma Y, Huang HD, Yao JG, Qu de Y, Lu YL. Polymorphism of XRCC1 and the frequency of mutation in codon 249 of the p53 gene in hepatocellular carcinoma among Guangxi population, China. Molecular Carcinogenesis. 2008;**47**:295-300. DOI: 10.1002/mc.20384

[8] Hsieh LL, Hsieh TT. Detection of aflatoxin B1-DNA adducts in human placenta and cord blood. Cancer Research. 1993;**53**:1278-1280. DOI: PMID.8383006

[9] Tulayakul P, Dong KS, Li JY, Manabe N, Kumagai S. The effect of feeding piglets with the diet containing green tea extracts or coumarin on in vitro metabolism of aflatoxin B1 by their tissues. Toxicon. 2007;**50**:339-348. DOI: 10.1016/j.toxicon.2007.04.005

[10] Zhang YJ, Chen S, Tsai WY, Ahsan H, Lunn RM, Wang L, et al. Expression of cytochrome P450 1A1/2 and 3A4 in liver tissues of hepatocellular carcinoma cases and controls from Taiwan and their relationship to hepatitis B virus and aflatoxin B1-and 4-aminobiphenyl-DNA adducts. Biomarkers. 2000;**5**:295-306. DOI: 10.1080/135475000413845

[11] Long XD, Zhao D, Wang C, Huang XY, Yao JG, Ma Y, et al. Genetic polymorphisms in DNA repair genes XRCC4 and XRCC5 and aflatoxin B1-related hepatocellular carcinoma. Epidemiology. 2013;**24**:671-681. DOI: 10.1097/EDE.0b013e31829d2744

[12] Long XD, Yao JG, Huang YZ, Huang XY, Ban FZ, Yao LM, et al. DNA repair gene XRCC7 polymorphisms (rs#7003908 and rs#10109984) and hepatocellular carcinoma related to AFB1 exposure among Guangxi population, China. Hepatology Research. 2011;**41**:1085-1093. DOI: 10.1111/j.1872-034X.2011.00866.x

[13] Wu XM, Ma Y, Deng ZL, Long XD. The polymorphism at codon

939 of xeroderma pigmentosum C gene and hepatocellular carcinoma among Guangxi population. Zhonghua Xiaohua Neijing Zazhi. 2010;**30**:846-848. DOI: 10.3760/cma.j.issn.0254-1432.2010.11.018

[14] Long XD, Ma Y, Zhou YF, Ma AM, Fu GH. Polymorphism in xeroderma pigmentosum complementation group C codon 939 and aflatoxin B1-related hepatocellular carcinoma in the Guangxi population. Hepatology. 2010;**52**:1301-1309. DOI: 10.1002/hep.23807

[15] Long XD, Ma Y, Zhou YF, Yao JG, Ban FZ, Huang YZ, et al. XPD codon 312 and 751 polymorphisms, and AFB1 exposure, and hepatocellular carcinoma risk. BMC Cancer. 2009;**9**:400. DOI: 10.1186/1471-2407-9-400

[16] Long XD, Ma Y, Deng ZL. GSTM1 and XRCC3 polymorphisms: Effects on levels of aflatoxin B1-DNA adducts. Chinese Journal of Cancer Research. 2009;**21**:177-184. DOI: 10.1007/s11670-009-0177-6

[17] Long XD, Ma Y, Qu de Y, Liu YG, Huang ZQ, Huang YZ, et al. The polymorphism of XRCC3 codon 241 and AFB1-related hepatocellular carcinoma in Guangxi population, China. Annals of Epidemiology. 2008;**18**:572-578. DOI: 10.1016/j.annepidem.2008.03.003

[18] Long XD, Yao JG, Zeng Z, Ma Y, Huang XY, Wei ZH, et al. Polymorphisms in the coding region of X-ray repair complementing group 4 and aflatoxin B1-related hepatocellular carcinoma. Hepatology. 2013;**58**:171-181. DOI: 10.1002/hep.26311

[19] Wang JS, Groopman JD. DNA damage by mycotoxins. Mutation Research. 1999;**424**:167-181. DOI: 10.1016/S0027-5107(99)00017-2

[20] Zuberi Z, Eeza MNH, Matysik J, Berry JP, Alia A. NMR-based metabolic profiles of intact Zebrafish embryos exposed to aflatoxin B1 recapitulates hepatotoxicity and supports possible neurotoxicity. Toxins (Basel). 2019;**11**:258. DOI: 10.3390/toxins11050258

[21] Zhou Y, Jin Y, Yu H, Shan A, Shen J, Zhou C, et al. Resveratrol inhibits aflatoxin B1-induced oxidative stress and apoptosis in bovine mammary epithelial cells and is involved the Nrf2 signaling pathway. Toxicon. 2019;**164**:10-15. DOI: 10.1016/j.toxicon.2019.03.022

[22] Zhou X, Gan F, Hou L, Liu Z, Su J, Lin Z, et al. Aflatoxin B1 induces immunotoxicity through the DNA methyltransferase-mediated JAK2/STAT3 pathway in 3D4/21 cells. Journal of Agricultural and Food Chemistry. 2019;**67**:3772-3780. DOI: 10.1021/acs.jafc.8b07309

[23] Zhou J, Tang L, Wang JS. Assessment of the adverse impacts of aflatoxin B1 on gut-microbiota dependent metabolism in F344 rats. Chemosphere. 2019;**217**:618-628. DOI: 10.1016/j.chemosphere.2018.11.044

[24] Zhao L, Feng Y, Deng J, Zhang NY, Zhang WP, Liu XL, et al. Selenium deficiency aggravates aflatoxin B1-induced immunotoxicity in chick spleen by regulating 6 selenoprotein genes and redox/inflammation/apoptotic signaling. The Journal of Nutrition. 2019;**149**:894-901. DOI: 10.1093/jn/nxz019

[25] Zhao F, Tian Y, Shen Q, Liu R, Shi R, Wang H, et al. A novel nanobody and mimotope based immunoassay for rapid analysis of aflatoxin B1. Talanta. 2019;**195**:55-61. DOI: 10.1016/j.talanta.2018.11.013

[26] Li S, Muhammad I, Yu H, Sun X, Zhang X. Detection of aflatoxin adducts as potential markers and the role of curcumin in alleviating AFB1-induced liver damage in chickens.

Ecotoxicology and Environmental Safety. 2019;**176**:137-145. DOI: 10.1016/j.ecoenv.2019.03.089

[27] Engin AB, Engin A. DNA damage checkpoint response to aflatoxin B1. Environmental Toxicology and Pharmacology. 2019;**65**:90-96. DOI: 10.1016/j.etap.2018.12.006

[28] Coskun E, Jaruga P, Vartanian V, Erdem O, Egner PA, Groopman JD, et al. Aflatoxin-guanine DNA adducts and oxidatively induced DNA damage in aflatoxin-treated mice in vivo as measured by liquid chromatography-tandem mass spectrometry with isotope dilution. Chemical Research in Toxicology. 2019;**32**:80-89. DOI: 10.1021/acs.chemrestox.8b00202

[29] Liang TJ. p53 proteins and aflatoxin B1: The good, the bad, and the ugly. Hepatology. 1995;**22**:1330-1332. PMID: 7557889

[30] Poapolathep S, Imsilp K, Machii K, Kumagai S, Poapolathep A. The effects of curcumin on aflatoxin B1-induced toxicity in rats. Biocontrol Science. 2015;**20**:171-177. DOI: 10.4265/bio.20.171

[31] Bayram S, Rencuzogullari E, Almas AM, Genc A. Effect of p53 Arg72Pro polymorphism on the induction of micronucleus by aflatoxin B1 in in vitro in human blood lymphocytes. Drug and Chemical Toxicology. 2016;**39**:331-337. DOI: 10.3109/01480545.2015.1121275

[32] Qi LN, Bai T, Chen ZS, Wu FX, Chen YY, De Xiang B, et al. The p53 mutation spectrum in hepatocellular carcinoma from Guangxi, China : Role of chronic hepatitis B virus infection and aflatoxin B1 exposure. Liver International. 2015;**35**:999-1009. DOI: 10.1111/liv.12460

[33] Chittmittrapap S, Chieochansin T, Chaiteerakij R, Treeprasertsuk S, Klaikaew N, Tangkijvanich P, et al. Prevalence of aflatoxin induced p53 mutation at codon 249 (R249s) in hepatocellular carcinoma patients with and without hepatitis B surface antigen (HBsAg). Asian Pacific Journal of Cancer Prevention. 2013;**14**:7675-7679. DOI: PMID24460352

[34] Gursoy-Yuzugullu O, Yuzugullu H, Yilmaz M, Ozturk M. Aflatoxin genotoxicity is associated with a defective DNA damage response bypassing p53 activation. Liver International. 2011;**31**:561-571. DOI: 10.1111/j.1478-3231.2011.02474.x

[35] Van Vleet TR, Watterson TL, Klein PJ, Coulombe RA Jr. Aflatoxin B1 alters the expression of p53 in cytochrome P450-expressing human lung cells. Toxicological Sciences. 2006;**89**:399-407. DOI: 10.1093/toxsci/kfj039

[36] Chan KT, Hsieh DP, Lung ML. In vitro aflatoxin B1-induced p53 mutations. Cancer Letters. 2003;**199**:1-7. DOI: 10.1016/S0304-3835(03)00337-9

[37] Shirabe K, Toshima T, Taketomi A, Taguchi K, Yoshizumi T, Uchiyama H, et al. Hepatic aflatoxin B1-DNA adducts and TP53 mutations in patients with hepatocellular carcinoma despite low exposure to aflatoxin B1 in southern Japan. Liver International. 2011;**31**:1366-1372. DOI: 10.1111/j.1478-3231.2011.02572.x

[38] Long XD, Yao JG, Zeng Z, Huang CH, Huang ZS, Huang YZ, et al. DNA repair capacity-related to genetic polymorphisms of DNA repair genes and aflatoxin B1-related hepatocellular carcinoma among Chinese population. In: Kruman I, editor. DNA Repair. Rijeka: InTech; 2011. pp. 505-524. DOI: 10.5772/20792

Section 3

The Toxification Effects of Aflatoxin B1

Chapter 7

The Toxic Effects of Aflatoxin B1: An Update

Yuhua Shan

Abstract

Aflatoxin B1 (AFB1) is the most toxic in aflatoxin family. It is well known for its involvement in hepatic carcinogenesis. Other adverse effects include immune weakness, reproduction deficiency, malnutrition, and growth impairment. The key mechanism of AFB1 carcinogenesis is supposed to be epoxidation, which produce the AFB1-8,9-epoxide (AFBO) strongly adductive to DNA molecules. Other metabolites like AFM1, AFH1, and AFL, which retain DNA adductive capability, extend its toxicity. Scientists now found that AFB1 also affected epigenetic regulation, which might shed new light into AFB1 toxicity mechanism researches. The detoxification of AFB1 has always been a hot spot in AFB1-related studies. The major methods can be categorized into physical treatment, biological treatment, chemical treatment, combination strategy, and sorbent additives. None of the methods is 100% perfect, however considering economic factors, simplicity, effectiveness, safety, and preservation of the food nutrition. This review will discuss the toxicity and toxic mechanisms of AFB1. Also, detoxification of AFB1 will be reviewed.

Keywords: AFB1, carcinogenesis, DNA adductive capability, epigenetic mutation, detoxification

1. Introduction

Aflatoxins are fungal metabolites majorly produced by *Aspergillus flavus* and *A. parasiticus* [1]. They are recognized as a family of toxic contaminants in a variety of crops, especially promoted by hot and humid climates as well as improper harvesting and storage process [2]. Among these toxins, aflatoxin B1 (AFB1) is the most hazardous, widely known for its "acute intoxication" targeting the liver featured by acute liver failure and death at a short yet high dosage exposure. Other major adverse effects include carcinogenicity and immunosuppression capacity in a chronic way.

2. Toxic effects of AFB1

AFB1 is well known to be hepatotoxic, causing degeneration and necrosis of the liver as well as proliferation of the bile duct and infiltration of inflammatory cells in many species. In recent studies, AFB1 is reported to lead to apoptosis of hepatocytes via an extrinsic mechanism because of high expression of death receptor pathway [3]. Moreover, in 2002, AFB1 has been classified into Group 1 of carcinogens, considering its direct contribution to hepatocellular carcinoma (HCC) [4]. In fact, as early as in the 1970s, its hepatocarcinogenic property has been testified in animal models [5], and there since, several epidemiological studies from Asia and Africa areas monitored intersection of high HCC incidence and AFB1 contamination, with 4.6–28.2% of HCC cases globally attributed to AFB1 exposure [6]. Moreover, hepatitis B virus (HBV) that cooperates with AFB1 can drastically increase the risk of HCC by 30-fold [7]. Recent researches also find evidences that hepatitis C virus (HCV) also has a synergistic role with AFB1 in hepatocarcinogenesis. Jeannot et al. found that the incidence of tumorous or pretumorous lesions was elevated by 2.5-fold in AFB1-treated HCV transgenic mice compared with wild-type mice [8]. Recently, a 20-year clinical follow-up study in Taiwan investigated HCC risk associated with AFB1 exposure in HCV-positive and HBV-HCV-negative individuals. HCV and AFB1 exposure were both found as independent risk factors for HCC development. Elevated serum AFB1-albumin adduct levels were significantly associated with an increased risk of HCC newly developed within 8 years of follow-up in non-HBV-non-HCV participants with habitual alcohol consumption [crude OR (95% CI) for high vs. low/undetectable levels, 4.22 (1.16–15.37)], and HCV-infected participants [3.39 (1.31–8.77)], but not in non-HBV-non-HCV participants without alcohol drinking habit. Therefore, it indicated that AFB1 exposure contributes to the development of HCC in participants with significant risk factors for cirrhosis including alcohol and HCV infection [9]. What's more, AFB1 exposure can induce the increased levels of blood glucose in mice and, also, the high probability to develop liver cancer [10].

Liver is not the only target organ of AFB1 toxification. Its impairment on the immune system has been established in both humans and animals. Several studies linked AFB1 exposure with reduced levels or functions of immunological factors, such as decreased T or B lymphocyte activity [11, 12], suppressed macrophage or neutrophil effector functions [13], modified synthesis of inflammatory cytokines [14, 15], impaired NK cell-mediated cytolysis [16], and thus increasing risk to infectious diseases. A study on Gambian children found that those children were generally exposed to high levels of aflatoxin (as much as 93%). The exposure significantly decreases sIgA in their saliva [17]. In another study, Jiang et al. reported that Ghanaians with higher serum aflatoxin-albumin adducts (AF-ALB) level had lower percentages of CD8+ T cells, perforin, and granzyme A than those with the lower level [18]. By comparing HIV-infected individuals exposed to high and low AF-ALB levels with HIV-negative counterparts, experts found that high AF-ALB appeared to accelerate HIV-associated changes in T-cell phenotypes and B cells in HIV-positive participants [19]. This result was in accordance with the observation of Hendrickse et al. long back in 1989 that heroin addicts often experienced rapid progression of HIV infection, while street heroin was often contaminated with aflatoxin and that aflatoxin derivatives were commonly found in the body fluids of the addicts [20]. Recent researches also show that when exposed to a low dose of AFB1, people were more vulnerable to SIV infection and suffered increased severity [21].

Another chronic adverse effect of AFB1 is malnutrition and growth impairment. Several observations in developing countries have pointed out the accordance of kwashiorkor occurrence with high AFB1 concentration in sera [22–24]. Animal models and in vitro methods have also been used to investigate the mechanism of AFB1-induced malnutrition. AFB1 is supposed to alter metal absorption and bioavailability. Long back in the 1990s, broiler chicks exposed to AFB1 were found to have lowered serum concentrations of vitamin D and calcium possibly due to impairing renal function and altering parathyroid metabolism [25]. AFB1 had toxicity toward the vitamin D receptors, interfering with the actions of vitamin D on calcium-binding gene expression in the kidney and intestine, which increase the risk of rickets. Experimental data indicated a 58 and 86% decrease if the cells were exposed to 5 and 50 ng/mL of AFB1, respectively [26]. Dietary intake of AFB1 also leads to vitamin A depletion in young broiler chicks, which could be attenuated by additional feeding of NovaSil PLUS, an AFB1-binding agent [27]. Other adverse effects included inactivating enzymes in liver lipid metabolism [28] and redistribution of various metal ions in the central nervous system and genital glands [29]. Mechanistically, it is unclear how AFB1 alters nutrient levels. Existing hypothesis includes impairment of liver, absorption deficiency, and insulin-like growth factor modulation. Ubagai et al. found that AFB1 could modulate the insulin-like growth factor (IGF)-2 signaling axis [30]. Furthermore, Castelino et al. found that Kenyan schoolchildren that exhibited high levels of AFB1-albumin were shorter and had lower levels of IGF1 and IGFBP3 than groups with lower levels of the AFB1 biomarker [31]. Additionally, AFB1 may affect nutrient absorption through intestinal toxicity. Enteropathy features decreases in intestinal density and increases in fibrosis/necrosis, which has been shown in poultry experimental models [32]. The disruption of intestinal function by AFB1 is due to the destruction of epithelial cells and their organization due to the inhibition of protein synthesis or cytotoxicity due to DNA and protein binding. This tissue damage can alter the structure of intestinal epithelial cells, affecting the efficiency of nutrient absorption [33, 34]. Recent studies also found that lack of protein [35] and vitamins A, C, and E [36] together with aflatoxicosis worsened hepatic oxidative stress. These findings gave rise to the theory that toxification and malnutrition can form a vicious circle, which add up to the damage of AFB1.

AFB1 is not likely to be limited by the physical barrier. Aflatoxin metabolites and biomarkers can be tested in breastmilk and cord blood, which means this toxin can affect fetuses and neonates. Levels of aflatoxins in pregnant women have also been linked to poor birth outcomes in humans. An early Kenyan study indicated that newborns birthed from aflatoxin-positive mothers had significantly lower birth weights. The relation between AFB1 maternal exposure and growth impairment was significant and may even lead to stillbirth [37]. Another study found a strong negative correlation between aflatoxin levels and birth weights in Gambian infants [38]. Also, Shuaib et al. reported that mothers in the highest quartile of serum AFB1-albumin levels were highly likely to have lower birthrates than mothers with lower concentrations [39].

AFB1 not only interferes with the reproductive process after embryo forms. The findings of the current study repeatedly demonstrate direct effects of dietary toxin intaking on spermatozoa, oocytes, and in vitro fertilization while exploring the potential hazards associated with AFB1 exposure [40]. Low dose of AFB1 exposure was reported to cause follicular atresia in ovaries in animal models [41]. AFB1 was also testified to impair sperm quality and fertilization competence in animal and in vitro models, although the mechanism underlying cellular damage has not been fully elucidated. In summary the alterations include impairment of (1) membrane integrity, (2) mitochondrial function, (3) DNA integrity, and (4) fertilization competence. Exposure of fresh semen to 10 μM AFB1 prefertilization resulted in sperm DNA damage and impaired fertilization competence, featured by reduced proportion of oocytes that are divided to early-stage embryos after fertilization [42]. Exposure of sperm to low concentrations of AFB1 for a few hours also resulted in decreased sperm viability and hyperpolarization of the mitochondrial membrane, which was most remarkable in ejaculated sperm, suggesting that later stages of spermatogenesis were affected. AFB1 may adversely affect the spermatogenesis through mitochondria-dependent apoptosis via inducing oxidative stress, diminishing cellular mitochondrial content, and enhancing pro-apoptotic Bax, caspase-3, and p53 expression [43].

Besides all mentioned above, AFB1 also induces damage to the heart [44–46], kidney [45], and even central nervous systems by direct toxicity to both the neural cells and blood-brain barrier [47–49]. It is of great importance to better understand how this toxin functions in order to discriminate its threats to public health.

3. The metabolism and toxic mechanism of AFB1

It is well established that AFB1 epoxidation is the key step in the genotoxic process leading to carcinogenesis. The predominant place of epoxidation is in the liver by the P450 family before transforming into the final carcinogen aflatoxin B1-8,9-epoxide (AFBO), which has two isomers: endo-8,9-epoxide and exo-8,9-epoxide [50]. CYP3A4 is the major producer of AFBO formation at high AFB1 concentrations, producing primarily the exo isomer of AFBO [51], while lower concentration of AFB1 exposure makes CYP1A2 the main producer of AFBO in turn. Additionally, CYP1A2 was found to produce more of the exo isomer than CYP3A4 at these low concentrations [52, 53]. The highly electrophilic nature of AFBO allows it to form adducts to amines in proteins or nucleic acids and then interrupt the function of these biological molecules. Since the exo isomer has a much higher affinity for guanine residues than the endo isomer, AFB1-exo-8,9 epoxide, which has the highest concentration in the liver, is therefore considered to be the major carcinogenic metabolite [54, 55].

AFB1 is also metabolized into a number of hydroxylation products through the P450 system. These include aflatoxin Q1 (AFQ1), aflatoxin P1 (AFP1), aflatoxin B2a (AFB2a), aflatoxin M1 (AFM1), aflatoxicol (AFL), and aflatoxicol H1 (AFH1), and among them, AFQ1, AFP1, and AFB2a were traditionally considered detoxification products of AFB1 due to their much lower DNA-binding potential [56–58]. In the recent decades, AFQ1 was found to have a potential as a biomarker for AFB1 exposure indication. AFQ1 consists of 1–11% of the AFB1 hydroxylation products indicating that in humans, AFQ1 production occurs frequently and at high enough levels to detect [59]. In 2005, a study evaluated fecal and urinary excretion of AFM1, AFQ1, and AFB1-N7-guanine in 83 Chinese males. The study demonstrated that AFQ1 is excreted in urine and feces at higher levels than AFM1, especially in feces, since fecal samples contained approximately 60 times more AFQ1 than AFM1. Additionally, fecal concentrations of AFM1 and AFQ1 were higher than in urine, indicating the usefulness of feces as a predictive marker for AFB1 exposure [60]. However, as the most prominent metabolite of AFB1, AFB2a has an interesting property as compared to many of the other metabolites which has the ability to bind to cellular proteins through the formation of a pyrrole ring. Additionally, this binding only occurs on primary amines that is favored in alkaline pHs. This adduction can also occur on phosphoethanolamine head groups on phospholipids, forming a unique structurally characterized aflatoxin-lipid adduct [61]. The protein-binding capability of AFB2a is thought to contribute to other potential cellular toxicities. For example, AFB2a binding has been shown to inhibit the activity of deoxyribonucleases, demonstrating the ability of AFB2a to alter enzymatic activities of target proteins [62]. Chen et al. recently observed mitochondria-mediated apoptosis and PI3K/Akt/mTOR-mediated autophagy induced by AFB2 in hepatocytes of broilers [63]. AFB2a has been found in high levels in poultry eggs possibly as a result of avian metabolism, providing a potential source of dietary exposure [64]. AFM1 is a major metabolite produced by CYP1A2 and is the most carcinogenic of the hydroxylated metabolites. This is supported by the DNA-binding effect of AFM1 which has been demonstrated in rat, mouse, and pig and has even been identified to form an N7-guanine adduct similar to AFB1 [65]. Just like AFB1, AFM1 can be excreted in cattle or human milk [66]. AFM1 is also excreted in high levels in urine following AFB1 exposure and thus has become an additional biomarker of AFB1 exposure [67]. AFL is found in the cytosolic fractions of liver preparations and is formed by an NADPH reductase, usually in the cytosol [68, 69]. AFL retains its DNA-binding activity and has been shown to be enzymatically reconverted back into AFB1 acting as a reservoir for AFB1, extending its toxic effects [69]. Despite excretion in breast milk and urine, AFL is the sole metabolite that is able to be transferred through the human placenta, and, furthermore, AFL is the only metabolite that is formed from AFB1 by the placenta itself. This indicates that AFL may play a large role in developmental toxicities of AFB1 [69]. AFH1 has a structure similar to AFL which contains an additional hydroxy group on the terminal cyclopentenone ring, which implies a similar toxicity. The metabolic formation of AFH1 was found to be dependent on two enzyme systems: the microsomal hydroxylase and cytoplasmic reductase systems [70].

By firmly binding to purine bases (usually at the N7 position on guanine) of DNA, epoxide intermediate forms AFB1-N7-guanine (AFB1-N7-Gua) adduct, and thus promoting mutations in nucleotide sequence. The charged adduct causes depurination and thus apurinic site formation [71]. The predominant mutation caused by AFB1-N7-Gua adduct has been identified to be the G → T transversion on the site of the original adduct [72]. Moreover, the mutation has a favor for specific base pair locations. Mace et al. reported a selective affinity for guanine bases with a guanine or a cytosine as 50 bases and more specifically at the third base of codon 249 of the p53 tumor suppressor gene [73]. This mutation was found really common in a great number of epidemiological studies on HCC patients from regions of high aflatoxin exposure, strengthening the association between HCC incidence and aflatoxin exposure [74].

Interestingly, AFB1 can be activated by other biotransformation aside from the principal pathway involving CYP. As early as in 1985, Battista et al. have described the epoxidation catalyzed by prostaglandin H (PGH) synthase [75], whereas Weng et al. hypothesized that lipid peroxidase (LPO) was one of the mechanisms behind AFB1 carcinogenesis, triggering the production of cyclic α-methyl-γ-hydroxy-1,N2-propano-dG (meth-OH-PdG) adduct and inhibiting DNA repair [76]. Another important role in DNA damage and thus carcinogenesis is played by oxidative stress. A recent study showed that the AFB1 treatment resulted in a significant and concentration-dependent increase in intracellular ROS production, whereas mitochondrial functions such as glutamate/malate and succinate-driven respiration were significantly uncoupled. Those oxidative stress effects activated mitochondrial ROS-dependent signal pathways, which induced apoptosis through the mitochondrial signal pathway [77]. What's more, there are some proteins modulated by AFB1 like CYP1A2, CYP1A5, CYP3A4, TP53, GSMT1, MDM2, CAT, OGG1, IRS1, IRS2, SRC, AKT1, MAPK1, MAPK3, and PDK1. These proteins are involved in important metabolic pathways such as FoxO signaling pathway, PI3K-Akt signaling pathway, AMPK signaling pathway, MAPK signaling pathway, and VEGF signaling pathway [65]. In fact, those modulations induce both tumor progression and chemotherapy resistance as well as in other pathogenetic procedures.

To further investigate the mechanism behind nuclei damage, epigenetic changes cannot be omitted. Accumulating evidence also indicates that epigenetic modifications play a vital role in AFB1-induced carcinogenesis and more attention is being paid to them [78]. It is believed that epigenetic aberrations play important roles in tumorigenesis, pathways, and development of carcinogenesis including tumor invasion, initiation, and plasticity [79, 80]. Those alterations include oncogene activation, tumor suppressor gene inactivation, and chromosomal instability (CIN), which then interfere with the critical signaling pathways. Epigenetic alterations include three kinds of modifications, DNA methylation, histone modifications, and regulation of noncoding RNA (specifically small noncoding RNAs, microRNAs) [81, 82].

DNA methylation, which regulates the gene expression level, is one of the frequent epigenetic events in cancer development. The formation of AFB1 adducts is believed to cause methylation alteration of some important genes regulating the mutagenesis of AFB1 in the carcinogenetic development of HCC. In in vitro studies, Rieswijk investigated the persistent AFB1-induced impact on the DNA methylation footprint in relation to the transcriptome in HCC for the first time. By comparing the transcription level and DNA methylation degree, a number of persistent hypomethylated and upregulated genes named PCNA, RAB27A, TXNRD1, DIAPH3, HIST1H2BF, and CCNK were identified to have an alteration on the transcriptome level. PCNA acts as a scaffold to recruit proteins involved in DNA replication and DNA repair including mismatch repair, cell cycle, apoptosis, chromatin remodeling, and preservation of epigenetic marks [83, 84]. RAB27A expression was closely correlated with tumor progression [85]. Upregulation of TXNRD1 decreases the expression of AFB1 aldehyde reductase (AFAR) and glutathione-S-transferase (GST) that are responsible for the detoxification of AFB1-8,9-epoxide via glutathione conjugation into less active metabolites, thereby promoting the formation of AFB1 adducts with macromolecules in the liver [86]. CCNK can bind with CDK12 to form the complex CCNK/CDK12 and regulate the expression of several DNA damage response genes and some critical regulators of genomic stability [87]. Moreover, Zhang et al. conducted a number of human studies about AFB1-induced methylation alterations in HCC. By investigating promoter methylation status in tumor suppressor and other cancer-related genes such as p16, RASSF1A [88], O6-methylguanine-DNA methyltransferase (MGMT) [89], glutathione-S-transferase p1 (GSTP1) [90], and the level of AFB1-DNA adducts in HCC tissue samples from Taiwan, they found that frequent aberrant methylation in the CpG islands of promoters of the genes mentioned above is closely related to hepatocarcinogenesis. In addition, the correlation between AFB1-DNA adducts and hypermethylation of these genes was found to be statistically significant. Since AFB1 plays an important role in the development of HCC, it can be speculated that AFB1 may bind preferentially to methylated CpG sites or specific structures in chromatin, inducing damage to DNA that may impact methylation [91]. Furthermore, according to the analysis of progression from the normal liver to HCC proposed by Herath et al. [92], under the aflatoxin exposure, methylation appears to precede cirrhosis in a subset of tumors, while tumors appear to be able to progress in the absence of cirrhosis, which may be a consequence of hypomethylation. The association between AFB1-DNA adducts and RASSF1A methylation in HCC was statistically significant. Multivariate analyses including the mRNA, protein expression, and methylation status of RASSF1A in HCC showed that RASSF1A hypermethylation was related to AFB1-DNA adducts. Besides, there seemed to be little effect of RASSF1A methylation on patient survival [93]. In whole-animal studies, Baik investigated the DNA methylation status of the rat gamma-glutamyl transpeptidase (GGT) gene in embryonic, adult, and neoplastic liver using rats treated with AFB1-contaminated peanuts in 1991. The methylation patterns of the GGT gene were investigated in AFB1-induced HCC tumors, and hypermethylation was observed. However, the regulatory mechanism of GGT methylation after AFB1 exposure was not clear [94]. In addition, it was observed to be more than partial hypermethylation in the analyzed CpG sites of the p19Arf promoter, and methylation of transcription factor-binding sites or consensus sequences was confirmed in lung tumors of mice [95]. Wu assessed the relationship between AFB1 exposure and global DNA methylation. The methylation status of DNA in white blood cells from cancer-free participants was investigated through pyrosequencing, and the results showed that decreased Sat2 or LINE-1 methylation was associated with dietary exposure to AFB1, supporting the hypothesis that AFB1 might play an important role in HCC by altering the global DNA methylation status and that exposure to AFB1 induces global DNA hypomethylation [96] .

AFB1 exposure and DNA methylation are reported to be associated with embryonic development as well. In vivo, when pregnant women are exposed to AFB1, the DNA methylation status of their infants may be constantly influenced until 2–8 years old. Exposure to AFB1 gives rise to methylation alterations of some important genes including growth factor genes, such as IGF1 and FGF12, and immune-related genes, TGFBI, TLR2, and CCL28 [97]. In vitro porcine models and oocyte exposure to AFB1 (50 μM) were revealed to appear increasing DNA methylation levels and oxidative stress, which may explain the excessive autophagy and apoptosis [98].

Histone, known as the chromatin-related protein, plays an important role in posttranslational modification. So, it is reasonable to speculate that AFB1-induced epigenetic mutation in histone is another mechanism of carcinogenesis. As early as in 1980, Groopman and Wogan used radiolabeled [3H] to mark the in vivo footprint of AFB1 residues in the rat liver. They observed that after 36 h of feeding marked AFB1, approximately 5–10% of the total nuclear-bound aflatoxin residues distributed in histones. Among all the histones, histone H1 was the major protein target for nuclear AFB1 binding, with an adduct level of three to four times higher than other companions [99]. Studies focusing on AFB1-induced reproductive toxicity also had a positive finding in histone. When investigating the relationship between AFB1-induced epigenetic modifications and mammalian oocyte maturation, in 2015, Liu observed toxic epigenetic modifications in porcine oocyte of exposure to 50 μM AFB1. Results indicated that the levels of transcription marks H3K27me3 and H3K4me2 decreased, while the level of H3K9me3 increased [98]. H3K27me3 is responsible for silencing the expression of key developmental genes during embryonic stem cell differentiation [100]. H3K4me2/H3K4me3 and H3K9me3 are supposed to play an important role in the efficient reprogramming of pluripotency genes in somatic nuclei and thus determine cell fate [101, 102]. Another similar research study on mice gave up to the similar conclusion. Mice were fed with mycotoxin-contaminated maize and observed for histone change in their oocytes. According to the fluorescence intensity analysis, the levels of H4K20me3 and H3K9me3 increased, while the levels of H4K20me2 and H3K27me3 decreased [103]. The results indicated that mycotoxins including AFB1 may improve the transcriptional activity of the oocyte genome by reducing the H3K27me3 levels and may affect the chromatin configuration and cell cycle progression in oocytes via altering the H3K9me3 levels, reducing H4K20me2 levels, and increasing H4K20me3 levels. In addition, the DNA methylation level of oocyte in these two findings was both found to be increased. Ghufran et al. investigated AFB1-induced effects on an epigenetic regulatory protein, arginine methyltransferase 5 (PRMT5), in human cell lines for the first time in 2016 [104]. Upregulation of PRMT5 was observed after AFB1 treatment, which might play an important role in AFB1-induced tumorigenesis. However, the mechanism of upregulation of PRMT5 in AFB1-induced cancer remains obscure. Furthermore, besides histone methylation, AFB1 was also found to affect histone acetylation and deacetylation in the liver. Results showed that AFB1 exposure increases the rate of deacetylation of histone fractions F2A1 and F3 [105].

MicroRNA (miRNA) is a kind of short-chain noncoding RNA which plays an important role in gene expression modulation. The previous research mainly focused on the regulation of miRNAs in AFB1-induced disease and tumorigenesis. In a study detecting the level of AFB1-DNA adducts and the expression of miRNA-429 [106] and miRNA-24 [107] in tumor tissues, miR-429 and miR-24 were found to be upregulated in HCC tumor tissues with high AFB1 exposure, and their high expression was significantly correlated with larger tumor size. Importantly, overexpression of these two miRNAs inhibits apoptosis, induces progression of tumor cell growth, and had a positive correlation with the levels of AFB1-DNA adducts, indicating the potency as biomarkers for AFB1-related HCC prognosis and tumorigenesis of those two miRNAs [106, 107]. Further, polymorphisms in pre-miRNAs were investigated for the potential as risk factors or prognostic biomarkers of AFB1-induced HCC in a large case-control hospital research in China, in which rs28599926 in miR-1268a was identified as one candidate [108]. Later, several studies about the mechanisms underlying the signaling pathway involved in these processes were conducted. Liu et al. found that in vivo upregulation of rno-miR-34a-5p leads to cell cycle arrest by downregulating the expression of the cell cycle-related genes MET, CCNE2, and CCND1. It also facilitated p53 repair of DNA damage in the liver of AFB1-treated rats. Thus, miR-34a-5p might be considered as a sensitive biomarker of AFB1-induced DNA damage in the liver [107]. Zeng hypothesized that the dysfunction of a novel GSK-3b-C/EBPa-miR-122-IGF-1R regulatory circuitry was the mechanism behind the development of HCC [109]. In vitro studies on different expression profiles of miRNAs identified several cancer-related microRNAs and the predicted target genes involved in cancer-related pathways. Zhu et al. found that upregulation of miR-34a might suppress the Wnt/β-catenin signaling pathway in HepG2 cells anticipated by AFB1 [110]. Another functional studies revealed that miR-138-1* inhibited proliferation, colony formation, migration, and invasion of P50 B-2A13 cells and might affect AFB1-induced malignant transformation through targeting PDK1 [111].

The majority of these studies investigated the regulation of miRNAs. One study, however, reported the changes of lncRNA expression in AFB1-induced HCC formation. The upregulation of H19 gene encoding lncRNA was found to promote cell growth and invasion in human HepG2 cells after AFB1 treatment [112]. Since lncRNA is a novel hot spot of noncoding RNA researches, the information is limited. More detailed studies are required to establish the signaling pathway involved in this process to understand the mechanism.

4. Detoxification strategies

It is reported that carry-over of AFB1 as AFM1 in the milk of dairy cows has been established to range from 0.3 to 6.2% [113]. In consideration of this high prevalence of AFB1 in food, it is of great priority to find effective strategies to prevent or remove contamination in order to restore the safety and edibility of food products. Prevention of *Aspergillus* infection can stop the contamination from the source. The control strategies include the use of genetically altered crops that are resistant to *Aspergillus* and environmental stressors, pesticide usage, crop rotation, and timing of planting, together with proper drying, packaging, storage, and preservative/pesticide usage to suppress fungal reproduction. These strategies however are not enough to fully inhibit contamination, so further postharvest techniques are being developed to detoxify contaminated foods. These then involve the knowledge of physical and chemical characteristics of AFB1. The characteristic frame of AFB1 is the fusion of a cyclopentenone ring to the lactone ring of the coumarin structure. The toxin favors polar organic solvents and is barely soluble in nonpolar solvents and slightly soluble in water. AFB1 remains stable even at high temperature (>100°C), so that regular thermal procession cannot detoxicate it during food manufacturing. This thermal stability makes a great obstacle in the reduction of aflatoxin in milk and dairy products, since the wild used sterilization such as pasteurization, etc. all belonging to thermal treatment. Other physical or chemical properties led to the development of other methods of decontamination in order to assure a good level of decontamination without disruption of the nutritional properties or safety of feed. Those strategies can be classified into physical treatment, biological treatment, chemical treatment, combination strategy, and sorbent additives.

Physical means of removing AFB1 from foods are most commonly heating comparatively to a higher temperature or for a longer time and irradiation using gamma (γ) rays. AFB1 is reported almost completely degraded at harsh heating temperatures as high as 160°C and above [114]. Prolonging of heating time and additional humidity can help the detoxification [115]. However, such a strategy may disrupt the integrity of product after heating/roasting is complete. This advantage inhibits the popularity of the maximum temperature that can be used, resulting in incomplete removal of AFB1. The other most commonly reported physical decontamination method is γ radiation. This technique has been widely tested in a variety of food substrates, with an average percent reduction of 65%. The fundamental of γ radiation is production of ionizing radiation. According to a recent study, the effective concentration ranged from 6 to 60 kGy [115].

Biological-based interventions have also been investigated for their potential in reducing AFB1 levels. Lact microbes such as lactobacillus, saccharomyces, cellulosimicrobium, and others have been identified to enzymatically convert aflatoxin, zearalenone, ochratoxin, patulin, fumonisin, deoxynivalenol, and T-2 toxin to less toxic products [116]. The reduction averaged approximately 86% across recent studies. Despite microbe degradation, herbal extract incubation is another biological strategy. Dissolving AFB1 in aqueous extracts of various plant species is also highly effective. For example, according to the reported data, extracts from *Adhatoda vasica* Ness and *Corymbia citriodora* both achieved >95% degradation of AFB1 [117]. Treatment time using those two approaches however is very long, usually requiring several days to carry out [118]. It would allow an increasing efficiency of those processes by further identification of the active components responsible for the degradation. Therefore, the use of purified enzymes from various biological sources has been investigated for AFB1 degradation potential. Those agents have included laccases, manganese peroxidase, and the recently identified *Bacillus* aflatoxin-degrading enzyme. The efficacy of these approaches has been high, but more information based on further practice on real food substrates is necessary. As is the case with all the biological control methods, the time of treatment is still long, taking several days to complete which may not be feasible in large-scale applications [119–121]. Another disadvantage lies in an uncertainty of the end products of the treatments, which makes the safety of treated foods hard to determine.

Chemical additives are also widely used to detoxify contaminated foods in the food industry. Acidification, including citric, lactic, tartaric, and hydrochloric acid, has shown high efficiency in reducing toxicity of AFB1-contaminated foods. These methods have been observed to have high reduction rate in less than 24 h even at room temperature. The conducting process is also simple, just requiring to soak contaminated foods in acidic solutions for a given amount of time [61, 122, 123]. Unlike biological degradation, the detoxification product of AFB1 in acid is AFB2a as mentioned above, which is widely recognized as a far less toxic metabolite of AFB1. On the other hand, ammoniation which refers to breaking down AFB1 in an alkaline environment is also effective in detoxification. When foods are treated with either gaseous or liquid ammonia (usually 1.5–2%), the degradation rate can sometimes reach above 99% in comparatively long time, ranging from 24 h to 15 days [124, 125]. The degradation product due to ammoniation is a less mutagenic metabolite of AFB1, known as aflatoxin D1 (AFD1), formed through hydrolysis and decarboxylation, though risking a reversion back into AFB1 if reset in an acidified environment [126]. Finally, ozonation is another commonly used chemical control method. Ozonolysis at a concentration of 6–90 mg/L has been shown to quickly degrade AFB1 by 86.75% in as little as 20 min in wheat. Other recent studies have treatment time range from 30 min to 96 h, mostly under 180 min, and all have seen >65% reductions. Additionally, ozone has been investigated in a variety of foodstuffs, indicating a stable effectiveness and reliable safety [115, 127, 128]. According to an analysis of the breakdown products of AFB1 after ozonolysis by Diao et al., the moieties responsible for mutagenicity disappeared, indicating that these products are likely less toxic, although it has not been verified using mutagenicity assays [115].

All those methods mentioned above solely have had moderate to high success in reducing AFB1 levels; nevertheless, the highest efficacies are seen when they are combined with one another. The combination of ammonia and heat has been shown to drastically reduce treatment time from several days to 15–120 min and repeatedly manifested >99% reduction of AFB1 in a series of studies [129–131]. Proctor et al. reported that heating along with ozonation turned out to have reduced treatment time and lower effective temperature while remaining as high as 77% reduction of AFB1 in peanuts at 75°C after only 10 min [132]. Treatment of contaminated foods with alkaline substances (other than ammonia) along with heat is another effective method. Nixtamalization, the tortilla-making process employing heat and alkaline calcium hydroxide, has been shown to decrease AFB1 by approximately 84 and 90% in two separate studies [133, 134]. The applications of high temperatures (80–120°C) together with acidification such as HCl, citric acid, and lactic acid were also reported to have high degrading potential (85–100%). The addition of citric acid can help degrade 98% of AFB1 at 100°C in 20 min [135–137]. The combination of heat and acidification is attractive with the fact that those two methods separately have already been widely used in food manufacturing industry, so that no specialized or expensive equipment is needed additionally. A unique combination has recently been performed by Rushing and Selim where acidification has been used with heat and arginine. This causes AFB1 to form a stable pyrrole ring with the amino acid, which is completely non-genotoxic and inabsorbable across the intestinal tract. This method was able to completely converse AFB1-contaminated corn in 20 min. This result advocates for adding amino acids to the previous acidification treatments to form stable, nontoxic forms of AFB1 [137].

Another unique approach to solving AFB1 contamination is the addition of sorbents to food. This method is different from the degradation methods because it prevents the hepatotoxic effects of AFB1 by acting as binding agents to prevent absorption of AFB1 across the intestinal tract after ingestion rather than destroying or reducing the amount of AFB1 in the food as mentioned above. Chlorophyllin and chlorophyll as the most well-studied of those agents were observed to reduce AFB1-DNA adduct by 37% in rainbow trout and in turn reduce tumor incidence by 77%, when added to the contaminated feed [138]. Simonich et al. reported that when AFB1-contaminated feed was added with chlorophyllin and chlorophyll, AFB1-DNA adducts, AFB1-albumin, and urinary AFM1 levels in rat reduced by 42, 65, and 90% compared with 55, 51, and 92%, respectively. Accordingly, the tumor incidence in these rats was reduced by 74 and 77%, respectively [139]. Egner et al. found that, by introducing chlorophyllin into the diets of humans in high-risk areas for AFB1 exposure, AFB1-N7-guanine levels in those subjects reduced by 55% compared to that in individuals who were not fed with this agent [140]. In another clinical study, four volunteers were given a single dose of 30 ng of AFB1 with either the co-administration of chlorophyll and chlorophyllin or not. Results showed that chlorophyllin and chlorophyll reduced urinary AFM1 levels by 28 and 41%, respectively [140]. Those data above show that sorbents or binding agents in diets in high-risk areas can partially alleviate the toxic effects of AFB1.

Clay is another commonly studied enterosorbent. With a mechanism similar to that of chlorophyllin and chlorophyll, clays have been shown to protect against AFB1 toxicities in multiple animal models by reducing AFB1 absorption and reducing AFM1 levels in milk. NovaSil (a calcium montmorillonite clay) is particularly successful in reducing the toxic effects of aflatoxin-contaminated feed and AFB1 biomarkers in humans [141]. In long-term animal study, no overt toxicities were observed when rats were fed up to 2.0% of NovaSil in their diet for 28 weeks, indicating the safety of using this substance [142]. In a clinical trial, Ghanaians in high risk for AFB1 exposure were given an oral bolus of placebo, low dose, or high dose of NovaSil. Participants in the low and high dose had significantly lower AFB1 biomarkers such as urinary AFM1 and serum AFB1-albumin after a period of 3 months. Additionally, during the observation, only mild, infrequent adverse effects were reported (such as nausea, diarrhea, heartburn, and dizziness), and no significant side effects were monitored by evaluating liver, kidney, or hematological parameters of all the individuals [143, 144]. These results indicate that the addition of NovaSil into the diet can be a safe and effective method to reduce AFB1 toxicity.

5. Future direction and conclusions

In the past decade, several studies have emphasized the important role of AFB1 in public dietary health. The high frequency and levels of AFB1 recently found in food supplies of various countries, particularly in Africa and Asia, indicate that exposure of populations to this toxin still remains largely uncontrolled. The toxin is then well known for its strong carcinogenesis potential. In fact, when further investigations were made, AFB1 was found to cause function feebleness of nearly all organs and systems. Furthermore, AFB1 has become an occupational hazard for those working in the food industry, leading to some particularly high rates of exposure. Evidence that has been gathered over the last several decades has shown the clear carcinogenic effect of AFB1. Also, the negative effect of AFB1 on nutritive status, growth/development, and immune system function is becoming clearer.

So as to disrupt or reverse AFB1-related pathobiological process, it is necessary to have a better understanding of the mechanism of AFB1 toxicity. Instead of stating AFB1 impairment to individual organ, a further exploration into the genotoxicity and epigenetic toxicity should be more proper, which has become a future trend in novel toxicity testing. However, researches focus on the relationship between histone modifications and AFB1 exposure, and the regulation of other noncoding RNAs except for miRNAs in AFB1 toxic mechanisms is rare. More effort is needed in related research. The network between epigenetic and genetic mechanisms in AFB1 toxicity needs further exploration, since genetic changes and epigenetic changes influence each other in most of the pathobiological process [92]. In addition, in the past few years, a variety of single-cell technologies have shed light on the extraordinary variability and accuracy of AFB1 toxicity. These technologies provide more opportunities to study the mechanism of AFB1 toxicity at the single-cell level, which is the central theme of recently raised concept precision toxicology [145].

In conclusion, AFB1 contamination remains an unneglectable threat to public health in developing countries. Its effect on malformation and other health problems may have been underestimated due to data deficiency. Despite the effectiveness of existing detoxification methods mentioned above, those methods are far from being popularized. Perhaps over time, these methods will see increased usage in order to provide cleaner foods worldwide.

Acknowledgements

We thank Prof. Xi-Dai Long for his writing help.

Conflicts of interest and source of funding

The authors declare no competing financial interests. This study was supported in part by the National Natural Science Foundation of China

(Nos. 81,860,489; 81,760,502; 81,572,353; and 81,660,495), the Natural Science Foundation of Guangxi (Nos. 2018GXNSFAA281043, 2017GXNSFAA198002, and 2017GXNSFGA198002), the Research Program of Guangxi "Zhouyue Scholar" (No. 2017-2038), the Research Program of Guangxi Specially-invited Expert (No. 2017-6th), the "12th Five" Planning Program of Guangxi Education Science (No. 2015C397), the Innovative Program of Guangxi Graduate Education (No. JGY2015139), the Research Program of Guangxi Clinic Research Center of Hepatobiliary Diseases (No. AD17129025), and the Open Research Program from Molecular Immunity Study Room Involving in Acute and Severe Diseases in Guangxi Colleges and Universities (Nos. kfkt20160062 and kfkt20160063).

Author details

Yuhua Shan[1,2]

1 Department of Surgery, Shanghai Children's Medical Center Affiliated to Shanghai Jiaotong University School of Medicine, Shanghai, China

2 The Affiliated Hospital of Youjiang Medical University for Medical University for National, Baise, China

*Address all correspondence to: danyuhua@scmc.com.cn

References

[1] Kew MC. Aflatoxins as a cause of hepatocellular carcinoma. Journal of Gastrointestinal and Liver Diseases. 2013;**22**(3):305-310

[2] Klich MA. Aspergillus flavus: The major producer of aflatoxin. Molecular Plant Pathology. 2007;**8**(6):713-722

[3] Mughal MJ, Xi P, Yi Z, Jing F. Aflatoxin B1 invokes apoptosis via death receptor pathway in hepatocytes. Oncotarget. 2017;**8**(5):8239-8249

[4] Nugraha A, Khotimah K, Rietjens I. Risk assessment of aflatoxin B1 exposure from maize and peanut consumption in Indonesia using the margin of exposure and liver cancer risk estimation approaches. Food and Chemical Toxicology. 2018;**113**:134-144

[5] Alpert ME, Hutt MS, Wogan GN, Davidson CS. Association between aflatoxin content of food and hepatoma frequency in Uganda. Cancer. 1971;**28**(1):253-260

[6] Liu Y, Wu F. Global burden of aflatoxin-induced hepatocellular carcinoma: A risk assessment. Environmental Health Perspectives. 2010;**118**(6):818-824

[7] Kucukcakan B, Hayrulai-Musliu Z. Challenging role of dietary aflatoxin B1 exposure and hepatitis B infection on risk of hepatocellular carcinoma. Open Access Macedonian Journal of Medical Sciences. 2015;**3**(2):363-369

[8] Jeannot E, Boorman GA, Kosyk O, et al. Increased incidence of aflatoxin B1-induced liver tumors in hepatitis virus C transgenic mice. International Journal of Cancer. 2012;**130**(6):1347-1356

[9] Chu YJ, Yang HI, Wu HC, et al. Aflatoxin B1 exposure increases the risk of hepatocellular carcinoma associated with hepatitis C virus infection or alcohol consumption. European Journal of Cancer. 2018;**94**:37-46

[10] Tsai FJ, Chen SY, Liu YC, Liao HY, Chen CJ. The comparison of CHCA solvent compositions for improving LC-MALDI performance and its application to study the impact of aflatoxin B1 on the liver proteome of diabetes mellitus type 1 mice. PLoS One. 2017;**12**(7):e0181423

[11] Reddy RV, Taylor MJ, Sharma RP. Studies of immune function of CD-1 mice exposed to aflatoxin B1. Toxicology. 1987;**43**(2):123-132

[12] Pier AC. Effects of aflatoxin on immunity. Journal of the American Veterinary Medical Association. 1973;**163**(11):1268-1269

[13] Cusumano V, Rossano F, Merendino RA, et al. Immunobiological activities of mould products: Functional impairment of human monocytes exposed to aflatoxin B1. Research in Microbiology. 1996;**147**(5):385-391

[14] Bossou YM, Serssar Y, Allou A, et al. Impact of mycotoxins secreted by aspergillus molds on the inflammatory response of human corneal epithelial cells. Toxins (Basel). 2017;**9**(7):197

[15] Meissonnier GM, Pinton P, Laffitte J, et al. Immunotoxicity of aflatoxin B1: Impairment of the cell-mediated response to vaccine antigen and modulation of cytokine expression. Toxicology and Applied Pharmacology. 2008;**231**(2):142-149

[16] Reddy RV, Sharma RP. Effects of aflatoxin B1 on murine lymphocytic functions. Toxicology. 1989;**54**(1):31-44

[17] Turner PC, Moore SE, Hall AJ, Prentice AM, Wild CP. Modification of immune function through exposure to

dietary aflatoxin in Gambian children. Environmental Health Perspectives. 2003;**111**(2):217-220

[18] Jiang Y, Jolly PE, Ellis WO, Wang JS, Phillips TD, Williams JH. Aflatoxin B1 albumin adduct levels and cellular immune status in Ghanaians. International Immunology. 2005;**17**(6):807-814

[19] Jiang Y, Jolly PE, Preko P, et al. Aflatoxin-related immune dysfunction in health and in human immunodeficiency virus disease. Clinical and Developmental Immunology. 2008;**2008**:790309

[20] Hendrickse RG, Maxwell SM. Heroin addicts, AIDS, and aflatoxins. British Medical Journal (Clinical Research Ed.). 1988;**296**(6631):1257

[21] Sun Y, Liu Z, Liu D, Chen J, Gan F, Huang K. Low-level aflatoxin B1 promotes influenza infection and modulates a switch in macrophage polarization from M1 to M2. Cellular Physiology and Biochemistry. 2018;**49**(3):1110-1126

[22] Watson S, Gong YY, Routledge M. Interventions targeting child undernutrition in developing countries may be undermined by dietary exposure to aflatoxin. Critical Reviews in Food Science and Nutrition. 2017;**57**(9):1963-1975

[23] McMillan A, Renaud JB, Burgess KMN, et al. Aflatoxin exposure in Nigerian children with severe acute malnutrition. Food and Chemical Toxicology: An International Journal Published for the British Industrial Biological Research Association. 2018;**111**:356-362

[24] Mupunga I, Mngqawa P, Katerere DR. Peanuts, aflatoxins and undernutrition in children in Sub-Saharan Africa. Nutrients. 2017;**9**(12):1287

[25] Glahn RP, Beers KW, Bottje WG, Wideman RF Jr, Huff WE, Thomas W. Aflatoxicosis alters avian renal function, calcium, and vitamin D metabolism. Journal of Toxicology and Environmental Health. 1991;**34**(3):309-321

[26] Costanzo P, Santini A, Fattore L, Novellino E, Ritieni A. Toxicity of aflatoxin B1 towards the vitamin D receptor (VDR). Food and Chemical Toxicology: An International Journal Published for the British Industrial Biological Research Association. 2015;**76**:77-79

[27] Pimpukdee K, Kubena LF, Bailey CA, Huebner HJ, Afriyie-Gyawu E, Phillips TD. Aflatoxin-induced toxicity and depletion of hepatic vitamin a in young broiler chicks: Protection of chicks in the presence of low levels of NovaSil PLUS in the diet. Poultry Science. 2004;**83**(5):737-744

[28] Bryden WL, Cumming RB, Balnave D. The influence of vitamin a status on the response of chickens to aflatoxin B1 and changes in liver lipid metabolism associated with aflatoxicosis. The British Journal of Nutrition. 1979;**41**(3):529-540

[29] Ikegwuonu FI. Zinc, copper, manganese and iron in rat organs after the administration and withdrawal of aflatoxin B1. Journal of Applied Toxicology. 1984;**4**(5):241-245

[30] Ubagai T, Kikuchi T, Fukusato T, Ono Y. Aflatoxin B1 modulates the insulin-like growth factor-2 dependent signaling axis. Toxicology In Vitro. 2010;**24**(3):783-789

[31] Castelino JM, Routledge MN, Wilson S, et al. Aflatoxin exposure is inversely associated with IGF1 and IGFBP3 levels in vitro and in Kenyan schoolchildren. Molecular Nutrition and Food Research. 2015;**59**(3):574-581

[32] Yunus AW, Razzazi-Fazeli E, Bohm J. Aflatoxin B(1) in affecting

broiler's performance, immunity, and gastrointestinal tract: A review of history and contemporary issues. Toxins (Basel). 2011;**3**(6):566-590

[33] Maresca M, Fantini J. Some food-associated mycotoxins as potential risk factors in humans predisposed to chronic intestinal inflammatory diseases. Toxicon: Official Journal of the International Society on Toxinology. 2010;**56**(3):282-294

[34] Smith LE, Stoltzfus RJ, Prendergast A. Food chain mycotoxin exposure, gut health, and impaired growth: A conceptual framework. Advances in Nutrition. 2012;**3**(4):526-531

[35] Rotimi OA, Rotimi SO, Oluwafemi F, Ademuyiwa O, Balogun EA. Coexistence of Aflatoxicosis with protein malnutrition worsens hepatic oxidative damage in rats. Journal of Biochemical and Molecular Toxicology. 2016;**30**(6):269-276

[36] Alpsoy L, Yalvac ME. Key roles of vitamins a, C, and E in aflatoxin B1-induced oxidative stress. Vitamins and Hormones. 2011;**86**:287-305

[37] Abdulrazzaq YM, Osman N, Yousif ZM, Trad O. Morbidity in neonates of mothers who have ingested aflatoxins. Annals of Tropical Paediatrics. 2004;**24**(2):145-151

[38] Turner PC, Collinson AC, Cheung YB, et al. Aflatoxin exposure in utero causes growth faltering in Gambian infants. International Journal of Epidemiology. 2007;**36**(5):1119-1125

[39] Shuaib FM, Jolly PE, Ehiri JE, et al. Association between birth outcomes and aflatoxin B1 biomarker blood levels in pregnant women in Kumasi, Ghana. Tropical Medicine and International Health. 2010;**15**(2):160-167

[40] Ibeh IN, Saxena DK, Uraih N. Toxicity of aflatoxin: Effects on spermatozoa, oocytes, and in vitro fertilization. Journal of Environmental Pathology, Toxicology and Oncology. 2000;**19**(4):357-361

[41] Hafez AH, Megalla SE, Abdel-Fattah HM, Kamel YY. Aflatoxin and aflatoxicosis. II. Effects of aflatoxin on ovaries and testicles in mature domestic fowls. Mycopathologia. 1982;**77**(3):137-139

[42] Komsky-Elbaz A, Saktsier M, Roth Z. Aflatoxin B1 impairs sperm quality and fertilization competence. Toxicology. 2018;**393**:42-50

[43] Yasin M, Mazdak R. Aflatoxin B1 impairs spermatogenesis: An experimental study for crosslink between oxidative stress and mitochondria-dependent apoptosis. Environmental Toxicology. 2018;**33**(11):1204-1213

[44] Ge J, Yu H, Li J, et al. Assessment of aflatoxin B1 myocardial toxicity in rats: Mitochondrial damage and cellular apoptosis in cardiomyocytes induced by aflatoxin B1. The Journal of International Medical Research. 2017;**45**(3):1015-1023

[45] Yilmaz S, Kaya E, Karaca A, Karatas O. Aflatoxin B1 induced renal and cardiac damage in rats: Protective effect of lycopene. Research in Veterinary Science. 2018;**119**:268-275

[46] Wang WJ, Xu ZL, Yu C, Xu XH. Effects of aflatoxin B1 on mitochondrial respiration, ROS generation and apoptosis in broiler cardiomyocytes. Animal Science Journal = Nihon Chikusan Gakkaiho. 2017;**88**(10):1561-1568

[47] Mehrzad J, Malvandi AM, Alipour M, Hosseinkhani S. Environmentally relevant level of aflatoxin B1 elicits toxic pro-inflammatory response in murine CNS-derived cells. Toxicology Letters. 2017;**279**:96-106

[48] Linardaki ZI, Lamari FN, Margarity M. Saffron (*Crocus sativus* L.) tea intake prevents learning/memory defects and Neurobiochemical alterations induced by aflatoxin B1 exposure in adult mice. Neurochemical Research. 2017;**42**(10):2743-2754

[49] Qureshi H, Hamid SS, Ali SS, Anwar J, Siddiqui AA, Khan NA. Cytotoxic effects of aflatoxin B1 on human brain microvascular endothelial cells of the blood-brain barrier. Medical Mycology. 2015;**53**(4): 409-416

[50] Raney KD, Shimada T, Kim DH, Groopman JD, Harris TM, Guengerich FP. Oxidation of aflatoxins and sterigmatocystin by human liver microsomes: Significance of aflatoxin Q1 as a detoxication product of aflatoxin B1. Chemical Research in Toxicology. 1992;**5**(2):202-210

[51] Ueng YF, Shimada T, Yamazaki H, Guengerich FP. Oxidation of aflatoxin B1 by bacterial recombinant human cytochrome P450 enzymes. Chemical Research in Toxicology. 1995;**8**(2):218-225

[52] Gallagher EP, Kunze KL, Stapleton PL, Eaton DL. The kinetics of aflatoxin B1 oxidation by human cDNA-expressed and human liver microsomal cytochromes P450 1A2 and 3A4. Toxicology and Applied Pharmacology. 1996;**141**(2):595-606

[53] Gallagher EP, Wienkers LC, Stapleton PL, Kunze KL, Eaton DL. Role of human microsomal and human complementary DNA-expressed cytochromes P4501A2 and P4503A4 in the bioactivation of aflatoxin B1. Cancer Research. 1994;**54**(1):101-108

[54] Guengerich FP, Johnson WW, Shimada T, Ueng YF, Yamazaki H, Langouet S. Activation and detoxication of aflatoxin B1. Mutation Research. 1998;**402**(1-2):121-128

[55] Wang JS, Groopman JD. DNA damage by mycotoxins. Mutation Research. 1999;**424**(1-2):167-181

[56] McLean M, Dutton MF. Cellular interactions and metabolism of aflatoxin: An update. Pharmacology and Therapeutics. 1995;**65**(2):163-192

[57] Holeski CJ, Eaton DL, Monroe DH, Bellamy GM. Effects of phenobarbital on the biliary excretion of aflatoxin P1-glucuronide and aflatoxin B1-S-glutathione in the rat. Xenobiotica. 1987;**17**(2):139-153

[58] Lillehoj EB, Ciegler A. Biological activity of aflatoxin B2a. Applied Microbiology. 1969;**17**(4):516-519

[59] Yourtee DM, Bean TA, Kirk-Yourtee CL. Human aflatoxin B1 metabolism: An investigation of the importance of aflatoxin Q1 as a metabolite of hepatic post-mitochondrial fraction. Toxicology Letters. 1987;**38**(3):213-224

[60] Mykkanen H, Zhu H, Salminen E, et al. Fecal and urinary excretion of aflatoxin B1 metabolites (AFQ1, AFM1 and AFB-N7-guanine) in young Chinese males. International Journal of Cancer. 2005;**115**(6):879-884

[61] Rushing BR, Selim MI. Effect of dietary acids on the formation of aflatoxin B2a as a means to detoxify aflatoxin B1. Food Additives and Contaminants. Part A: Chemistry, Analysis, Control, Exposure and Risk Assessment. 2016;**33**(9):1456-1467

[62] Pitout MJ, McGee HA, Schabort JC. The effect of aflatoxin B1, aflatoxin B 2 and sterigmatocystin on nuclear deoxyribonucleases from rat and mouse livers. Chemico-Biological Interactions. 1971;**3**(5):353-361

[63] Chen B, Li D, Li M, et al. Induction of mitochondria-mediated apoptosis and PI3K/Akt/mTOR-mediated autophagy

by aflatoxin B2 in hepatocytes of broilers. Oncotarget. 2016;**7**(51):84989-84998

[64] Tchana AN, Moundipa PF, Tchouanguep FM. Aflatoxin contamination in food and body fluids in relation to malnutrition and cancer status in Cameroon. International Journal of Environmental Research and Public Health. 2010;7(1):178-188

[65] Marchese S, Polo A, Ariano A, Velotto S, Costantini S. Aflatoxin B1 and M1: Biological properties and their involvement in cancer development. 2018;**10**(6):214

[66] Giovati L, Magliani W, Ciociola T, Santinoli C, Conti S, Polonelli L. AFM(1) in milk: Physical, biological, and prophylactic methods to mitigate contamination. Toxins (Basel). 2015;**7**(10):4330-4349

[67] Ross RK, Yuan JM, Yu MC, et al. Urinary aflatoxin biomarkers and risk of hepatocellular carcinoma. Lancet. 1992;**339**(8799):943-946

[68] Lozano MC, Diaz GJ. Microsomal and cytosolic biotransformation of aflatoxin B1 in four poultry species. British Poultry Science. 2006;**47**(6):734-741

[69] Partanen HA, El-Nezami HS, Leppanen JM, Myllynen PK, WoodhouseHJ,VahakangasKH.Aflatoxin B1 transfer and metabolism in human placenta. Toxicological Sciences. 2010;**113**(1):216-225

[70] Salhab AS, Hsieh DP. Aflatoxicol H1: A major metabolite of aflatoxin B1 produced by human and rhesus monkey livers in vitro. Research Communications in Chemical Pathology and Pharmacology. 1975;**10**(3):419-429

[71] Wild CP, Turner PC. The toxicology of aflatoxins as a basis for public health decisions. Mutagenesis. 2002;**17**(6):471-481

[72] Bailey EA, Iyer RS, Stone MP, Harris TM, Essigmann JM. Mutational properties of the primary aflatoxin B1-DNA adduct. Proceedings of the National academy of Sciences of the United States of America. 1996;**93**(4):1535-1539

[73] Mace K, Aguilar F, Wang JS, et al. Aflatoxin B1-induced DNA adduct formation and p53 mutations in CYP450-expressing human liver cell lines. Carcinogenesis. 1997;**18**(7):1291-1297

[74] Li D, Cao Y, He L, Wang NJ, Gu JR. Aberrations of p53 gene in human hepatocellular carcinoma from China. Carcinogenesis. 1993;**14**(2):169-173

[75] Battista JR, Marnett LJ. Prostaglandin H synthase-dependent epoxidation of aflatoxin B1. Carcinogenesis. 1985;**6**(8):1227-1229

[76] Weng MW, Lee HW, Choi B, et al. AFB1 hepatocarcinogenesis is via lipid peroxidation that inhibits DNA repair, sensitizes mutation susceptibility and induces aldehyde-DNA adducts at p53 mutational hotspot codon 249. Oncotarget. 2017;**8**(11):18213-18226

[77] Liu Y, Wang W. Aflatoxin B1 impairs mitochondrial functions, activates ROS generation, induces apoptosis and involves Nrf2 signal pathway in primary broiler hepatocytes. Animal Science Journal. 2016;**87**(12):1490-1500

[78] Chappell G, Pogribny IP, Guyton KZ, Rusyn I. Epigenetic alterations induced by genotoxic occupational and environmental human chemical carcinogens: A systematic literature review. Mutation Research, Reviews in Mutation Research. 2016;**768**:27-45

[79] Carmona FJ, Esteller M. Epigenomics of human colon cancer. Mutation Research. 2010;**693**(1-2):53-60

[80] Murtha M, Esteller M. Extraordinary cancer epigenomics: Thinking outside the classical coding and promoter box. Trends Cancer. 2016;**2**(10):572-584

[81] Sandoval J, Esteller M. Cancer epigenomics: Beyond genomics. Current Opinion in Genetics and Development. 2012;**22**(1):50-55

[82] Vaissiere T, Sawan C, Herceg Z. Epigenetic interplay between histone modifications and DNA methylation in gene silencing. Mutation Research. 2008;**659**(1-2):40-48

[83] Alenzi FQ, El-Nashar EM, Al-Ghamdi SS, et al. Original article: Investigation of Bcl-2 and PCNA in hepatocellular carcinoma: Relation to chronic HCV. Journal of the Egyptian National Cancer Institute. 2010;**22**(1):87-94

[84] Moldovan GL, Pfander B, Jentsch S. PCNA, the maestro of the replication fork. Cell. 2007;**129**(4):665-679

[85] Dong WW, Mou Q, Chen J, Cui JT, Li WM, Xiao WH. Differential expression of Rab27A/B correlates with clinical outcome in hepatocellular carcinoma. World Journal of Gastroenterology. 2012;**18**(15):1806-1813

[86] McLeod R, Ellis EM, Arthur JR, et al. Protection conferred by selenium deficiency against aflatoxin B1 in the rat is associated with the hepatic expression of an aldo-keto reductase and a glutathione S-transferase subunit that metabolize the mycotoxin. Cancer Research. 1997;**57**(19):4257-4266

[87] Blazek D, Kohoutek J, Bartholomeeusen K, et al. The cyclin K/Cdk12 complex maintains genomic stability via regulation of expression of DNA damage response genes. Genes and Development. 2011;**25**(20):2158-2172

[88] Zhang YJ, Ahsan H, Chen Y, et al. High frequency of promoter hypermethylation of RASSF1A and p16 and its relationship to aflatoxin B1-DNA adduct levels in human hepatocellular carcinoma. Molecular Carcinogenesis. 2002;**35**(2):85-92

[89] Zhang L, Lu W, Miao X, Xing D, Tan W, Lin D. Inactivation of DNA repair gene O6-methylguanine-DNA methyltransferase by promoter hypermethylation and its relation to p53 mutations in esophageal squamous cell carcinoma. Carcinogenesis. 2003;**24**(6):1039-1044

[90] Zhang YJ, Chen Y, Ahsan H, et al. Silencing of glutathione S-transferase P1 by promoter hypermethylation and its relationship to environmental chemical carcinogens in hepatocellular carcinoma. Cancer Letters. 2005;**221**(2):135-143

[91] Zhang YJ, Wu HC, Yazici H, Yu MW, Lee PH, Santella RM. Global hypomethylation in hepatocellular carcinoma and its relationship to aflatoxin B(1) exposure. World Journal of Hepatology. 2012;**4**(5):169-175

[92] Herath NI, Leggett BA, MacDonald GA. Review of genetic and epigenetic alterations in hepatocarcinogenesis. Journal of Gastroenterology and Hepatology. 2006;**21**(1 Pt 1):15-21

[93] Feng Y, Xue WJ, Li P, et al. RASSF1A hypermethylation is associated with aflatoxin B1 and polycyclic aromatic hydrocarbon exposure in hepatocellular carcinoma. Hepato-Gastroenterology. 2012;**59**(118):1883-1888

[94] Baik JH, Griffiths S, Giuili G, Manson M, Siegrist S, Guellaen G. DNA methylation patterns of the rat gamma-glutamyl transpeptidase gene in embryonic, adult and neoplastic liver. Carcinogenesis. 1991;**12**(6):1035-1039

[95] Tam AS, Devereux TR, Patel AC, Foley JF, Maronpot RR, Massey TE. Perturbations of the Ink4a/Arf gene locus in aflatoxin B1-induced mouse lung tumors. Carcinogenesis. 2003;**24**(1):121-132

[96] Wu HC, Wang Q, Yang HI, Tsai WY, Chen CJ, Santella RM. Global DNA methylation in a population with aflatoxin B1 exposure. Epigenetics. 2013;**8**(9):962-969

[97] Hernandez-Vargas H, Castelino J, Silver MJ, et al. Exposure to aflatoxin B1 in utero is associated with DNA methylation in white blood cells of infants in the Gambia. International Journal of Epidemiology. 2015;**44**(4):1238-1248

[98] Liu J, Wang QC, Han J, Xiong B, Sun SC. Aflatoxin B1 is toxic to porcine oocyte maturation. Mutagenesis. 2015;**30**(4):527-535

[99] Groopman JD, Busby WF Jr, Wogan GN. Nuclear distribution of aflatoxin B1 and its interaction with histones in rat liver in vivo. Cancer Research. 1980;**40**(12):4343-4351

[100] Park KE, Magnani L, Cabot RA. Differential remodeling of mono- and trimethylated H3K27 during porcine embryo development. Molecular Reproduction and Development. 2009;**76**(11):1033-1042

[101] Murata K, Kouzarides T, Bannister AJ, Gurdon JB. Histone H3 lysine 4 methylation is associated with the transcriptional reprogramming efficiency of somatic nuclei by oocytes. Epigenetics and Chromatin. 2010;**3**(1):4

[102] Becker JS, Nicetto D, Zaret KS. H3K9me3-dependent heterochromatin: Barrier to cell fate changes. Trends in Genetics (TIG). 2016;**32**(1):29-41

[103] Zhu CC, Hou YJ, Han J, et al. Effect of mycotoxin-containing diets on epigenetic modifications of mouse oocytes by fluorescence microscopy analysis. Microscopy and Microanalysis: The Official Journal of Microscopy Society of America, Microbeam Analysis Society, Microscopical Society of Canada. 2014;**20**(4):1158-1166

[104] Ghufran MS, Ghosh K, Kanade SR. Aflatoxin B1 induced upregulation of protein arginine methyltransferase 5 in human cell lines. Toxicon: Official Journal of the International Society on Toxinology. 2016;**119**:117-121

[105] Edwards GS, Allfrey VG. Aflatoxin B1 and actinomycin D effects on histone: Acetylation and deacetylation in the liver. Biochimica et Biophysica Acta. 1973;**299**(2):354-366

[106] Huang XY, Yao JG, Huang HD, et al. MicroRNA-429 modulates hepatocellular carcinoma prognosis and tumorigenesis. Gastroenterology Research and Practice. 2013;**2013**:804128

[107] Liu C, Yu H, Zhang Y, et al. Upregulation of miR-34a-5p antagonizes AFB1-induced genotoxicity in F344 rat liver. Toxicon: Official Journal of the International Society on Toxinology. 2015;**106**:46-56

[108] Long XD, Huang XY, Yao JG, et al. Polymorphisms in the precursor microRNAs and aflatoxin B1-related hepatocellular carcinoma. Molecular Carcinogenesis. 2016;**55**(6):1060-1072

[109] Zeng C, Wang R, Li D, et al. A novel GSK-3 beta-C/EBP alpha-miR-122-insulin-like growth factor 1 receptor regulatory circuitry in human hepatocellular carcinoma. Hepatology (Baltimore, MD). 2010;**52**(5):1702-1712

[110] Zhu L, Gao J, Huang K, Luo Y, Zhang B, Xu W. miR-34a screened by miRNA profiling negatively regulates Wnt/beta-catenin signaling pathway

in Aflatoxin B1 induced hepatotoxicity. Scientific Reports. 2015;**5**:16732

[111] Wang Y, Zhang Z, Wang H, et al. miR-138-1* regulates aflatoxin B1-induced malignant transformation of BEAS-2B cells by targeting PDK1. Archives of Toxicology. 2016;**90**(5):1239-1249

[112] Lv J, Yu YQ, Li SQ, Luo L, Wang Q. Aflatoxin B1 promotes cell growth and invasion in hepatocellular carcinoma HepG2 cells through H19 and E2F1. Asian Pacific Journal of Cancer Prevention : APJCP. 2014;**15**(6):2565-2570

[113] Shreeve BJ, Patterson DS, Roberts BA. The 'carry-over' of aflatoxin, ochratoxin and zearalenone from naturally contaminated feed to tissues, urine and milk of dairy cows. Food and Cosmetics Toxicology. 1979;**17**(2):151-152

[114] Raters M, Matissek R. Thermal stability of aflatoxin B1 and ochratoxin a. Mycotoxin Research. 2008;**24**(3):130-134

[115] Rushing BR, Selim MI. Aflatoxin B1: A review on metabolism, toxicity, occurrence in food, occupational exposure, and detoxification methods. Food and Chemical Toxicology. 2019;**124**:81-100

[116] McCormick SP. Microbial detoxification of mycotoxins. Journal of Chemical Ecology. 2013;**39**(7):907-918

[117] Iram W, Anjum T, Iqbal M, Ghaffar A, Abbas M. Structural elucidation and toxicity assessment of degraded products of aflatoxin B1 and B2 by aqueous extracts of Trachyspermum ammi. Frontiers in Microbiology. 2016;**7**:346

[118] Brana MT, Cimmarusti MT, Haidukowski M, Logrieco AF. Bioremediation of aflatoxin B1-contaminated maize by king oyster mushroom (*Pleurotus eryngii*). PLoS One. 2017;**12**(8):e0182574

[119] Loi M, Fanelli F, Zucca P, et al. Aflatoxin B(1) and M(1) degradation by Lac2 from *Pleurotus pulmonarius* and redox mediators. Toxins (Basel). 2016;**8**(9):245

[120] Xu L, Eisa Ahmed MF, Sangare L, et al. Novel aflatoxin-degrading enzyme from *Bacillus shackletonii* L7. Toxins (Basel). 2017;**9**(1):36

[121] Yehia RS. Aflatoxin detoxification by manganese peroxidase purified from *Pleurotus ostreatus*. Brazilian Journal of Microbiology. 2014;**45**(1):127-133

[122] Lee J, Her JY, Lee KG. Reduction of aflatoxins (B(1), B(2), G(1), and G(2)) in soybean-based model systems. Food Chemistry. 2015;**189**:45-51

[123] Safara M, Zaini F, Hashemi S, Mahmoudi M, Khosravi A, Shojai-Aliabadi F. Aflatoxin detoxification in Rice using citric acid. Iranian Journal of Public Health. 2010;**39**(2):24-29

[124] Bagley DM, Hayes JR. Xenobiotic imprinting of the hepatic monooxygenase system. Effects of neonatal phenobarbital administration. Biochemical Pharmacology. 1985;**34**(7):1007-1014

[125] Jorgensen KV, Park DL, Rua SM Jr, Price RL. Reduction of mutagenic potentials in milk: Effects of ammonia treatment on aflatoxin-contaminated cottonseed. Journal of Food Protection. 1990;**53**(9):777-778

[126] Grove MD, Plattner RD, Peterson RE. Detection of aflatoxin D1 in ammoniated corn by mass spectrometry-mass spectrometry. Applied and Environmental Microbiology. 1984;**48**(4):887-889

[127] Diao E, Hou H, Chen B, Shan C, Dong H. Ozonolysis efficiency and safety evaluation of aflatoxin B1 in peanuts. Food and Chemical Toxicology. 2013;**55**:519-525

[128] Chen R, Ma F, Li PW, et al. Effect of ozone on aflatoxins detoxification and nutritional quality of peanuts. Food Chemistry. 2014;**146**:284-288

[129] Gomaa MN, Ayesh AM, Abdel Galil MM, Naguib K. Effect of high pressure ammoniation procedure on the detoxification of aflatoxins. Mycotoxin Research. 1997;**13**(1):23-34

[130] Gardner HK Jr, Koltun SP, Dollear FG, Rayner ET. Inactivation of aflatoxins in peanut and cottonseed meals by ammoniation. Journal of the American Oil Chemists' Society. 1971;**48**(2):70-73

[131] Weng CY, Martinez AJ, Park DL. Efficacy and permanency of ammonia treatment in reducing aflatoxin levels in corn. Food Additives and Contaminants. 1994;**11**(6):649-658

[132] Proctor AD, Ahmedna M, Kumar JV, Goktepe I. Degradation of aflatoxins in peanut kernels/flour by gaseous ozonation and mild heat treatment. Food Additives and Contaminants. 2004;**21**(8):786-793

[133] Elias-Orozco R, Castellanos-Nava A, Gaytan-Martinez M, Figueroa-Cardenas JD, Loarca-Pina G. Comparison of nixtamalization and extrusion processes for a reduction in aflatoxin content. Food Additives and Contaminants. 2002;**19**(9):878-885

[134] Torres P, Guzman-Ortiz M, Ramirez-Wong B. Revising the role of pH and thermal treatments in aflatoxin content reduction during the tortilla and deep frying processes. Journal of Agricultural and Food Chemistry. 2001;**49**(6):2825-2829

[135] Aiko V, Edamana P, Mehta A. Decomposition and detoxification of aflatoxin B1 by lactic acid. Journal of the Science of Food and Agriculture. 2016;**96**(6):1959-1966

[136] Aly SE, Hathout AS. Fate of aflatoxin B(1) in contaminated corn gluten during acid hydrolysis. Journal of the Science of Food and Agriculture. 2011;**91**(3):421-427

[137] Rushing BR, Selim MI. Structure and oxidation of pyrrole adducts formed between aflatoxin B2a and biological amines. Chemical Research in Toxicology. 2017;**30**(6):1275-1285

[138] Breinholt V, Hendricks J, Pereira C, Arbogast D, Bailey G. Dietary chlorophyllin is a potent inhibitor of aflatoxin B1 hepatocarcinogenesis in rainbow trout. Cancer Research. 1995;**55**(1):57-62

[139] Simonich MT, Egner PA, Roebuck BD, et al. Natural chlorophyll inhibits aflatoxin B1-induced multi-organ carcinogenesis in the rat. Carcinogenesis. 2007;**28**(6):1294-1302

[140] Egner PA, Groopman JD, Wang JS, Kensler TW, Friesen MD. Quantification of aflatoxin-B1-N7-guanine in human urine by high-performance liquid chromatography and isotope dilution tandem mass spectrometry. Chemical Research in Toxicology. 2006;**19**(9):1191-1195

[141] Phillips TD, Afriyie-Gyawu E, Williams J, et al. Reducing human exposure to aflatoxin through the use of clay: A review. Food Additives and Contaminants. Part A: Chemistry, Analysis, Control, Exposure and Risk Assessment. 2008;**25**(2):134-145

[142] Afriyie-Gyawu E, Mackie J, Dash B, et al. Chronic toxicological evaluation of dietary NovaSil clay in Sprague-Dawley rats. Food Additives and Contaminants. 2005;**22**(3):259-269

[143] Wang P, Afriyie-Gyawu E, Tang Y, et al. NovaSil clay intervention in Ghanaians at high risk for aflatoxicosis: II. Reduction in biomarkers of aflatoxin exposure in blood and urine. Food Additives and Contaminants. Part A: Chemistry, Analysis, Control, Exposure and Risk Assessment. 2008;**25**(5):622-634

[144] Afriyie-Gyawu E, Ankrah NA, Huebner HJ, et al. NovaSil clay intervention in Ghanaians at high risk for aflatoxicosis. I. Study design and clinical outcomes. Food Additives and Contaminants. Part A: Chemistry, Analysis, Control, Exposure and Risk Assessment. 2008;**25**(1):76-87

[145] Zhang B, Huang K, Zhu L, Luo Y, Xu W. Precision toxicology based on single cell sequencing: An evolving trend in toxicological evaluations and mechanism exploration. Archives of Toxicology. 2017;**91**(7):2539-2549

Chapter 8

The Carcinogenicity of Aflatoxin B1

Jie Li and Mengxi Liu

Abstract

Aflatoxins are a class of carcinogenic mycotoxins, products of *Aspergillus* fungi, which are known contaminants in a large portion of the world's food supply. Aflatoxin B1 (AFB1) is the most potent toxin, which has been strongly linked to the development of hepatocellular carcinoma (HCC), especially given coinfection with hepatitis B virus (HBV). AFB1 is catalyzed by cytochrome P450 (CYP450) into aflatoxin B1-8,9-exo-epoxide to form DNA adducts, which leads to carcinogenesis by disrupting DNA repair. AFB1-induced DNA damage is also caused by the production of excessive ROS, leading to the oxidation of DNA bases. The majority of AFB1-related to HCC carry G-to-T transversion of p53 gene. When the p53 gene is mutated, it shows a "gain of oncogenic function." In addition, epigenetic alterations may potentially be beneficial for the treatment of HCC, because the epigenetic changes are reversible. This chapter will provide important information on the carcinogenicity of AFB1, including DNA damage checkpoint response and epigenetic alteration.

Keywords: aflatoxins, hepatocellular carcinoma, DNA adducts, carcinogenicity

1. Introduction

Aflatoxins were reported to be potent liver carcinogens for laboratory animals since the 1960s [1]. The International Agency for Research on Cancer (IARC) has identified aflatoxins as one of the most harmful human carcinogens [2]. There are four main kinds of aflatoxins, B1, B2, G1, and G2, which are classified based on UV-induced fluorescence color and chromatography retention time [3].

Among these aflatoxins, aflatoxin B1 (AFB1), which is synthesized by *Aspergillus* fungi, is the most common carcinogenic and can be found in foods, such as corn, peanuts, cereals, rice, etc. [4, 5]. AFB1 is chemically stable and resistant to various thermal processes such as boiling, autoclaving, cooking, and fermentation [6]. AFB1 is catalyzed by cytochrome P450 into aflatoxin B1-8,9-exo-epoxide to form DNA adducts, which leads to carcinogenesis by disrupting DNA repair [7]. Although most countries introduce strict regulations for the maximum permitted concentrations of aflatoxin in food, excess of AFB1-DNA adducts has remained in normal and tumorous tissues of individuals with hepatocellular carcinoma (HCC) [8, 9]. HCC is ranked as the second leading cause of death from cancer globally, with 700,000 annual deaths recorded worldwide in 2012 [10, 11]. There are about 4.5 billion people in the world that are exposed to AFB1 and may develop HCC [12]. The risks of AFB1 to induce HCC are dependent on populations and areas, e.g., urban populations are generally exposed to lower levels of aflatoxins than rural populations. Moreover, AFB1 exposure is altered by strong seasonal variation that is correlated with increased food availability. In addition, hepatitis B virus (HBV) infection is associated with AFB1 exposure [12, 13].

IntechOpen

Some studies reported that the detection of urinary AFB1-N7-guanine adduct, a good biomarker for AFB1 exposures and dietary AFB1 intake, has a significant association with HCC [13, 14]. The AFB1-DNA adduct is formed by the reactive intermediate of AFB1, AFB1-8,9-epoxide (AFB1-E), and binds to the DNA of hepatocytes. On the one hand, AFB1 is supposed to cause tumorigenesis by promoting the formation of DNA adducts, resulting in aberrant gene expression and genetic mutations, such as tumor suppressor gene p53, in targeted liver cells [15]. On the other hand, AFB1-developed HCC rat model presents various epigenetic (DNA methylation, histone modification, and noncoding RNA) alterations in hepatocytes [16, 17]. Therefore, this chapter focuses on the potential mechanisms of AFB1-induced development of HCC, including DNA damage checkpoint response and epigenetic alteration.

2. AFB1-DNA adduct formation

AFB1 is mainly absorbed in the small intestine after ingestion and transported from blood to the liver [18]. It passes through hepatocytes by nonionic diffusion, which is not dependent on metabolic energy status [19]. Although AFB1 cannot directly bind to DNA, it is metabolized into reactive epoxide named AFB1-E by cytochrome P450 (CYP450) in the liver [7]. AFB1-E can rapidly conjugate with N7 of guanine residues, resulting in the formation of highly mutagenic AFB1-E-deoxyguanosine or AFB1-formamidopyrimidine (AFB1-FaPy-dG) adducts [20]. In fact, AFB1-E can spontaneously and irreversibly conjugate with guanine residues to form 8,9-dihydro-8-(N7-guanyl)-9-hydroxyaflatoxin B1 (AFB1-E-N7-dG) adducts, leading to the occurrence of DNA damage and mutations [21, 22]. AFB1-E-N7-dG adduct may undergo imidazole ring opening or depurination spontaneously to yield AFB1-FaPy-dG, which has been found in many hepatocellular carcinoma cases [23]. Although both AFB1-FaPy and AFB1-E-N7-dG adducts have similar structures, they bind DNA in a different manner, which results in the differences in the lethality, mutagenicity, and repair capacity of these metabolites. In fact, enzymes involved in DNA repair pathways have higher affinity with AFB1-E-N7-dG than AFB1-FaPy analog. AFB1-FaPy-dG adduct block the replication more effectively than AFB1-E-N7-dG adduct, e.g., AFB1-FaPy-dG adducts induce at least six times more G-to-T transversion than AFB1-E-N7-dG [20]. Therefore, AFB1-FaPy-dG is recognized as the major adduct and the most lethal aflatoxin-induced replication block in vivo.

AFB1 is bioactivated by the predominant enzyme cytochrome P450 in human liver microsomes. Specifically, CYP1A2 is the major enzyme for AFB1-E-dG formation and DNA damage at the low dietary intake of AFB1, while CYP3A4 is the major enzyme at higher doses of exposure [24, 25]. In general, CYP1A2 contributes to 95% of AFB1-DNA adduct formation [26]. AFB1 exposure significantly affected the expression of almost 200 genes and exhibited a fivefold decrease in histone transcripts, which is revealed by microarray studies [27].

In addition, the formation of urinary AFB1-E-N7-guanine excretion and levels of AFB1-serum albumin adducts are highly associated to AFB1 intake [28]. Accordingly, AFB1-E-N7-dG adduct is closely related with the incidence of liver tumors [29, 30]. Then, AFB1-E-N7-dG adduct is rapidly removed from DNA and excreted solely in urine [30]. Actually, people who excreted AFB1-E-N7-dG adduct has 9.1 times more risk of developing HCC than the ones with no adducts [31]. These findings indicate that AFB1-DNA adducts have strong effects on HCC development [26, 27].

3. AFB1-induced oxidative stress

Besides the generation of AFB1-DNA adducts, AFB1-induced DNA damage is also caused by the production of excessive ROS, leading to the oxidation of DNA bases [32]. On the one hand, AFB1 increases ROS generation, superoxide dismutase (SOD), glutathione peroxidase (GPx), catalase (CAT), and glutathione reductase (GR); on the other hand, AFB1 decreases glutathione (GSH) while increasing nitric oxide, fragmented DNA-conjugated dienes, caspase-3, superoxide anion radicals, lipid hydroperoxides, and malondialdehyde (MDA) [11, 33]. It suggests that AFB1-induced hepatocarcinogenesis is partially due to the increase of oxidative stress biomarkers and DNA damage [34].

In addition, the lipid peroxidation contributes to the progression of hepatocarcinogenesis by enhancing the susceptibility to mutation and provokes aldehyde-DNA adducts at p53 mutational hotspot codon 249 [35]. To prevent the further formation of ROS/RNS, p53 modulates the transcription of antioxidant genes; however, the extensive DNA damage promotes apoptosis by activating the prooxidant genes. The elevated oxidative stress is well correlated with the induction of AFB1-induced apoptosis of splenic lymphocytes [36]. Therefore, TP53 mutation is considered as a reliable biomarker for evaluating the extent of AFB1 exposure [37]. Vital antioxidant enzymes alleviate oxidative damage through removing free radicals, e.g., selenium, as a cofactor, and promote cell survival by activating the antioxidant system in response to AFB1-induced mitochondrial damage [38]. The dietary intake of AFB1 is associated with the amount of pathological lesions and apoptosis rate of hepatocytes [39]. Therefore, AFB1 causes instability between antioxidant system activity and ROS production, resulting in excessive reactive species that lead to the apoptosis of hepatocytes [11]. It has been reported that AFB1-treatment increases 8-hydroxy-2′-deoxyguanosine (8-OHdG), which was enormously found in tissues exposed to AFB1 [32]. The 8-OHdG adduct, which is generated from the binding between the hydroxyl radicals and guanine residues of DNA, is considered as a valuable biomarker for the measurement of oxidative DNA damage [40].

In polluted food and water, especially in the regions that are warm and have high humidity, AFB1 coexists with microcystin-LR (MC-LR), a hepatotoxic toxin produced by *Cyanobacteria*. DNA damage is enhanced when cells are exposed to both AFB1 and MC-LR, compared to the exposure to AFB1 or MC-LR, alone, because exposure to both AFB1 and MC-LR further increases the release of ROS. In this case, AFB1 induces genotoxicity through increasing oxidative stress and inhibiting the activity of DNA base excision repair genes [41]. Thus, induction of oxidative DNA damage is responsible for AFB1-induced hepatocarcinogenesis besides the elevated number of AFB1-DNA adducts.

4. AFB1-induced DNA damage checkpoint response

DNA damage checkpoint response is critical for the genomic integrity and the survival of the organism in response to AFB1-induced genotoxicity, especially in the DNA that is actively replicating [42]. Mechanically, AFB1 activates critical proteins in response to DNA damage, such as ataxia telangiectasia and Rad3-related (ATR), ataxia telangiectasia mutated (ATM), Chk2 (serine/threonine protein kinase Chk2 or checkpoint kinase 2), DNA repair enzymes, and p53 [43]. In this context, AFB1-induced DNA double-strand breaks trigger the activation of ATM, which is one of the earliest activated kinases in response to double-strand breaks [44, 45]. Notably, the ATR/Chk1 pathway is not activated in response to AFB1-induced DNA double-strand breaks [26].

Cell cycle-dependent regulation plays an important role in the modulation of DNA repair, such as checkpoint activation, which slows down the cell cycle progression to facilitate DNA repair [46]. In this way, temporary DNA lesions are restrained to become inheritable mutations [47]. AFB1 induces the mutation of ATM kinase, which results in the defectiveness of cell cycle checkpoints [48]. On the one hand, the damaged cells with activated checkpoints can be eliminated by apoptosis if the DNA lesions are severe; on the other hand, damaged cell can continue the cell cycle progression upon checkpoint termination if the DNA lesions have been repaired [49]. Actually, AFB1 decreased the rate of DNA double-strand break repair and apoptosis, resulting in elevated risk of cancer [50].

Since ATM plays a critical role in the activation of cell cycle checkpoints [51], the damaged DNA activates ATM kinase to trigger the DNA repair signaling pathways. One of the substrates of ATM kinase is the structural maintenance of chromosome 1 (SMC1) protein, which plays key roles in regulating DNA replication forks and DNA repair in response to the damage [52, 53]. The ATM signaling inhibits the cell cycle progression from G1 to S (the G1/S checkpoint) or G2 to mitosis (the G2/M checkpoint) by activating p53 and inhibiting cyclin-dependent kinases [45, 54]. Ultimately, ATM is involved in the regulation of G2/M checkpoint, which has a crucial role in the maintenance of genomic integrity [50, 55]. In addition, ATM activates Chk2 by promoting its phosphorylation in response to DNA damage [56]. Subsequently, phosphorylated Chk2 (pChk2) induces G2/M cell cycle checkpoint by activating p53 signal pathway [57, 58]. Indeed, AFB1 activates ATM-Chk2-p53 axis, leading to G2/M phase arrest via cdc25-cyclin B/cdc2 route [59]. In this signaling pathway, Mdm2 is an E3 ubiquitin ligase that facilitates the ubiquitination of p53 and proteasome-mediated degradation [60, 61]. Thus, ATM-Chk2-p53 axis plays a critical role in AFB1-induced DNA damage response.

5. AFB1 exposure and genetic mutation

More than 50% of HCC patients are from the regions where the daily food is contaminated by excess amount of AFB1 [62]. In these cases, the AFB1 exposure is associated partly with the genetic mutations [20]. For example, high frequent mutation of p53 gene at codon 249 with G-to-T transversion has been found in HCC patients who are exposed to excess dietary aflatoxin [30].

AFB1 preferentially induces G-to-T transversion in exon 7 of p53 tumor suppressor gene, so as to the frequency of G-to-T transversion of p53 significantly associated with AFB1-DNA adducts [63]. Thus, HCC patients who have AFB1-DNA adducts also have AGG-to-AGT mutation at codon 249 of p53 gene [64]. In addition, AFB1 also promotes G-to-T transversion of ras genes, which can enhance the malignant transformation of normal cells. AFB1-FaPy-dG adduct that is a highly persistent DNA lesion in the liver is associated with the lethality and mutagenicity potential [65]. Indeed, the metabolically activated AFB1-E and its cationic metabolite, AFB1-E-N7-dG, are highly related with the genotoxicity of AFB1 [66]. Additionally, there are at least 80% of HCC patients who have chronic infection with hepatitis B virus (HBV) or hepatitis C virus (HCV) [67]. Although AFB1 exposure slows down the replication of HBV, AFB1-mediated DNA damage and p53 induction are not associated with virus infection [68].

6. AFB1 and epigenetic alteration

Epigenetic alterations are heritable phenotype changes that do not include alteration of the DNA sequences [17]. AFB1 exposure induces various kinds of epigenetic alterations, such as DNA methylation and histone modifications, leading to the development of HCC.

DNA methylation is an enzymatic process that a methyl group is conjugated into the CpG site of DNA, where a cytosine (C) is found next to a guanine (G) separated by a single phosphate (p) [69]. AFB1-induced change of DNA methylation is considered as one of the major mechanisms that are associated with AFB1-induced hepatocarcinogenesis [70]. The global hypomethylation of DNA has been identified as one of the most common biomarkers in human cancer [71]. It can lead to the silencing of critical tumor suppressor genes, such as p53 [72]. AFB1 exposure interferes DNA methylation patterns, resulting in an interruption of the methylation machinery associated with HCC development.

A nucleosome is composed of a segment of DNA, which is wrapped around an octamer of histone protein cores composed of two copies of each of the protein histones H2A, H2B, H3, and H4 [73, 74]. Thousands of nucleosome units highly compact into a structure called chromatin [17, 75]. Several translational modifications occur at the N-terminal domains of the histones, e.g., acetylation, methylation, phosphorylation, and ubiquitination, which regulate important cellular processes, including DNA repair, chromatin structure, gene expression, and DNA replication [74]. AFB1 exposure can alter the pattern of modifications in histones, resulting in an increase or repression of genes, facilitating the development of cancer, such as HCC [76].

The most common modifications in histones regulated by AFB1 are methylation and acetylation [74]. Methylation is catalyzed by enzymes called histone methyltransferases, which add the methyl group into the lysine of the histones H3 and H4, occurring as three different forms, including mono-, di-, or trimethylation. Additionally, histone demethylase can remove the methyl group. AFB1-induced histone methylation causes conformational changes of chromatin, leading to gene silencing [77, 78]. In contrast to methylation, acetylation leads to a relaxation of chromatin, resulting in the activation of the gene transcription. Histone acetyltransferases, which catalyze the addition of the acetyl group, and the histone deacetylase (HDAC) enzymes, which remove the acetyl group, are the major enzymes involved in this dynamic process [73, 79]. The increased expression of HDACs causes the hypoacetylation of histone H3, leading to the repression of the silencing of specific tumor suppressor genes, such as p21, inducing the differentiation and proliferation of liver tumor cells [74, 80, 81].

7. Conclusion

Aflatoxin B1 (AFB1), which is synthesized by *Aspergillus* fungi, is the most common carcinogenic type of aflatoxins and can be found in human diet, such as corn, peanuts, cereals, rice, etc. Although AFB1 cannot directly conjugate with DNA, its metabolite, AFB1-E, can form carcinogenic AFB1-E-N7-dG and AFB1-FaPy-dG adducts spontaneously and irreversibly. Besides the generation of AFB1-DNA adducts, AFB1-induced DNA damage is also caused by the production of excessive ROS, leading to the oxidation of DNA bases. The majority of AFB1-related HCC carry G-to-T transversion of p53 gene. When the p53 protein is mutated, it shows a "gain of oncogenic function." In addition, epigenetic alterations may potentially be beneficial for the treatment of HCC, because the epigenetic changes are reversible.

Author details

Jie Li* and Mengxi Liu
Laura and Isaac Perlmutter Cancer Center, Department of Biochemistry and Molecular Pharmacology, New York University School of Medicine, New York, USA

*Address all correspondence to: jie.li@nyumc.org

References

[1] Stoloff L. Aflatoxin is not a probably human carcinogen: The published evidence is sufficient. Regulatory Toxicology and Pharmacology. 1989;**10**(3):272-283

[2] Ostry V, Malir F, Toman J, Grosse Y. Mycotoxins as human carcinogens—The IARC monographs classification. Mycotoxin Research. 2017;**33**(1):65-73

[3] Bennett JW, Klich M. Mycotoxins. Clinical Microbiology Reviews. 2003;**16**(3):497-516

[4] Kumar P, Mahato DK, Kamle M, Mohanta TK, Kang SG. Aflatoxins: A global concern for food safety, human health and their management. Frontiers in Microbiology. 2016;7:2170

[5] Gross-Steinmeyer K, Eaton DL. Dietary modulation of the biotransformation and genotoxicity of aflatoxin B(1). Toxicology. 2012;**299**(2-3):69-79

[6] Wang Y et al. Effective biodegradation of aflatoxin B1 using the *Bacillus licheniformis* (BL010) strain. Toxins (Basel). 2018;**10**(12):497

[7] Rushing BR, Selim MI. Aflatoxin B1: A review on metabolism, toxicity, occurrence in food, occupational exposure, and detoxification methods. Food and Chemical Toxicology. 2019;**124**:81-100

[8] Harrison JC, Carvajal M, Garner RC. Does aflatoxin exposure in the United Kingdom constitute a cancer risk? Environmental Health Perspectives. 1993;**99**:99-105

[9] Turner PC, Flannery B, Isitt C, Ali M, Pestka J. The role of biomarkers in evaluating human health concerns from fungal contaminants in food. Nutrition Research Reviews. 2012;**25**(1):162-179

[10] Ferlay J et al. Cancer incidence and mortality worldwide: Sources, methods and major patterns in GLOBOCAN 2012. International Journal of Cancer. 2015;**136**(5):E359-E386

[11] Mughal MJ, Xi P, Yi Z, Jing F. Aflatoxin B1 invokes apoptosis via death receptor pathway in hepatocytes. Oncotarget. 2017;**8**(5):8239-8249

[12] Liu Y, Wu F. Global burden of aflatoxin-induced hepatocellular carcinoma: A risk assessment. Environmental Health Perspectives. 2010;**118**(6):818-824

[13] Asim M, Sarma MP, Thayumanavan L, Kar P. Role of aflatoxin B1 as a risk for primary liver cancer in North Indian population. Clinical Biochemistry. 2011;**44**(14-15):1235-1240

[14] Yu MW, Chiang YC, Lien JP, Chen CJ. Plasma antioxidant vitamins, chronic hepatitis B virus infection and urinary aflatoxin B1-DNA adducts in healthy males. Carcinogenesis. 1997;**18**(6):1189-1194

[15] Hamid AS, Tesfamariam IG, Zhang Y, Zhang ZG. Aflatoxin B1-induced hepatocellular carcinoma in developing countries: Geographical distribution, mechanism of action and prevention. Oncology Letters. 2013;**5**(4):1087-1092

[16] Kew MC. Aflatoxins as a cause of hepatocellular carcinoma. Journal of Gastrointestinal and Liver Diseases. 2013;**22**(3):305-310

[17] Dai Y, Huang K, Zhang B, Zhu L, Xu W. Aflatoxin B1-induced epigenetic alterations: An overview. Food and Chemical Toxicology. 2017;**109**(Pt 1): 683-689

[18] Kumagai S. Intestinal absorption and excretion of aflatoxin in rats.

Toxicology and Applied Pharmacology. 1989;**97**(1):88-97

[19] Muller N, Petzinger E. Hepatocellular uptake of aflatoxin B1 by non-ionic diffusion. Inhibition of bile acid transport by interference with membrane lipids. Biochimica et Biophysica Acta. 1988;**938**(3):334-344

[20] Smela ME et al. The aflatoxin B(1) formamidopyrimidine adduct plays a major role in causing the types of mutations observed in human hepatocellular carcinoma. Proceedings of the National Academy of Sciences of the United States of America. 2002;**99**(10):6655-6660

[21] Eaton DL, Gallagher EP. Mechanisms of aflatoxin carcinogenesis. Annual Review of Pharmacology and Toxicology. 1994;**34**:135-172

[22] Shimada T, Guengerich FP. Evidence for cytochrome P-450NF, the nifedipine oxidase, being the principal enzyme involved in the bioactivation of aflatoxins in human liver. Proceedings of the National Academy of Sciences of the United States of America. 1989;**86**(2):462-465

[23] Lin YC et al. DNA polymerase zeta limits chromosomal damage and promotes cell survival following aflatoxin exposure. Proceedings of the National Academy of Sciences of the United States of America. 2016;**113**(48):13774-13779

[24] Gallagher EP, Kunze KL, Stapleton PL, Eaton DL. The kinetics of aflatoxin B1 oxidation by human cDNA-expressed and human liver microsomal cytochromes P450 1A2 and 3A4. Toxicology and Applied Pharmacology. 1996;**141**(2):595-606

[25] Kamdem LK, Meineke I, Godtel-Armbrust U, Brockmoller J, Wojnowski L. Dominant contribution of P450 3A4 to the hepatic carcinogenic activation of aflatoxin B1. Chemical Research in Toxicology. 2006;**19**(4):577-586

[26] Gursoy-Yuzugullu O, Yuzugullu H, Yilmaz M, Ozturk M. Aflatoxin genotoxicity is associated with a defective DNA damage response bypassing p53 activation. Liver International. 2011;**31**(4):561-571

[27] Guo Y et al. Analysis of cellular responses to aflatoxin B(1) in yeast expressing human cytochrome P450 1A2 using cDNA microarrays. Mutation Research. 2006;**593**(1-2):121-142

[28] Groopman JD, DeMatos P, Egner PA, Love-Hunt A, Kensler TW. Molecular dosimetry of urinary aflatoxin-N7-guanine and serum aflatoxin-albumin adducts predicts chemoprotection by 1,2-dithiole-3-thione in rats. Carcinogenesis. 1992;**13**(1):101-106

[29] Lin YC et al. Error-prone replication bypass of the primary aflatoxin B1 DNA adduct, AFB1-N7-Gua. The Journal of Biological Chemistry. 2014;**289**(26):18497-18506

[30] Wang JS, Groopman JD. DNA damage by mycotoxins. Mutation Research. 1999;**424**(1-2):167-181

[31] Poirier MC. DNA adducts as exposure biomarkers and indicators of cancer risk. Environmental Health Perspectives. 1997;**105**(Suppl 4):907-912

[32] Guindon KA, Bedard LL, Massey TE. Elevation of 8-hydroxydeoxyguanosine in DNA from isolated mouse lung cells following in vivo treatment with aflatoxin B(1). Toxicological Sciences. 2007;**98**(1):57-62

[33] Ajiboye TO, Yakubu MT, Oladiji AT. Lophirones B and C prevent aflatoxin B1-induced oxidative stress and DNA fragmentation in rat

hepatocytes. Pharmaceutical Biology. 2016;**54**(10):1962-1970

[34] Ajiboye TO, Yakubu MT, Oladiji AT. Lophirones B and C extenuate AFB1-mediated oxidative onslaught on cellular proteins, lipids, and DNA through Nrf-2 expression. Journal of Biochemical and Molecular Toxicology. 2014;**28**(12):558-567

[35] Weng MW et al. AFB1 hepatocarcinogenesis is via lipid peroxidation that inhibits DNA repair, sensitizes mutation susceptibility and induces aldehyde-DNA adducts at p53 mutational hotspot codon 249. Oncotarget. 2017;**8**(11):18213-18226

[36] Chen J et al. Effects of aflatoxin B1 on oxidative stress markers and apoptosis of spleens in broilers. Toxicology and Industrial Health. 2016;**32**(2):278-284

[37] Hussain SP, Schwank J, Staib F, Wang XW, Harris CC. TP53 mutations and hepatocellular carcinoma: Insights into the etiology and pathogenesis of liver cancer. Oncogene. 2007;**26**(15):2166-2176

[38] Shi D et al. Protective effects of selenium on aflatoxin B1-induced mitochondrial permeability transition, DNA damage, and histological alterations in duckling liver. Biological Trace Element Research. 2015;**163**(1-2):162-168

[39] Yang J et al. Effects of feeding corn naturally contaminated with aflatoxin B1 and B2 on hepatic functions of broilers. Poultry Science. 2012;**91**(11):2792-2801

[40] Shen HM, Ong CN, Lee BL, Shi CY. Aflatoxin B1-induced 8-hydroxydeoxyguanosine formation in rat hepatic DNA. Carcinogenesis. 1995;**16**(2):419-422

[41] Liu W et al. Microcystin-LR increases genotoxicity induced by aflatoxin B1 through oxidative stress and DNA base excision repair genes in human hepatic cell lines. Environmental Pollution. 2018;**233**:455-463

[42] Fasullo M, Sun M, Egner P. Stimulation of sister chromatid exchanges and mutation by aflatoxin B1-DNA adducts in Saccharomyces cerevisiae requires MEC1 (ATR), RAD53, and DUN1. Molecular Carcinogenesis. 2008;**47**(8):608-615

[43] Yang X et al. Cytochrome P450 2A13 enhances the sensitivity of human bronchial epithelial cells to aflatoxin B1-induced DNA damage. Toxicology and Applied Pharmacology. 2013;**270**(2):114-121

[44] Burma S, Chen BP, Murphy M, Kurimasa A, Chen DJ. ATM phosphorylates histone H2AX in response to DNA double-strand breaks. The Journal of Biological Chemistry. 2001;**276**(45):42462-42467

[45] Sancar A, Lindsey-Boltz LA, Unsal-Kacmaz K, Linn S. Molecular mechanisms of mammalian DNA repair and the DNA damage checkpoints. Annual Review of Biochemistry. 2004;**73**:39-85

[46] Warmerdam DO, Kanaar R. Dealing with DNA damage: Relationships between checkpoint and repair pathways. Mutation Research. 2010;**704**(1-3):2-11

[47] Yang XH, Zou L. Checkpoint and coordinated cellular responses to DNA damage. Results and Problems in Cell Differentiation. 2006;**42**:65-92

[48] Branzei D, Foiani M. Regulation of DNA repair throughout the cell cycle. Nature Reviews. Molecular Cell Biology. 2008;**9**(4):297-308

[49] Bartek J, Lukas J. DNA damage checkpoints: From initiation to recovery or adaptation. Current Opinion in Cell Biology. 2007;**19**(2):238-245

[50] Lavin MF, Kozlov S. ATM activation and DNA damage response. Cell Cycle. 2007;**6**(8):931-942

[51] Kurz EU, Lees-Miller SP. DNA damage-induced activation of ATM and ATM-dependent signaling pathways. DNA Repair (Amst). 2004;**3**(8-9):889-900

[52] Kitagawa R, Kastan MB. The ATM-dependent DNA damage signaling pathway. Cold Spring Harbor Symposia on Quantitative Biology. 2005;**70**:99-109

[53] Lee JH, Paull TT. Activation and regulation of ATM kinase activity in response to DNA double-strand breaks. Oncogene. 2007;**26**(56):7741-7748

[54] Niida H, Nakanishi M. DNA damage checkpoints in mammals. Mutagenesis. 2006;**21**(1):3-9

[55] Kudoh A et al. *Epstein-Barr* virus lytic replication elicits ATM checkpoint signal transduction while providing an S-phase-like cellular environment. The Journal of Biological Chemistry. 2005;**280**(9):8156-8163

[56] Wilson KA, Stern DF. NFBD1/MDC1, 53BP1 and BRCA1 have both redundant and unique roles in the ATM pathway. Cell Cycle. 2008;**7**(22):3584-3594

[57] Hirao A et al. DNA damage-induced activation of p53 by the checkpoint kinase Chk2. Science. 2000;**287**(5459):1824-1827

[58] Yu Q et al. UCN-01 inhibits p53 up-regulation and abrogates gamma-radiation-induced G(2)-M checkpoint independently of p53 by targeting both of the checkpoint kinases, Chk2 and Chk1. Cancer Research. 2002;**62**(20):5743-5748

[59] Yin H et al. The molecular mechanism of G2M cell cycle arrest induced by AFB1 in the jejunum. Oncotarget. 2016;**7**(24):35592-35606

[60] Chen X et al. MDM2 promotes invasion and metastasis in invasive ductal breast carcinoma by inducing matrix metalloproteinase-9. PLoS ONE. 2013;**8**(11):e78794

[61] Noon AP et al. p53 and MDM2 in renal cell carcinoma: Biomarkers for disease progression and future therapeutic targets? Cancer. 2010;**116**(4):780-790

[62] Shen HM, Ong CN. Mutations of the p53 tumor suppressor gene and ras oncogenes in aflatoxin hepatocarcinogenesis. Mutation Research. 1996;**366**(1):23-44

[63] Aguilar F, Hussain SP, Cerutti P. Aflatoxin B1 induces the transversion of G-->T in codon 249 of the p53 tumor suppressor gene in human hepatocytes. Proceedings of the National Academy of Sciences of the United States of America. 1993;**90**(18):8586-8590

[64] Shirabe K et al. Hepatic aflatoxin B1-DNA adducts and TP53 mutations in patients with hepatocellular carcinoma despite low exposure to aflatoxin B1 in southern Japan. Liver International. 2011;**31**(9):1366-1372

[65] Croy RG, Wogan GN. Quantitative comparison of covalent aflatoxin-DNA adducts formed in rat and mouse livers and kidneys. Journal of the National Cancer Institute. 1981;**66**(4):761-768

[66] Brown KL et al. Unraveling the aflatoxin-FAPY conundrum: Structural basis for differential replicative processing of isomeric forms of the formamidopyrimidine-type DNA adduct of aflatoxin B1. Journal of the American Chemical Society. 2006;**128**(47):15188-15199

[67] McGlynn KA, London WT. The global epidemiology of hepatocellular

carcinoma: Present and future. Clinics in Liver Disease. 2011;**15**(2):223-243, vii-x

[68] Lereau M et al. Interactions between hepatitis B virus and aflatoxin B(1): Effects on p53 induction in HepaRG cells. The Journal of General Virology. 2012;**93**(Pt 3):640-650

[69] Goel N, Karir P, Garg VK. Role of DNA methylation in human age prediction. Mechanisms of Ageing and Development. 2017;**166**:33-41

[70] Udali S, Guarini P, Moruzzi S, Choi SW, Friso S. Cardiovascular epigenetics: From DNA methylation to microRNAs. Molecular Aspects of Medicine. 2013;**34**(4):883-901

[71] Udali S et al. Hepcidin and DNA promoter methylation in hepatocellular carcinoma. European Journal of Clinical Investigation. 2018;**48**(2):e12870

[72] You JS, Jones PA. Cancer genetics and epigenetics: Two sides of the same coin? Cancer Cell. 2012;**22**(1):9-20

[73] Ma L, Chua MS, Andrisani O, So S. Epigenetics in hepatocellular carcinoma: An update and future therapy perspectives. World Journal of Gastroenterology. 2014;**20**(2):333-345

[74] Chrun ES, Modolo F, Daniel FI. Histone modifications: A review about the presence of this epigenetic phenomenon in carcinogenesis. Pathology, Research and Practice. 2017;**213**(11):1329-1339

[75] Anestopoulos I et al. Epigenetic therapy as a novel approach in hepatocellular carcinoma. Pharmacology & Therapeutics. 2015;**145**:103-119

[76] Chappell G, Pogribny IP, Guyton KZ, Rusyn I. Epigenetic alterations induced by genotoxic occupational and environmental human chemical carcinogens: A systematic literature review. Mutation Research, Reviews in Mutation Research. 2016;**768**:27-45

[77] Rieswijk L et al. Aflatoxin B1 induces persistent epigenomic effects in primary human hepatocytes associated with hepatocellular carcinoma. Toxicology. 2016;**350-352**:31-39

[78] Valinluck V et al. Oxidative damage to methyl-CpG sequences inhibits the binding of the methyl-CpG binding domain (MBD) of methyl-CpG binding protein 2 (MeCP2). Nucleic Acids Research. 2004;**32**(14):4100-4108

[79] Zhao N et al. Expression of microRNA-195 is transactivated by Sp1 but inhibited by histone deacetylase 3 in hepatocellular carcinoma cells. Biochimica et Biophysica Acta. 2016;**1859**(7):933-942

[80] Buurman R, Sandbothe M, Schlegelberger B, Skawran B. HDAC inhibition activates the apoptosome via Apaf1 upregulation in hepatocellular carcinoma. European Journal of Medical Research. 2016;**21**(1):26

[81] Lai YC, Cheng CC, Lai YS, Liu YH. Cytokeratin 18-associated histone 3 modulation in hepatocellular carcinoma: A mini review. Cancer Genomics Proteomics. 2017;**14**(4):219-223

Chapter 9

X-Ray Repair Cross Complementing 4 (XRCC4) Genetic Single Nucleotide Polymorphisms and the Liver Toxicity of AFB1 in Hepatocellular Carcinoma

Yan Deng, Xue-Min Wu, Xiao-Ying Huang and Xi-Dai Long

Abstract

Our previous reports have shown that the genetic single-nucleotide polymorphisms (GSNPs) in the DNA repair gene X-ray repair cross complementing 4 (XRCC4) are involved in the carcinogenesis of hepatocellular carcinoma (HCC) induced by aflatoxin B1 (AFB1). However, the effects of GSNPs in the coding regions of XRCC4 on hepatic toxicity of AFB1 have been less investigated. We conducted a hospital-based clinic tissue samples with pathologically diagnosed HCC (n = 380) in a high AFB1 exposure area to explore the possible roles of GSNPs in the coding regions of XRCC4 in AFB1-induced HCC using liver toxicity assays. A total of 143 GSNPs were included in the present study and genotyped using the SNaPshot method, whereas the liver toxicity of AFB1 was evaluated using AFB1-DNA adducts in the tissues with HCC. In the clinicopathological samples with HCC, the average adduct amount is 2.27 ± 1.09 μmol/mol DNA. Among 143 GSNPs of XRCC4, only rs1237462915, rs28383151, rs762419679, rs766287987, and rs3734091 significantly increased the levels of AFB1-DNA adducts. Furthermore, XRCC4 GSNPs (including rs28383151, rs766287987, and rs3734091) also increased cumulative hazard for patients with HCC. These results suggest that the liver toxicity of AFB1 may be modified by XRCC4 GSNPs.

Keywords: AFB1, liver toxicity, XRCC4, genetic single-nucleotide polymorphism, hepatocellular carcinoma

1. Introduction

Aflatoxin B1 (AFB1) is an important type I chemical toxicant mainly produced by the toxigenic strains of *Aspergillus flavus* (*A. flavus*) and *Aspergillus parasiticus* (*A. parasiticus*) [1, 2]. This carcinogen is often taken into human body via contaminating human foods such as nuts and cereals and displays its toxic effects, especially hepatic toxicity [1–8]. AFB1-induced hepatic effects consist of acute toxic damages (such as severe DNA damage, severe liver degeneration and necrosis, and the failure of hepatic function) and chronic cumulative damages (such as a series of cumulative DNA damage, slight hepatocellular degeneration and necrosis, chronic inflammation, liver cirrhosis, and liver cancer) [3–5]. Increasing evidence has shown that under the same exposure of AFB1, some individuals feature severe hepatic damage; others have no noticeable damage [9–14]. This suggests that different individuals have different responses to the toxic effects of AFB1 and genetic factors may play a central role in the AFB1-induced hepatic toxicity.

X-ray repair cross complementing 4 (XRCC4), an important DNA repair gene involved in nonhomologous end-joining (NHEJ) repair pathway, plays a scaffold function via stabilizing and localizing DNA repair enzymes LIG IV, Ku70/80 heterodimer, and the DNA-dependent protein kinase (DNA-PK) catalytic subunit (DNA-PKcs) in the ends of DNA double-stranded breaks (DSBs) during NHEJ [15, 16]. In the past decades, growing reports have exhibited that the abnormal structures and functions of XRCC4 may alter the capacity of DNA repair and ultimately result in human diseases [17–22]. Several recent studies have also shown that the genetic alterations in the coding regions of XRCC4 can modify hepatocellular carcinoma (HCC) risk and prognosis [23–27]. However, the effects of this genetic alteration on the hepatic toxicity of AFB1 is unclear. Here, we conducted a clinical sample study exposure to explore whether the genetic single-nucleotide polymorphisms (GSNPs, a type of genetic alterations) in the coding regions of XRCC4 modified the effects of AFB1 on hepatic damage.

2. Materials and methods

2.1 Study population

This was a hospital-based molecular epidemiological study conducted in high AFB1 exposure area, Guangxi Zhuang Region, China. All participants were newly diagnosed HCC cases and recruited from the Affiliated Hospitals of Youjiang Medical University for Nationalities (located at Bose region, a major AFB1 exposure area) between January 2010 and January 2013 inclusively. The inclusive criteria of cases consisted of (a) cases with ultimately histopathologically confirmed HCC; (b) cases without any evidence of hepatitis virus infection; (c) cases with the history of AFB1 exposure which was defined according to positive history of peripheral serum AFB1-albumin adducts [5, 24]; and (d) cases with available tumor tissue samples and clinicopathological data.

According to the criteria, a total of 380 cases with HCC were recruited in this study during the period. With informed consent, the tissue samples with HCC for all patients and clinicopathological data were collected. Additionally, survival follow-up information was also collected through cases themselves or their family contact. In this study, the last follow-up date was set on January 31, 2019. The protocol for clinical samples was approved by Youjiang Medical University for Nationalities Medical Ethics Committee.

2.2 The evaluation of AFB1-related hepatic toxicity

Hepatic toxicity of AFB1 was evaluated using AFB1-DNA adducts in the tissue samples with HCC, and the amounts of AFB1-DNA adducts were tested by the previously described enzyme-linked immunosorbent assay (ELISA).

2.3 GSNP selection

All GSNPs of XRCC4 gene were first screened from the SNPdatabase (http://asia.ensembl.org/Homo_sapiens/Gene/Variation_Gene/Table?db=core;g=ENSG00000152422;r=5:83077498-83353787). According to the data from SNPdatabase, a total of 143 GSNPs can result in missense mutations and the change of amino acids in XRCC4 protein, and thus they were ultimately selected for final analyses.

2.4 Genotypic analyses

Genomic DNA in all tumor tissue samples with HCC was standard phenol-chloroform extraction binding with proteinase K. The GSNPs of XRCC4 were genotyped using SNaPshot method (Applied Biosystems [ABI], Foster City, CA) as previously described [28]. For quality control, all laboratory personnel were blind to the status of every sample with hepatocarcinoma, and controls were also included in each analysis.

2.5 Statistical analysis

The test for genotypic distribution of XRCC4 GSNPs among HCC cases featuring different AFB1-DNA adducts was accomplished using student *t*-test or one-way analysis of variance (ANOVA) test. Multiple tests were adjusted using a *Bonferroni* correction, and the threshold for GSNP screening was defined as $\alpha = 3.53 \times 10^{-4}$. Kaplan-Meier survival model with log-rank test and Cox regression model (the selection of significant varies based on forward-step method with likelihood ratio test) was used to analyze the association between XRCC4 GSNPs and HCC outcomes. Cumulative hazard value for the effects of XRCC4 GSNPs on the hepatic toxicity for AFB1 and corresponding 95% confidence interval (CI) were calculated using hazard ratio (HR) from significant multivariate Cox regression model (including all significant variates). All statistical analyses were performed with SPSS statistical package (Version 18, SPSS Institute, Chicago, IL, USA).

3. Results

3.1 The characteristics of subjects

All subjects suffered from hepatic carcinoma, and **Table 1** summarized their characteristics. The mean age of all participants was 50.74 ± 11.55 years, and more than 70% of them are male. For these cancer patients, 70.3% (267/380) and 26.3% (100/380) cases featured TNM II and III stages of tumor, and they also had an average AFB1 exposure value of 2.27 ± 1.09 μmol/mol DNA.

3.2 XRCC4 GSNPs increased AFB1-DNA adducts

A total of 143 GSNPs in the coding regions of XRCC4 gene were selected in our final analyses, and **Table 2** showed the genotypic distribution of all GSNPs. To evaluate the effects of these potential GSNPs on AFB1-DNA adducts, the role of each GSNP in the coding regions of XRCC4 gene was tested using Student *t*-test or ANOVA test with the adjustment of multiple test. Among these GSNPs, only rs1237462915 (cat#SNP016, at codon 38), rs28383151 (cat#SNP026, at codon 56), rs762419679 (cat#SNP069, at codon 127), rs766287987 (cat#SNP112, at codon 203),

	n	%
Total	380	100.0
Age (years)		
≤35	53	13.9
36–40	38	10.0
41–45	55	14.5
46–50	43	11.3
51–55	56	14.7
56–60	42	11.1
61–65	49	12.9
≥66	44	11.6
Gender		
Male	271	71.3
Female	109	28.7
Race		
Han	221	58.2
Zhuang	159	41.8
TNM stage		
I–II	13	3.4
III	267	70.3
IV	100	26.3

Table 1.
The characteristics of subjects.

and rs3734091 (cat#SNP138, at codon 247) significantly affected the levels of AFB1-DNA adducts in the tumor tissues with HCC. The adduct amounts of their wild genotypes (defined as XX genotype) were 2.15 ± 0.97 μmol/mol DNA, 2.07 ± 0.99 μmol/mol DNA, 2.12 ± 0.86 μmol/mol DNA, 2.11 ± 0.89 μmol/mol DNA, and 2.09 ± 0.97 μmol/mol DNA, respectively. For their mutant heterozygotic genotypes (defined as XY genotype), the amounts of AFB-DNA adduct were from 2.64 to 4.33 μmol/mol DNA, whereas the adduct levels were from 3.04 to 5.78 for the mutant homozygotic genotypes (defined as YY genotype) (**Table 2**).

Additionally, mutant genotypes of several other GSNPs, including rs761695470 (SNP008, at codon 18), rs758779099 (SNP018, at codon 40), rs144653114 (SNP054, at codon 103), rs1277864722 (SNP085, at codon 153), and rs777195630 (SNP100, at codon 180), also increased the amounts of AFB1-DNA adducts; however, they had no statistical significance according to screening threshold value.

3.3 XRCC4 GSNPs modified the AFB1-related HCC prognosis

Because the poor prognosis of patients with HCC has been associated with the toxicity of AFB1, we followed up the survival information of all patients and explored whether positive GSNPs of XRCC4 modified HCC outcomes, including overall survival (OS) and disease recurrence-free survival (RFS) (**Figures 1** and **2**). Results from Kaplan-Meier survival model (based on the cumulative risk models) and Cox regression model analyses showed that compared with their wild

No.	SNP ID	Chr: bp	Alleles (x/y)[a]	Genotypes (xx/xy/yy)[b]	Amino acid position	Amino acid change	$N_{xx/xy/yy}$[c]	Adducts (mean ± SD)	P^d
SNP001	rs142575170	5:83104923	G/A	GG/GA/AA	2	E/K	323/54/3	2.28 ± 1.09/2.21 ± 1.08/ 2.36 ± 1.05	0.23
SNP002	rs1449631425	5:83104929	A/G	AA/AG/GG	4	K/E	377/3/0	2.27 ± 1.09/2.21 ± 0.54/–	0.99
SNP003	rs1166890864	5:83104930	A/G	AA/AG/GG	4	K/R	378/2/0	2.27 ± 1.09/1.57 ± 0.03/–	0.99
SNP004	rs1425642930	5:83104933	T/G	TT/TG/GG	5	I/R	376/4/0	2.27 ± 1.09/2.10 ± 0.61/–	0.96
SNP005	rs1252823908	5:83104946	C/A	CC/CA/AA	9	H/Q	376/4/0	2.27 ± 1.09/2.16 ± 0.56/–	0.94
SNP006	rs28383138	5:83104954	C/G	CC//CG/GG	12	S/C	319/47/14	2.26 ± 1.09/2.41 ± 1.06/ 2.00 ± 1.07	0.23
SNP007	rs774071130	5:83104966	T/C	TT/TC/CC	16	I/T	370/10/0	2.28 ± 1.09/2.05 ± 0.94/–	0.99
SNP008	rs761695470	5:83104971	C/T	CC/CT/TT	18	H/Y	371/6/3	2.24 ± 1.03/2.87 ± 2.00/ 4.42 ± 2.93	0.04
SNP009	rs755776572	5:83104983	G/A	GG/GA/AA	22	V/I	380/0/0	2.27 ± 1.09/–/–	—
SNP010	rs1271180927	5:83104986	T/A	TT/TA/AA	23	S/T	364/13/3	2.26 ± 1.09/2.52 ± 1.04/ 2.44 ± 0.77	0.89
SNP011	rs1288681786	5:83104992	G/A	GG/GA/AA	25	E/K	354/26/0	2.28 ± 1.10/2.16 ± 0.96/–	0.56
SNP012	rs550773308	5:83104999	C/T	CC/CT/TT	27	T/I	367/13/0	2.26 ± 1.06/2.51 ± 1.80/–	0.63
SNP013	rs1484250582	5:83105006	A/C	AA/AC/CC	29	E/D	376/4/0	2.27 ± 1.09/2.18 ± 1.42/–	0.87
SNP014	rs1305679408	5:83105013	T/A	TT/TA/AA	32	F/I	350/30/0	2.27 ± 1.08/2.26 ± 1.14/–	0.96
SNP015	rs1232077487	5:83105022	A/G	AA/AG/GG	35	T/A	380/0/0	2.27 ± 1.09/–/–	—
SNP016	rs1237462915	5:83105031	G/T	GG/GT/TT	38	D/Y	352/19/9	2.15 ± 0.97/3.62 ± 1.40/ 4.21 ± 0.93	2.96×10^{-5}
SNP017	rs748540743	5:83105032	A/T	AA/AT/TT	38	D/V	380/0/0	2.27 ± 1.09/–/–	—
SNP018	rs758779099	5:83105039	T/G	TT/TG/GG	40	H/Q	353/25/2	2.23 ± 1.03/2.78 ± 1.61/ 2.63 ± 0.01	0.04

No.	SNP ID	Chr: bp	Alleles (x/y)[a]	Genotypes (xx/xy/yy)[b]	Amino acid position	Amino acid change	$N_{xx/xy/yy}$[c]	Adducts (mean ± SD)	P^d
SNP019	rs587779351	5:83105046	T/C	TT/TC/CC	43	W/R	380/0/0	2.27 ± 1.09/−/−	—
SNP020	rs771111816	5:83105050	C/T	CC/CT/TT	44	T/I	362/25/3	2.26 ± 1.08/2.33 ± 1.23/ 2.68 ± 0.07	0.78
SNP021	rs1460004120	5:83105053	G/C	GG/GC/CC	45	G/A	375/5/0	2.27 ± 1.09/2.21 ± 0.82/−	0.91
SNP022	rs1248835327	5:83111031	C/T	CC/CT/TT	48	S/F	370/10/0	2.27 ± 1.09/2.21 ± 1.01/−	0.87
SNP023	rs1326359694	5:83111033	G/A	GG/GA/AA	49	E/K	355/25/0	2.28 ± 1.11/2.16 ± 0.76/−	0.61
SNP024	rs868207005	5:83111039	G/A	GG/GA/AA	51	E/K	380/0/0	2.27 ± 1.09/−/−	—
SNP025	rs945155269	5:83111049	A/C	AA/AC/CC	54	Q/P	364/26/0	2.29 ± 1.07/2.02 ± 1.04/−	0.24
SNP026	rs28383151	5:83111054	G/A	GG/GA/AA	56	A/T	277/63/40	2.07 ± 0.99/2.64 ± 1.33/ 3.04 ± 0.78	2.83×10^{-55}
SNP027	rs1245127767	5:83111063	A/G	AA/AG/GG	59	M/V	354/25/1	2.27 ± 1.10/2.18 ± 0.92/2.78*	0.67*
SNP028	rs748124509	5:83111066	G/T	GG/GT/TT	60	A/S	354/23/3	2.25 ± 1.11/2.36 ± 0.74/2.78 ± 1.01	0.66
SNP029	rs760546308	5:83111070	T/C	TT/TC/CC	61	M/T	352/28/0	2.27 ± 1.04/2.25 ± 1.56/−	0.91
SNP030	rs1369565470	5:83111071	G/C	GG/GC/CC	61	M/I	380/0/0	2.27 ± 1.09/−/−	—
SNP031	rs867574505	5:83111072	G/A	GG/GA/AA	62	E/K	380/0/0	2.27 ± 1.09/−/−	—
SNP032	rs1285557699	5:83111073	A/G	AA/AG/GG	62	E/G	380/0/0	2.27 ± 1.09/−/−	—
SNP033	rs1248297453	5:83111085	A/G	AA/AG/GG	66	Y/C	351/29/0	2.26 ± 1.07/2.36 ± 1.25/−	0.63
SNP034	rs776362814	5:83111087	G/A	GG/GA/AA	67	V/I	350/30/0	2.26 ± 1.11/2.31 ± 0.84/−	0.83
SNP035	rs1423928075	5:83111090	G/A	GG/GA/AA	68	G/S	380/0/0	2.27 ± 1.09/−/−	—
SNP036	rs1478505961	5:83111093	G/A	GG/GA/AA	69	E/K	250/28/2	2.27 ± 1.07/2.24 ± 1.28/2.69 ± 1.16	0.86
SNP037	rs759064378	5:83111097	T/C	TT/TC/CC	70	L/P	354/26/0	2.28 ± 1.09/2.15 ± 1.01/−	0.58
SNP038	rs371307071	5:83111100	G/C	GG/GC/CC	71	R/T	380/0/0	2.27 ± 1.09/−/−	—

No.	SNP ID	Chr: bp	Alleles (x/y)[a]	Genotypes (xx/xy/yy)[b]	Amino acid position	Amino acid change	$N_{xx/xy/yy}$[c]	Adducts (mean ± SD)	P^d
SNP039	rs61762970	5:83111112	T/C	TT/TC/CC	75	L/S	356/24/0	2.29 ± 1.10/1.99 ± 0.89/–	0.20
SNP040	rs763501478	5:83111117	G/A	GG/GA/AA	77	G/R	361/29/0	2.27 ± 1.09/–/–	—
SNP041	rs764572419	5:83111120	G/T	GG/GT/TT	78	A/S	349/31/0	2.26 ± 1.09/2.39 ± 1.09/–	0.52
SNP042	rs528259464	5:83111121	C/T	CC/CT/TT	78	A/V	376/4/0	2.26 ± 1.09/2.77 ± 0.44/–	0.36
SNP043	rs757644947	5:83111126	C/T	CC/CT/TT	80	P/S	369/11/0	2.26 ± 1.07/2.51 ± 1.51/–	0.46
SNP044	rs572613361	5:83111138	T/C	TT/TC/CC	84	Y/H	351/27/2	2.27 ± /2.24 ± 1.02/3.09 ± 0.47	0.57
SNP045	rs1398927737	5:83111141	A/C	AA/AC/CC	85	T/P	380/0/0	2.27 ± 1.09/–/–	—
SNP046	rs756247552	5:83111142	C/T	CC/CT/TT	85	T/M	374/6/0	2.26 ± 1.08/2.56 ± 1.35/–	0.50
SNP047	rs149355996	5:83111147	A/T	AA/AT/TT	87	N/Y	371/9/0	2.27 ± 1.10/2.36 ± 0.70/–	0.81
SNP048	rs1049631686	5:83111162	T/A	TT/TA/AA	92	S/T	364/26/0	2.27 ± 1.09/–/–	—
SNP049	rs772190420	5:83111169	A/G	AA/AG/GG	94	Y/C	354/26/0	2.28 ± 1.08/2.08 ± 1.23/–	0.36
SNP050	rs1239084198	5:83111171	T/G	TT/TG/GG	95	F/V	356/24/0	2.26 ± 1.07/2.36 ± 1.34/–	0.68
SNP051	rs1184763400	5:83111174	T/A	TT/TA/AA	96	F/I	380/0/0	2.27 ± 1.09/–/–	—
SNP052	rs1236326383	5:83111177	T/C	TT/TC/CC	97	F/L	366/14/0	2.28 ± 1.09/1.92 ± 0.92/–	0.24
SNP053	rs1472843465	5:83111180	G/A	GG/GA/AA	98	E/K	377/3/0	2.27 ± 1.09/2.58 ± 0.84/–	0.63
SNP054	rs144653114	5:83111195	G/A	GG/GA/AA	103	N/D	240/127/13	2.17 ± 1.09/2.48 ± 1.08/2.11 ± 0.84	0.03
SNP055	rs79561451	5:83195782	T/C	TT/TC/CC	110	S/P	352/25/3	2.28 ± 1.11/2.20 ± 0.84/1.82 ± 0.37	0.74
SNP056	rs757113391	5:83195787	C/G	CC//CG/GG	111	F/L	380/0/0	2.27 ± 1.09/–/–	—
SNP057	rs1378785946	5:83195794	G/C	GG/GC/CC	114	E/Q	360/20/0	2.277 ± 1.10/2.227 ± 0.84/–	0.83
SNP058	rs1240771489	5:83195795	A/G	AA/AG/GG	114	E/G	281/80/19	2.297 ± 1.09/2.197 ± 1.06/–	0.75

No.	SNP ID	Chr: bp	Alleles (x/y)[a]	Genotypes (xx/xy/yy)[b]	Amino acid position	Amino acid change	$N_{xx/xy/yy}$[c]	Adducts (mean ± SD)	P^d
SNP059	rs769556494	5:83195797	A/G	AA/AG/GG	115	K/E	340/40/0	2.277 ± 1.09/2.277 ± 1.04/–	0.99
SNP060	rs1056939125	5:83195798	A/C	AA/AC/CC	115	K/T	380/0/0	2.27 ± 1.09/–/–	—
SNP061	rs1301137729	5:83195800	G/C	GG/GC/CC	116	V/L	359/21/0	2.27 ± 1.09/2.19 ± 0.99/–	0.74
SNP062	rs550178738	5:83195807	A/T	AA/AT/TT	118	N/I	341/39/0	2.27 ± 1.10/2.28 ± 1.00/–	0.93
SNP063	rs375157105	5:83195809	C/A	CC/CA/AA	119	P/T	352/28/0	2.29 ± 1.102.06 ± 0.83/–	0.28
SNP064	rs768175717	5:83195810	C/T	CC/CT/TT	119	P/L	380/0/0	2.27 ± 1.09/–/–	—
SNP065	rs369641536	5:83195816	A/G	AA/AG/GG	121	E/G	380/0/0	2.27 ± 1.09/–/–	—
SNP066	rs1395194011	5:83195819	T/A	TT/TA/AA	122	V/D	289/81/10	2.24 ± 1.07/2.62 ± 1.22/–	0.05
SNP067	rs1198491910	5:83195821	A/G	AA/AG/GG	123	I/V	348/32/0	2.27 ± 1.09/2.25 ± 1.13/–	0.95
SNP068	rs1159852376	5:83195824	A/G	AA/AG/GG	124	R/G	369/11/0	2.26 ± 1.10/2.40 ± 0.88/–	0.64
SNP069	rs762419679	5:83195834	T/C	TT/TC/CC	127	I/T	359/15/6	2.12 ± 0.86/4.33 ± 1.99/5.99 ± 1.12	1.17×10^{-43}
SNP070	rs1412506484	5:83195840	A/G	AA/AG/GG	129	Y/C	349/31/0	2.27 ± 1.10/2.26 ± 1.32/–	0.96
SNP071	rs1178870682	5:83195848	G/C	GG/GC/CC	132	D/H	365/15/0	2.27 ± 1.10/2.26 ± 0.78/–	0.98
SNP072	rs1484047716	5:83195852	C/G	CC//CG/GG	133	T/S	374/6/0	2.26 ± 1.07/2.71 ± 1.90/–	0.32
SNP073	rs28360135	5:83195855	T/C	TT/TC/CC	134	I/T	304/64/12	2.31 ± 1.13/2.12 ± 0.90/ 2.12 ± 0.69	0.39
SNP074	rs1335801774	5:83195856	T/G	TT/TG/GG	134	I/M	380/0/0	2.27 ± 1.09/–/–	—
SNP075	rs372774793	5:83195857	G/C	GG/GC/CC	135	A/P	358/22/0	2.27 ± 1.06/2.25 ± 1.46/–	0.92
SNP076	rs1384832919	5:83195863	A/G	AA/AG/GG	137	N/D	368/12/0	2.27 ± 1.10/2.00 ± 0.59/–	0.38
SNP077	rs56334522	5:83195865	T/G	TT/TG/GG	137	N/K	366/13/1	2.26 ± 1.10/2.53 ± 0.80/1.34b	0.89
SNP078	rs370037164	5:83195869	G/A	GG/GA/AA	139	A/T	292/84/4	2.28 ± 1.06/2.23 ± 1.18/ 2.49 ± 0.83	0.89

No.	SNP ID	Chr: bp	Alleles (x/y)[a]	Genotypes (xx/xy/yy)[b]	Amino acid position	Amino acid change	$N_{xx/xy/yy}$[c]	Adducts (mean ± SD)	P^d
SNP079	rs374892515	5:83195876	A/G	AA/AG/GG	141	N/S	380/0/0	2.27 ± 1.09/−/−	—
SNP080	rs28360136	5:83195878	G/C	GG/GC/CC	142	E/Q	254/111/15	2.33 ± 1.10/2.12 ± 1.02/2.35 ± 1.26	0.21
SNP081	rs553111266	5:83195883	C/A	CC/CA/AA	143	H/Q	373/7/0	2.26 ± 1.09/2.75 ± 1.07/−	0.24
SNP082	rs1022211508	5:83195897	A/G	AA/AG/GG	148	N/S	342/38/0	2.30 ± 1.11/2.03 ± 0.79/−	0.15
SNP083	rs757278630	5:83195903	G/A	GG/GA/AA	150	R/K	378/12/0	2.27 ± 1.09/1.99 ± 1.01/−	0.36
SNP084	rs1375107569	5:83195905	C/T	CC/CT/TT	151	L/F	380/0/0	2.27 ± 1.09/−/−	—
SNP085	rs1277864722	5:83195912	G/A	GG/GA/AA	153	R/K	355/25/0	2.29 ± 1.01/1.93 ± 0.72/−	0.02
SNP086	rs745751715	5:83195922	T/G	TT/TG/GG	156	N/K	289/89/2	2.28 ± 1.04/2.25 ± 1.23/2.12 ± 1.83	0.97
SNP087	rs1201811742	5:83195924	A/C	AA/AC/CC	157	D/A	353/26/1	2.24 ± 1.07/2.67 ± 1.22/2.72[e]	0.13
SNP088	rs369499884	5:83195930	A/G	AA/AG/GG	159	Q/R	367/13/0	2.28 ± 1.09/2.03 ± 1.08/−	0.42
SNP089	rs372493882	5:83195933	G/T	GG/GT/TT	160	G/V	250/30/0	2.29 ± 1.10/2.07 ± 0.97/−	0.30
SNP090	rs1156689163	5:83203553	T/G	TT/TG/GG	162	F/V	380/0/0	2.27 ± 1.09/−/−	—
SNP091	rs1325151692	5:83203554	T/A	TT/TA/AA	162	F/Y	345/95/0	2.26 ± 1.04/2.39 ± 1.46/−	0.49
SNP092	rs375731584	5:83203566	T/G	TT/TG/GG	166	V/G	355/25/0	2.25 ± 1.09/2.48 ± 0.97/−	0.32
SNP093	rs1359488275	5:83203568	A/T	AA/AT/TT	167	S/C	380/0/0	2.27 ± 1.09/−/−	—
SNP094	rs753605351	5:83203575	A/C	AA/AC/CC	169	K/T	385/15/0	2.26 ± 1.10/2.40 ± 0.89/−	0.64
SNP095	rs1376295451	5:83203587	A/T	AA/AT/TT	173	E/V	340/40/0	2.28 ± 1.10/2.18 ± 0.98/−	0.58
SNP096	rs778422015	5:83203595	C/T	CC/CT/TT	176	L/F	380/0/0	2.27 ± 1.09/−/−	—
SNP097	rs777300742	5:83203599	A/G	AA/AG/GG	177	Y/C	354/26/0	2.26 ± 1.08/2.39 ± 1.24/−	0.57
SNP098	rs140143447	5:83203604	C/T	CC/CT/TT	179	R/W	372/8/0	2.28 ± 1.09/1.69 ± 0.56/−	0.13
SNP099	rs771544881	5:83203605	G/A	GG/GA/AA	179	R/Q	380/0/0	2.27 ± 1.09/−/−	—

No.	SNP ID	Chr: bp	Alleles (x/y)[a]	Genotypes (xx/xy/yy)[b]	Amino acid position	Amino acid change	$N_{xx/xy/yy}$[c]	Adducts (mean ± SD)	P[d]
SNP100	rs777195630	5:83203607	T/C	TT/TC/CC	180	F/L	354/26/0	2.22 ± 1.04/2.89 ± 1.51/–	0.04
SNP101	rs1379408635	5:83203610	A/T	AA/AT/TT	181	I/F	338/41/1	2.26 ± 1.07/2.37 ± 1.22/2.98[e]	0.67
SNP102	rs1199884817	5:83203611	T/C	TT/TC/CC	181	I/T	345/35/–	2.27 ± 1.08/2.26 ± 1.20/–	0.96
SNP103	rs1018879495	5:83203623	A/T	AA/AT/TT	185	N/I	366/14/0	2.27 ± 1.09/2.18 ± 0.94/–	0.76
SNP104	rs1482288279	5:83203635	C/T	CC/CT/TT	189	T/I	380/0/0	2.27 ± 1.09/–/–	—
SNP105	rs770217916	5:83203641	T/A	TT/TA/AA	191	I/N	341/38/1	2.28 ± 1.10/2.10 ± 0.90/4.31b	0.11
SNP106	rs775587299	5:83203644	G/T	GG/GT/TT	192	R/I	351/24/5	2.28 ± 1.09/2.24 ± 1.16/ 1.94 ± 0.64	0.79
SNP107	rs763186148	5:83203652	C/T	CC/CT/TT	195	H/Y	328/50/2	2.28 ± 1.11/2.23 ± 0.97/2.18 ± 0.47	0.95
SNP108	rs1173748737	5:83203653	A/G	AA/AG/GG	195	H/R	380/0/0	2.27 ± 1.09/–/–	—
SNP109	rs764109844	5:83203654	T/G	TT/TG/GG	195	H/Q	380/0/0	2.27 ± 1.09/–/–	—
SNP110	rs1458486332	5:83203659	A/G	AA/AG/GG	197	K/R	380/0/0	2.27 ± 1.09/–/–	—
SNP111	rs1263079073	5:83203676	C/G	CC//CG/GG	203	Q/E	355/25/–	2.28 ± 1.09/2.18 ± 1.09/–	0.69
SNP112	rs766287987	5:83203678	A/T	AA/AT/TT	203	Q/H	357/16/7	2.11 ± 0.89/4.15 ± 0.77/5.78 ± 1.17	1.05×10^{-59}
SNP113	rs778723397	5:83203683	G/A	GG/GA/AA	205	R/Q	365/15/0	2.29 ± 1.09/1.87 ± 0.97/–	0.15
SNP114	rs777199609	5:83203691	G/C	GG/GC/CC	208	D/H	292/86/2	2.22 ± 1.05/2.43 ± 1.18/ 2.86 ± 1.40	0.20
SNP115	rs1224705261	5:83203694	A/G	AA/AG/GG	209	I/V	380/0/0	2.27 ± 1.09/–/–	—
SNP116	rs201604424	5:83203698	A/G	AA/AG/GG	210	K/R	300/72/8	2.29 ± 1.11/2.15 ± 0.97/2.77 ± 1.03	0.26
SNP117	rs1276157833	5:83203701	A/G	AA/AG/GG	211	Q/R	371/9/0	2.28 ± 1.08/1.82 ± 1.17/–	0.22
SNP118	rs1298401873	5:83203706	G/A	GG/GA/AA	213	G/R	359/21/0	2.29 ± 1.10/1.93 ± 0.87/–	0.14
SNP119	rs746407658	5:83204816	G/A	GG/GA/AA	214	E/K	291/79/10	2.30 ± 1.10/2.22 ± 1.09/1.72 ± 072	0.23

No.	SNP ID	Chr: bp	Alleles (x/y)[a]	Genotypes (xx/xy/yy)[b]	Amino acid position	Amino acid change	$N_{xx/xy/yy}$[c]	Adducts (mean ± SD)	P^d
SNP120	rs969467594	5:83204820	C/G	CC//CG/GG	215	T/S	380/0/0	2.27 ± 1.09/−/−	—
SNP121	rs780330653	5:83204823	C/A	CC/CA/AA	216	A/E	307/61/12	2.24 ± 1.08/2.46 ± 1.19/ 2.06 ± 0.72	0.28
SNP122	rs1348464342	5:83204825	A/G	AA/AG/GG	217	I/V	375/5/0	2.27 ± 1.09/2.46 ± 0.94/−	0.69
SNP123	rs749647860	5:83204828	T/G	TT/TG/GG	218	C/G	358/22/0	2.27 ± 1.08/2.22 ± 1.23/−	0.84
SNP124	rs908326126	5:83204840	A/G	AA/AG/GG	222	T/A	380/0/0	2.27 ± 1.09/−/−	—
SNP125	rs1347664669	5:83204847	A/G	AA/AG/GG	224	D/G	354/26/0	2.26 ± 1.09/2.38 ± 1.12/−	0.58
SNP126	rs866477694	5:83204848	C/A	CC/CA/AA	224	D/E	380/0/0	2.27 ± 1.09/−/−	—
SNP127	rs774555675	5:83204850	G/A	GG/GA/AA	225	R/Q	348/32/0	2.28 ± 1.10/2.11 ± 0.97/−	0.39
SNP128	rs748307585	5:83204852	G/A	GG/GA/AA	226	D/N	285/86/9	2.29 ± 1.09/2.20 ± 1.09/2.37 ± 1.12	0.77
SNP129	rs368106955	5:83204867	G/A	GG/GA/AA	231	E/K	380/0/0	2.27 ± 1.09/−/−	—
SNP130	rs140579916	5:83204874	C/A	CC/CA/AA	233	T/N	342/38/0	2.26 ± 1.07/2.39 ± 1.23/2.27 ± 1.09	0.46
SNP131	rs762812825	5:83204882	G/A	GG/GA/AA	236	E/K	357/21/2	2.26 ± 1.08/2.43 ± 1.33/ 2.23 ± 0.26	0.78
SNP132	rs574436773	5:83204897	A/T	AA/AT/TT	241	T/S	376/4/0	2.27 ± 1.09/1.96 ± 1.19/−	0.57
SNP133	rs542187236	5:83204901	A/G	AA/AG/GG	242	D/G	380/0/0	2.27 ± 1.09/−/−	—
SNP134	rs1013137284	5:83204904	T/A	TT/TA/AA	243	L/H	374/6/0	2.26 ± 1.09/3.00 ± 0.56/−	0.10
SNP135	rs1261641487	5:83204906	T/C	TT/TC/CC	244	S/P	380/0/0	2.27 ± 1.09/−/−	—
SNP136	rs767176080	5:83204907	C/T	CC/CT/TT	244	S/F	376/6/0	2.27 ± 1.09/1.71 ± 0.34/−	0.31
SNP137	rs371824973	5:83204910	G/A	GG/GA/AA	245	G/E	380/0/0	2.27 ± 1.09/−/−	—
SNP138	rs3734091	5:83204915	G/T	GG/GT/TT	247	A/S	296/46/38	2.09 ± 0.97/2.79 ± 1.49/ 3.08 ± 0.77	1.20×10^{-70}
SNP139	rs141122119	5:83258556	A/G	AA/AG/GG	258	I/V	363/17/0	2.28 ± 1.10/2.04 ± 0.82/−	0.37

No.	SNP ID	Chr: bp	Alleles (x/y)[a]	Genotypes (xx/xy/yy)[b]	Amino acid position	Amino acid change	$N_{xx/xy/yy}$[c]	Adducts (mean ± SD)	P^d
SNP140	rs138837678	5:83258665	A/C	AA/AC/CC	294	Q/P	372/8/0	2.28 ± 1.09/1.98 ± 0.79/–	0.45
SNP141	rs61749611	5:83353207	A/C	AA/AC/CC	324	N/H	348/30/2	2.27 ± 1.09/2.21 ± 1.14/2.53 ± 0.16	0.90
SNP142	rs148273490	5:83353231	G/C	GG/GC/CC	332	D/H	356/24/0	2.29 ± 1.10/2.02 ± 0.86/–	0.25
SNP143	rs141304949	5:83353238	T/C	TT/TC/CC	334	I/T	344/35/1	2.26 ± 1.07/2.39 ± 1.26/1.37[e]	0.58

[a]*x/y represents wild-type allele/ variant type allele.*
[b]*xx/xy/yy represents wild-type homozygote/heterozygote/variant-type homozygote.*
[c]*$N_{xx/xy/yy}$ represents the number of subjects with xx genotype, the number of subjects with xy genotype, and the number of subjects with yy genotype.*
[d]*P values are calculated using t-test or one-way analysis of variance.*
[e]*SD is not determined.*
** SD for genotype yy is not determined and P-value is used for genotypes xx and xy.*

Table 2.
The association between SNPs in the coding region of XRCC4 and AFB1-DNA adducts in tissues with hepatocellular carcinoma.

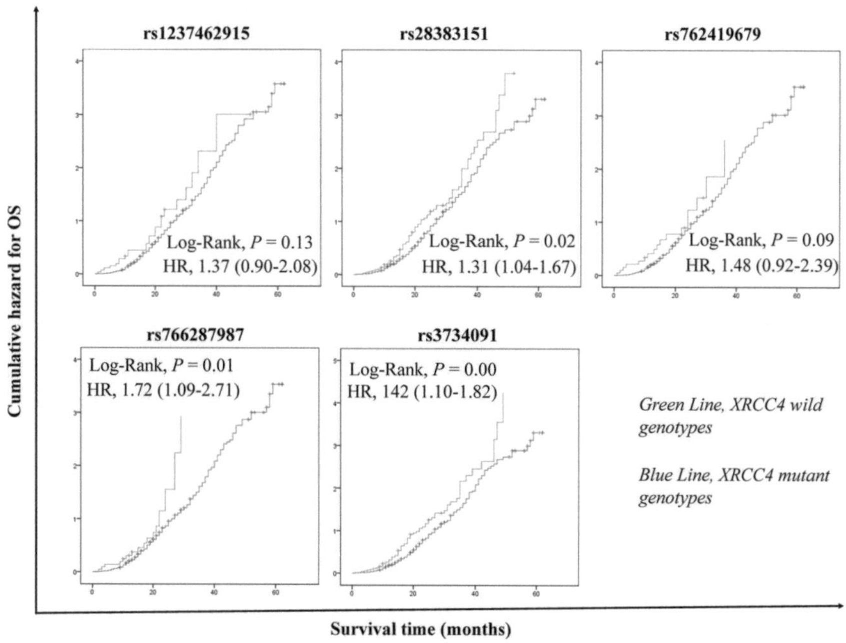

Figure 1.
XRCC4 GSNPs significantly correlating with the overall survival (OS) of hepatocellular carcinoma (HCC). Cumulative hazard function was plotted by Kaplan-Meier methodology, and P *value was calculated with two-sided log-rank tests. The relative hazard ratio (HR) values for genotypes were calculated using multivariable Cox regression models (with all significant variables) based on forward-step method with likelihood ratio test.*

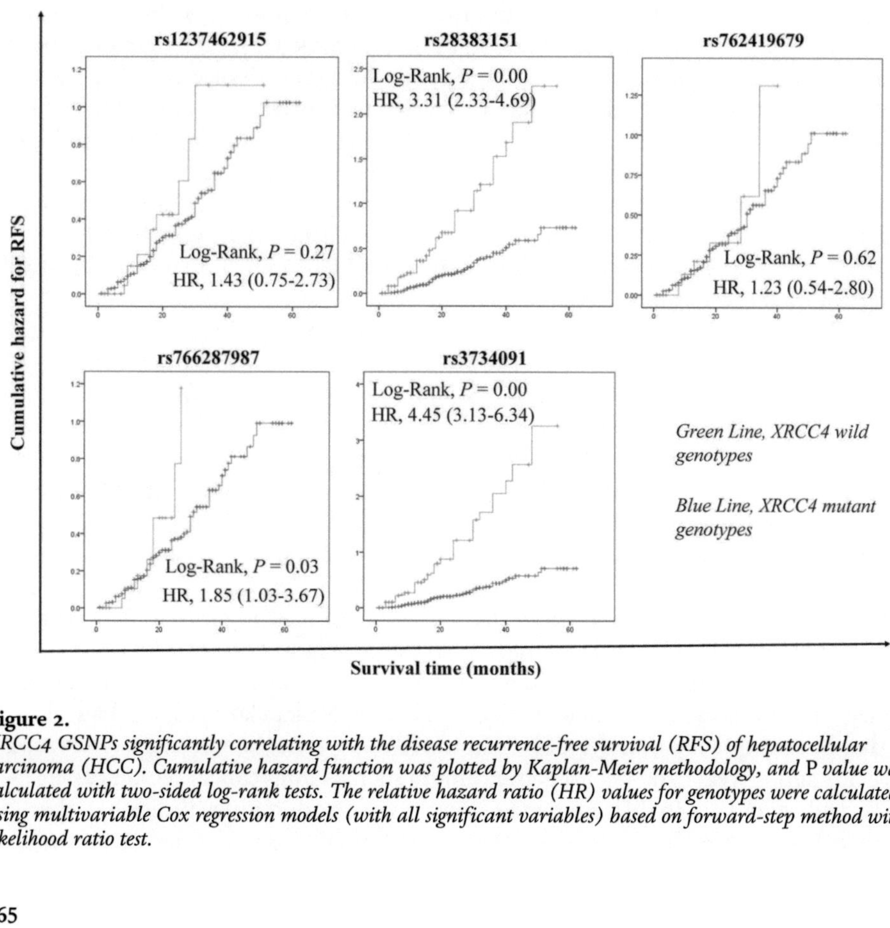

Figure 2.
XRCC4 GSNPs significantly correlating with the disease recurrence-free survival (RFS) of hepatocellular carcinoma (HCC). Cumulative hazard function was plotted by Kaplan-Meier methodology, and P *value was calculated with two-sided log-rank tests. The relative hazard ratio (HR) values for genotypes were calculated using multivariable Cox regression models (with all significant variables) based on forward-step method with likelihood ratio test.*

genotypes (XX genotypes), the mutant genotypes (including XY and YY genotypes) of rs28383151, rs766287987, and rs3734091 polymorphisms increased cumulative hazard for OS [HR = 1.31 (1.04–1.67), 1.72 (1.09–2.71), and 1.42 (1.10–1.82), respectively] (**Figure 1**). For RFS, the corresponding hazard values were 3.31 (2.33–4.69) for rs28383151, 1.85 (1.03–3.67) for rs766287987, and 4.45 (3.13–6.34) for rs3734091, respectively (**Figure 2**).

4. Discussion

In this study, we investigated the association between the GSNPs in the coding regions of XRCC4 gene and the toxic effects of AFB1 on the liver. We found that five XRCC4 GSNPs, including rs1237462915 (at codon 38), rs28383151 (at codon 56), rs762419679 (at codon 127), rs766287987 (at codon 203), and rs3734091 (at codon 247), significantly increased the amount of AFB1-DNA adducts in tissues with HCC (2.07–2.15 μmol/mol DNA for XY genotypes and 2.64–4.33 μmol/mol DNA for YY genotypes, respectively) and progressed the cumulative hazard of AFB1 hepatic toxicity.

AFB1 acts as a type of human chemical toxicant, and the toxic effects of this toxicant are characterized by organophilism (mainly causing hepatic damage), genic toxicity (mainly inducing DNA damages such as hotspot mutation at codon 249 of TP53 gene, AFB1-DNA adduct formation, and so on), and carcinogenicity (mainly resulting in HCC) [6–8]. Among the hepatic toxicity of AFB1, the formation of AFB1-DNA adducts in hepatic cells is a key step during the metabolism of this toxicant [9–14]. Evidence from molecular epidemiological studies and clinical studies has proved that the levels of AFB1-DNA adducts in the hepatic tissues are positively associated with the levels and time of AFB1 exposure [3, 24, 26–44]. This is indicative of AFB1-DNA adduct acting as the biomarker for AFB1's toxic capacity in the liver. In this study, AFB1-DNA adduct in the tumor tissues with HCC was used to evaluate hepatic toxicity related to AFB1, mainly because normal liver tissue samples cannot be obtained. Our results exhibited HCC tumor samples from high AFB1 exposure areas have an average adduct amount of 2.27 ± 1.09 μmol/mol DNA. Supporting our findings, several studies from high AFB1 exposure areas Nanning and Tiandong, China, have also shown the similar level of DNA adducts [4, 5, 26, 27, 37, 39, 45]. Taken together, the amount of AFB1-DNA adducts should be able to reflect the hepatic toxic potential of AFB1.

XRCC4, a key gene in the V(D)J recombination repair pathway, is located at 5q14.2 and consists of 13 exons (PubMed). Normally, XRCC4 is mainly expressed in genital meatus, alimentary tract, and lymphoid tissue; however, its expression will noticeably increase in other tissues such as the skin and liver under the condition of in vitro and in vivo injuries. This gene's encoding protein plays a vital role in both NHEJ and the completion of V(D)J recombination via acting as a scaffold protein for DNA ligase IV and DNA-PK in the repair of DNA DSBs [15, 19]. Mutations in XRCC4, including GSNPs and other non-GSNPs variants, can cause endocrine dysfunction, microcephaly, short stature, and diseases [16, 21]. With the development of human Geno projects, more than 1000 GSNPs are identified. Among these GSNPs, we focused on genetic alterations in the coding regions of XRCC4, mainly because they will result in missense mutations and ultimately cause the structure damage and function deficiency of XRCC4 protein. Molecular epidemiological studies have displayed that the GSNPs in the XRCC4 genes can increase DNA repair capacity and increase the risk of some tumors such as lung cancer, colon cancer, HCC, and so on [21, 46–51]. Evidence from in vitro and in vivo studies has also proved that XRCC4 GSNPs increase the amount of DNA damage and induce more gene mutations [23, 24, 26, 27]. In our study, we tested the genotypic distributions of all known GSNPs in the coding region of XRCC4 in liver tumor tissues. Five positive GSNPs were identified, and they result in the change of amino acid D to Y at codon 38 for rs1237462915, A to T at codon 56 for rs28383151, I to T at codon 127 for rs762419679, Q to H at codon 203 for rs766287987, and A to S at codon 247 for rs3734091, respectively. Although evidence that several other GSNPs, including rs761695470, rs758779099, rs144653114, rs1277864722, and rs777195630, increased the amounts of AFB1-DNA adducts was not statistically significant according to our defined threshold value, their effects should not be neglected because small-size samples may underestimate values.

Because the toxic effects of AFB1 also modify the prognosis of patients with HCC [26, 27, 33, 52, 53], we accomplished patients' survival analyses on the basis of the cumulative risk models and found only rs28383151, rs766287987, and rs3734091 polymorphisms shortened HCC cases' OS and RFS. Supporting our findings, several previous reports have proved that XRCC4 GSNPs can alter the levels of XRCC4 mRNA and protein expression and dysregulation of XRCC4 expression increasing the amount of AFB1-DNA adducts and mutative risk of TP53 gene [23, 24, 26, 27].

To conclude, this study is the first report investigating the modified function of XRCC4 GSNPs on AFB1's hepatic toxicity. Our findings suggest that the GSNPs in the coding regions of XRCC4 gene, like rs1237462915, rs28383151, rs762419679, rs766287987, and rs3734091, may alter the DNA repair capacity of DNA damage induced by AFB1. If these individuals with mutant genotypes of these GSNPs decrease their exposure to AFB1, they will be free from toxic effects of AFB1 on hepatic damage. Several limitations should be focused for our study. First, relatively small-size samples may underestimate the effects of XRCC4 GSNPs on AFB1 hepatic toxicity. Second, the hospital-based design may result in selective bias. Third, we only accomplished the cumulative risk analyses but not the cumulative survival analyses. Finally, we did not finish functional and mechanical analyses. Thus, XRCC4 GSNPs may be valuable biomarkers for predicting the toxic effects of AFB1 on the liver once the present findings were proved by larger samples and toxic function analyses.

Acknowledgements

We thank Dr. Qiu-Xiang Liang, Dr. Yun Yi, Dr. Yun Xia, Dr. Yong-Zhi Huang, and Dr. Yuan-Feng Zhou for sample collection and management and Dr. Hua Huang for molecular biochemical technique. We also thank all members of the Department of Medical Test and Infective Control, Affiliated Hospital of Youjiang Medical University for Nationalities for their help.

Conflicts of interest and source of funding

The authors declare no competing financial interests. This study was supported in part by the National Natural Science Foundation of China (Nos. 81860489, 81760502, 81572353, and 81660495), the Natural Science Foundation of Guangxi (Nos. 2018GXNSFAA281043, 2017GXNSFAA198002, and 2017GXNSFGA198002), Research Program of Guangxi "Zhouyue Scholar" (No. 2017-38), Research Program of Guangxi Specially Invited Expert (No. 2017-6th), "12th Five-Year" Planning Program of Guangxi Education Science (No. 2015C397), Innovative Program of Guangxi Graduate Education (No. JGY2015139), Research Program of Guangxi Clinic Research Center of Hepatobiliary Diseases (No. AD17129025), and Open

Research Program from Molecular Immunity Study Room Involving in Acute and Severe Diseases in Guangxi Colleges and Universities (Nos. kfkt20160062 and kfkt20160063).

Abbreviations

AFB1	aflatoxin B1
CI	confidence interval
GSNPs	the genetic single-nucleotide polymorphisms
HCC	hepatocellular carcinoma
HR	hazard ratio
OS	overall survival
RFS	disease recurrence-free survival
XRCC4	X-ray repair cross complementing 4

Author details

Yan Deng[1,2]†, Xue-Min Wu[1,3]†, Xiao-Ying Huang[1,3]† and Xi-Dai Long[1,3]*

1 Department of Pathology, The Affiliated Hospital of Youjiang Medical University for Nationalities, Baise, China

2 Department of Epidemiology, Youjiang Medical University for Nationalities, Baise, China

3 Centra of Pathological Diagnosis and Research, The Affiliated Tumor Hospital, Guangxi Medical University, Nanning, China

*Address all correspondence to: sjtulongxd@263.net

† These authors contributed equally.

References

[1] Rushing BR, Selim MI. Adduction to arginine detoxifies aflatoxin B1 by eliminating genotoxicity and altering in vitro toxicokinetic profiles. Oncotarget. 2018;**9**:4559-4570. DOI: 10.18632/oncotarget.23382

[2] Liu W, Wang L, Zheng C, Liu L, Wang J, Li D, et al. Microcystin-LR increases genotoxicity induced by aflatoxin B1 through oxidative stress and DNA base excision repair genes in human hepatic cell lines. Environmental Pollution. 2018;**233**: 455-463. DOI: 10.1016/j.envpol.2017.10.067

[3] Wang XZ, Huang XY, Yao JG, Wang C, Xia Q, Long XD. Genetic polymorphisms in ataxin-3 and liver cirrhosis risk related to aflatoxin B1. Oncotarget. 2018;**9**:27321-27332. DOI: 10.18632/oncotarget.24535

[4] Long XD, Deng Y, Huang XY, Yao JG, Su QY, Wu XM, et al. Molecular mechanisms of hepatocellular carcinoma related to aflatoxins: An update. In: Rodrigo L, editor. Liver Research and Clinical Management. 1st ed. Vol. 1. Rijeka: IntechOpen; 2018. pp. 113-136. DOI: 10.5772/intechopen.72883

[5] Wu XM, Xi ZF, Lu J, Wang XZ, Zhang TQ, Huang XY, et al. Genetic single nucleotide polymorphisms (GSNPs) in the DNA repair genes and hepatocellular carcinoma related to aflatoxin B1 among Guangxiese population. In: Parine NR, editor. Genetic Polymorphisms. Vol. 1. Rijeka: IntechOpen; 2017. pp. 97-119. DOI: 10.5772/intechopen.69530

[6] Ellis WO, Smith JP, Simpson BK, Oldham JH. Aflatoxins in food: Occurrence, biosynthesis, effects on organisms, detection, and methods of control. Critical Reviews in Food Science and Nutrition. 1991;**30**:403-439. DOI: 10.1080/10408399109527551

[7] Park DL, Rua SM Jr. Biological evaluation of aflatoxins and metabolites in animal tissues. Drug Metabolism Reviews. 1990;**22**:871-890. DOI: 10.3109/03602539008991476

[8] Schoental R. Aflatoxins. Annual Review of Pharmacology. 1967;**7**: 343-356. DOI: 10.1146/annurev.pa.07.040167.002015

[9] Zuberi Z, Eeza MNH, Matysik J, Berry JP, Alia A. NMR-based metabolic profiles of intact Zebrafish embryos exposed to aflatoxin B1 recapitulates hepatotoxicity and supports possible neurotoxicity. Toxins (Basel). 2019;**11**: 258. DOI: 10.3390/toxins11050258

[10] Zhou J, Tang L, Wang JS. Assessment of the adverse impacts of aflatoxin B1 on gut-microbiota dependent metabolism in F344 rats. Chemosphere. 2019;**217**:618-628. DOI: 10.1016/j.chemosphere.2018.11.044

[11] Singh C, Prakash C, Mishra P, Tiwari KN, Mishra SK, More RS, et al. Hepatoprotective efficacy of *Premna integrifolia* L. leaves against aflatoxin B1-induced toxicity in mice. Toxicon. 2019; **166**:88-100. DOI: 10.1016/j.toxicon.2019.05.014

[12] Rotimi OA, Rotimi SO, Goodrich JM, Adelani IB, Agbonihale E, Talabi G. Time-course effects of acute aflatoxin B1 exposure on hepatic mitochondrial lipids and oxidative stress in rats. Frontiers in Pharmacology. 2019; **10**:467. DOI: 10.3389/fphar.2019.00467

[13] Huang B, Mu P, Chen X, Tang S, Ye W, Zhu W, et al. Aflatoxin B1 induces S phase arrest by upregulating the expression of p21 via MYC, PLK1 and PLD1. Biochemical Pharmacology.

2019;**166**:108-119. DOI: 10.1016/j.bcp.2019.05.008

[14] Ferreira RG, Cardoso MV, de Souza Furtado KM, Espindola KMM, Amorim RP, Monteiro MC. Epigenetic alterations caused by aflatoxin b1: A public health risk in the induction of hepatocellular carcinoma. Translational Research. 2019;**204**:51-71. DOI: 10.1016/j.trsl.2018.09.001

[15] Wu CN, Liang SY, Tsai CW, Bau DT. The role of XRCC4 in carcinogenesis and anticancer drug discovery. Recent Patents on Anti-Cancer Drug Discovery. 2008;**3**: 209-219. DOI: 10.2174/157489208786242304

[16] Pastwa E, Blasiak J. Non-homologous DNA end joining. Acta Biochimica Polonica. 2003;**50**:891-908. DOI: 035004891

[17] Wen Y, Dai G, Wang L, Fu K, Zuo S. Silencing of XRCC4 increases radiosensitivity of triple-negative breast cancer cells. Bioscience Reports. 2019; **39**:BSR20180893. DOI: 10.1042/BSR20180893

[18] Nishikubo K, Izumi Y, Matsumoto Y, Fujii K, Matsuo K, Yokoya A. Structural analysis of DNA repair protein Xrcc4 applying circular dichroism in an aqueous solution. Radiation Protection Dosimetry. 2019; **183**:36-39. DOI: 10.1093/rpd/ncy275

[19] Liu F, Fan Z, Song N, Han M, Yan M, Guo LH, et al. XRCC4, which is inhibited by PFDA, regulates DNA damage repair and cell chemosensitivity. Journal of Cellular Biochemistry. 2019;**120**:12665-12676. DOI: 10.1002/jcb.28534

[20] Kitagawa M, Someya M, Hasegawa T, Mikami T, Asaishi K, Hasegawa T, et al. Influence of XRCC4 expression by breast cancer cells on ipsilateral recurrence after breast-conserving therapy. Strahlentherapie und Onkologie. 2019;**195**:648-658. DOI: 10.1007/s00066-019-01468-z

[21] Garcia JA, Kalacas NA, Sy Ortin T, Ramos MC, Albano PM. XRCC4 c.1394G>T single nucleotide polymorphisms and breast cancer risk among Filipinos. Asian Pacific Journal of Cancer Prevention. 2019;**20**: 1097-1101. DOI: 10.31557/APJCP.2019.20.4.1097

[22] Enguita-Marruedo A, Martin-Ruiz M, Garcia E, Gil-Fernandez A, Parra MT, Viera A, et al. Transition from a meiotic to a somatic-like DNA damage response during the pachytene stage in mouse meiosis. PLoS Genetics. 2019;**15**:e1007439. DOI: 10.1371/journal.pgen.1007439

[23] Lu J, Wang XZ, Zhang TQ, Huang XY, Yao JG, Wang C, et al. Prognostic significance of XRCC4 expression in hepatocellular carcinoma. Oncotarget. 2017;**8**:87955-87970. DOI: 10.18632/oncotarget.21360

[24] Yao JG, Huang XY, Long XD. Interaction of DNA repair gene polymorphisms and aflatoxin B1 in the risk of hepatocellular carcinoma. International Journal of Clinical and Experimental Pathology. 2014;**7**: 6231-6244. DOI: 10.2016/1936-2625.25337275

[25] Lin ZH, Chen JC, Wang YS, Huang TJ, Wang J, Long XD. DNA repair gene XRCC4 codon 247 polymorphism modified diffusely infiltrating astrocytoma risk and prognosis. International Journal of Molecular Sciences. 2014;**15**:250-260. DOI: 10.3390/ijms15010250

[26] Long XD, Zhao D, Wang C, Huang XY, Yao JG, Ma Y, et al. Genetic polymorphisms in DNA repair genes XRCC4 and XRCC5 and aflatoxin B1-related hepatocellular carcinoma.

Epidemiology. 2013;**24**:671-681. DOI: 10.1097/EDE.0b013e31829d2744

[27] Long XD, Yao JG, Zeng Z, Ma Y, Huang XY, Wei ZH, et al. Polymorphisms in the coding region of X-ray repair complementing group 4 and aflatoxin B1-related hepatocellular carcinoma. Hepatology. 2013;**58**: 171-181. DOI: 10.1002/hep.26311

[28] Huang XY, Yao JG, Huang BC, Ma Y, Xia Q, Long XD. Polymorphisms of a disintegrin and metalloproteinase with thrombospondin motifs 5 and aflatoxin B1-related hepatocellular carcinoma. Cancer Epidemiology, Biomarkers & Prevention. 2016;**25**:334-343. DOI: 10.1158/1055-9965.EPI-15-0774

[29] Wu XM, Xi ZF, Liao P, Huang HD, Huang XY, Wang C, et al. Diagnostic and prognostic potential of serum microRNA-4651 for patients with hepatocellular carcinoma related to aflatoxin B1. Oncotarget. 2017;**8**: 81235-81249. DOI: 10.18632/ oncotarget.16027

[30] Long XD, Huang XY, Yao JG, Liao P, Tang YJ, Ma Y, et al. Polymorphisms in the precursor microRNAs and aflatoxin B1-related hepatocellular carcinoma. Molecular Carcinogenesis. 2016;**55**:1060-1072. DOI: 10.1002/mc.22350

[31] Long XD, Huang HD, Huang XY, Yao JG, Xia Q. XPC codon 939 polymorphism is associated with susceptibility to DNA damage induced by aflatoxin B1 exposure. International Journal of Clinical and Experimental Medicine. 2015;**8**:1197-1204. DOI: PMC4358568

[32] Long XD, Huang HD, Xia Q. The polymorphism of XRCC3 codon 241 and the hotspot mutation in the TP53 gene in hepatocellular carcinoma induced by aflatoxin B1. Journal of Tumor. 2014;**2**:272-277. DOI: 10.6051/ j.issn.1819-6187.2014.02.57

[33] Liu YX, Long XD, Xi ZF, Ma Y, Huang XY, Yao JG, et al. MicroRNA-24 modulates aflatoxin B1-related hepatocellular carcinoma prognosis and tumorigenesis. BioMed Research International. 2014;**2014**:482926. DOI: 10.1155/2014/482926

[34] Long XD, Yao JG, Huang YZ, Huang XY, Ban FZ, Yao LM, et al. DNA repair gene XRCC7 polymorphisms (rs#7003908 and rs#10109984) and hepatocellular carcinoma related to AFB1 exposure among Guangxi population, China. Hepatology Research. 2011;**41**:1085-1093. DOI: 10.1111/j.1872-034X.2011.00866.x

[35] Long XD, Ma Y, Zhou YF, Ma AM, Fu GH. Polymorphism in xeroderma pigmentosum complementation group C codon 939 and aflatoxin B1-related hepatocellular carcinoma in the Guangxi population. Hepatology. 2010;**52**:1301-1309. DOI: 10.1002/ hep.23807

[36] Long XD, Ma Y, Zhou YF, Yao JG, Ban FZ, Huang YZ, et al. XPD codon 312 and 751 polymorphisms, and AFB1 exposure, and hepatocellular carcinoma risk. BMC Cancer. 2009;**9**:400. DOI: 10.1186/1471-2407-9-400

[37] Long XD, Ma Y, Deng ZL. GSTM1 and XRCC3 polymorphisms: Effects on levels of aflatoxin B1-DNA adducts. Chinese Journal of Cancer Research. 2009;**21**:177-184. DOI: DOI. DOI: 10.1007/s11670-009-0177-6

[38] Long XD, Ma Y, Qu de Y, Liu YG, Huang ZQ, Huang YZ, et al. The polymorphism of XRCC3 codon 241 and AFB1-related hepatocellular carcinoma in Guangxi population, China. Annals of Epidemiology. 2008;**18**:572-578. DOI: 10.1016/j.annepidem.2008.03.003

[39] Long XD, Ma Y, Huang HD, Yao JG, Qu de Y, Lu YL. Polymorphism of XRCC1 and the frequency of mutation in codon 249 of the p53 gene in

hepatocellular carcinoma among Guangxi population, China. Molecular Carcinogenesis. 2008;**47**:295-300. DOI: 10.1002/mc.20384

[40] Long XD, Ma Y, Deng ZL, Huang YZ, Wei NB. Association of the Thr241Met polymorphism of DNA repair gene XRCC3 with genetic susceptibility to AFB1-related hepatocellular carcinoma in Guangxi population. Zhonghua Yi Xue Yi Chuan Xue Za Zhi. 2008;**25**:268-271. DOI: 940625058

[41] Long XD, Ma Y, Wei YP, Deng ZL. The polymorphisms of GSTM1, GSTT1, HYL1*2, and XRCC1, and aflatoxin B1-related hepatocellular carcinoma in Guangxi population, China. Hepatology Research. 2006;**36**:48-55. DOI: 10.1016/j.hepres.2006.06.004

[42] Long XD, Ma Y, Wei YP, Deng ZL. X-ray repair cross-complementing group 1 (XRCC1) Arg 399 Gln polymorphism and aflatoxin B1 (AFB1)-related hepatocellular carcinoma (HCC) in Guangxi population. Chinese Journal of Cancer Research. 2005;**17**:17-21. DOI: 10.1007/s11670-005-0004-7

[43] Long XD, Ma Y, Wei YP, Deng ZL. A study about the association of detoxication gene GSTM1 polymorphism and the susceptibility to aflatoxin B1-related hepatocellular carcinoma. Zhonghua Gan Zang Bing Za Zhi. 2005;**13**:668-670. DOI: PMID16174455

[44] Long XD, Ma Y, Wei YP, Deng ZL. Study on the detoxication gene gstM1-gstT1-null and susceptibility to aflatoxin B1 related hepatocellular carcinoma in Guangxi. Zhonghua Liu Xing Bing Xue Za Zhi. 2005;**26**:777-781. DOI: PMID16536303

[45] Xia Q, Huang XY, Xue F, Zhang JJ, Zhai B, Kong DC, et al. Genetic polymorphisms of DNA repair genes and DNA repair capacity related to aflatoxin b1 (AFB1)-induced DNA damages. In: Chen C, editor. New Research Directions in DNA Repair. 1st ed. Rijeka: IntechOpen; 2013. pp. 377-412. DOI: 10.5772/53967

[46] Jin D, Zhang M, Hua H. Impact of polymorphisms in DNA repair genes XPD, hOGG1 and XRCC4 on colorectal cancer risk in a Chinese Han population. Bioscience Reports. 2019;**39**:BSR20181074. DOI: 10.1042/BSR20181074

[47] Makkoch J, Praianantathavorn K, Sopipong W, Chuaypen N, Tangkijvanich P, Payungporn S. Genetic variations in XRCC4 (rs1805377) and ATF6 (rs2070150) are not associated with hepatocellular carcinoma in Thai patients with hepatitis B virus infection. Asian Pacific Journal of Cancer Prevention. 2016;**17**:591-595. DOI: 10.7314/APJCP.2016.17.2.591

[48] Shao N, Li J, Xu B, Wang Y, Lu X, Feng N. Role of the functional variant (-652T>G) in the XRCC4 promoter in prostate cancer. Molecular Biology Reports. 2014;**41**:7463-7470. DOI: 10.1007/s11033-014-3636-1

[49] Jung SW, Park NH, Shin JW, Park BR, Kim CJ, Lee JE, et al. Polymorphisms of DNA repair genes in Korean hepatocellular carcinoma patients with chronic hepatitis B: Possible implications on survival. Journal of Hepatology. 2012;**57**:621-627. DOI: 10.1016/j.jhep.2012.04.039

[50] Yu H, Zhao H, Wang LE, Han Y, Chen WV, Amos CI, et al. An analysis of single nucleotide polymorphisms of 125 DNA repair genes in the Texas genome-wide association study of lung cancer with a replication for the XRCC4 SNPs. DNA Repair (Amst). 2011;**10**:398-407. DOI: 10.1016/j.dnarep.2011.01.005

[51] Long XD, Ma Y, Huang YZ, Yi Y, Liang QX, Ma AM, et al. Genetic polymorphisms in DNA repair genes XPC, XPD, and XRCC4, and

susceptibility to *Helicobacter pylori* infection-related gastric antrum adenocarcinoma in Guangxi population, China. Molecular Carcinogenesis. 2010; **49**:611-618. DOI: 10.1002/mc.20630

[52] Engin AB, Engin A. DNA damage checkpoint response to aflatoxin B1. Environmental Toxicology and Pharmacology. 2019;**65**:90-96. DOI: 10.1016/j.etap.2018.12.006

[53] Kensler TW, Roebuck BD, Wogan GN, Groopman JD. Aflatoxin: A 50-year odyssey of mechanistic and translational toxicology. Toxicological Sciences. 2011;**120**(Suppl 1):S28-S48. DOI: 10.1093/toxsci/kfq283

Section 4

The Detoxification of Aflatoxin B1

Chapter 10

Decontamination of Aflatoxin B1

Qian Yang

Abstract

Aflatoxins are a class of highly toxic carcinogenic mycotoxins by food contaminant *Aspergillus* fungi: *Aspergillus flavus* and *Aspergillus parasiticus*. Aflatoxins are classified into four compounds: aflatoxin B1 (AFB1), aflatoxin B2 (AFB2), aflatoxin G1 (AFG1), and aflatoxin G2 (AFG2), while AFB1 is the most potent carcinogenic agent associated with hepatocellular carcinoma (HCC). *Aspergillus* fungi is ubiquitously found in the soil and contaminates the crops such as maize, groundnuts, rice, and so on. Prevention of aflatoxin contamination, detection and degradation of *Aspergillus* fungi contamination, and the concentration of AFB1 in the foodstuffs are of the primary task to prevent health problems from aflatoxin. Here, the different ways are summarized to degrade or decontaminate the aflatoxins available with the foods. Traditional decontamination of aflatoxin includes physical (heat and irradiation), biological, and chemical treatments. However, these traditional aflatoxin decontamination technologies are not enough to remove the aflatoxin from the foods. Recently, some novel processing approached have been explored to achieve full degradation of the aflatoxin available with the foodstuffs, like microwave heating, gamma and electron beam irradiation, pulsed light, electrolyzed water, cold plasma, and so on. Decontamination mechanism, degradation efficiency, advantages, and limitations of these new technologies shall be discussed herein.

Keywords: aflatoxin B1, detoxification, toxicity, decontamination, biological degradation

1. Introduction

Mycotoxins are low-molecular-weight nature products as secondary metabolites by filamentous fungi or mold, which display overlapping toxicities to invertebrates, plants, and microorganism. The term mycotoxin was coined in 1962 in the aftermath of unusual veterinary crisis close to London, England, where nearly 100,000 turkey poultry died. It came out that was linked to peanut meal contaminated by aflatoxins. Now, more than 300 mycotoxins are found; however, only very few mycotoxins caught scientists' eyeball, which have been proven to be carcinogenic and toxic.

Human food can be contaminated with mycotoxins during storage. One of the principal classes of highly toxic carcinogenic mycotoxins is the metabolite of *Aspergillus flavus* and *Aspergillus parasiticus* aflatoxins [1]. Aflatoxins are classified into such four compounds as aflatoxin B1 (AFB1), aflatoxin B2 (AFB2), aflatoxin G1 (AFG1), and aflatoxin G2 (AFG2) based on their fluorescence under UV light (blue or green), and in the milk it was aflatoxin M1 (AFM1) and aflatoxin M2 (AFM2) which are the metabolites of AFB1 and AFB2, respectively [2–4]. The toxic effect upon the living organisms of aflatoxin decreases in an order B1, G1, B2, and G2 [5]. AFB1 is the most potent carcinogenic agent associated with hepatocellular carcinoma (HCC), one of the most lethal and common cancers in the world, especially in Asia and Africa. The mycotoxin aflatoxin B1 (AFB1), the most notorious liver carcinogen, has been proven to be genotoxic. Epidemiological studies have shown that chronic exposure to aflatoxin B1 in the diet is one of the important factors in the etiology of liver cancer in experimental animal models, including rats and rainbow trouts [6].

Discovery of practical and economical procedure to prevent aflatoxin contamination, detect and degrade *Aspergillus* fungi contamination, and lower the concentration of AFB1 in the foodstuffs is of the primary task to prevent or eliminate the aflatoxin risk.

Aspergillus fungi is ubiquitously found in the soil and contaminates the crops in the field and during storage, such as maize, groundnuts, rice, and so on. Mycotoxins are the low-molecular weight nature products as the secondary metabolites of molds that make the industrial factories lose money resulting from condemnation of contaminated crops. They have been detected in various commodities such as maize, wheat, barley, oilseed, peanut, and beverages made from contaminated grains and other foods. Thus direct exposure to aflatoxin-contaminated commodities may impose a great risk to the consumers.

Unquestionably, prevention is the best method to control mycotoxin contamination. As the result of the high prevalence of AFB1 in the foods, many strategies are being developed to prevent or remove AFB1 contamination. In general, two ways are available to prevent AFB1 from contamination: pre- and postharvest treatment. Pre-harvest techniques are the first barrier to prevent mycotoxin contamination in all kinds of grains or feed. Pre-harvest techniques include the use of genetically altered crops that are resistant to *Aspergillus* infection and environmental stressors, pesticide usage, crop rotation, and timing of planting. Postharvest strategies include physical methods (proper drying, packaging, storage, preservative/pesticide usage). These strategies play the roles as the preventative measures to reduce the chance and the amount of contaminations that are introduced to the crops. However, these strategies fail to prevent the contaminations fully and effectively; thus some postharvest techniques are being developed to degrade or reduce AFB1 contamination. In this review, we aimed to investigate AFB1 decontamination methods, including several traditional strategies, and update some new methods.

2. Physical treatment of aflatoxin removal and detoxification

2.1 Cleaning and segregation of aflatoxins

The first option to reduce aflatoxin is to physically separate the mold-contaminated grains or feed (kernel, seeds, and nuts) from the intact and apparently uncontaminated product. The physical procedure is the safe way not to alter the products significantly, including cleaning, sorting, and handpicking [7]. In the developing countries or economically underdeveloped areas, the people have little or no access to do mycotoxin testing of their foods. Hand sorting is still the primary method to remove AFB1. As compared with other methods including flotation and dehulling of the grains, hand sorting of maize grains boasts <6% of AFB1 and <5% of fumonisin B1. Thus hand sorting of maize grains is being recommended as a last line of defense against mycotoxin exposure among subsistence consumers [8].

2.2 Heating treatment

Aflatoxins are well known to be stable at high temperature. In modern food/feed manufacturing technology, heating treatment is always used to degrade mycotoxins to a certain extent during the processing. Recent studies have shown that AFB1 could be significantly removed at high humidity [9–12]. However, several possible facts are associated with the prediction of the extent of mycotoxin reduction, such as initial mycotoxin concentration, the extent of binding between mycotoxin and food or feed products, heat penetration, moisture content, and processing conditions. Nonetheless, heat treatment to partially reduce the mycotoxin concentration in the food/feed stuffs is still the feasible physiological method because heating technique can be carried out easily at low cost. Extrusion cooking is broadly used in the field of food industry, which is an efficient process in food/feed process. High temperature with short-time extrusion is commonly used in the industry [5].

2.3 Microwave heat treatment

Perez-Flores et al. [13] found that aflatoxin content could be significantly reduced by microwave thermal-alkaline treatment in the traditional Mexico food tortillas. Using extract acidification methods to mimic human stomach digestion procedure to quantify AFB1 concentration, the results indicated that the aflatoxin reduction was almost permanent. However, this thermal-alkaline treatment for tortilla-making could only remove most of AFB; thus some AFB would be left in the food.

2.4 Irradiation treatment

Another most commonly reported physical decontamination technology is γ radiation. The use of γ radiation has been reported on some kinds of food substrates including groundnuts, grains, palm juice, soybean, and animal feed. Irradiating the food products with a γ-ray source is moderately effective with an average percent reduction of 65% at high irradiation dose [14–20]. Gamma irradiation is a promising method to improve the safety and economy of moderately fungi-damaged feedstuffs.

2.5 Electrolyzed water (EOW) treatment

Electrolyzed water treatment is a sort of newly developing skill to treat AFB1-contaminated foods or feeds. The AFB1 was markedly reduced when treated with EOW, particularly with neutral electrolyzed oxidizing water (NEW). The levels of OH that exist in EOW could be the important reason that leads to significant fungicidal efficiencies against *A. flavus*. After 15 min treatment with EOW, AFB1 was mostly degraded [21, 22]. Another study performed by Fan et al. [23] showed that alkaline electrolyzed water (AIEW) could remove AFB1, and its best working condition was at pH 12.2. When 10 ml AIEW with pH 12.2 was added into 5.0 g peanut oil or olive oil, followed by oscillation for 5 min at 20°C, AFB1 removal could reach nearly 100%.

2.6 Pulsed light technology to remove AFB1

Pulsed light has been demonstrated to be an effective decontamination technique capable of destroying bacteria, viruses, fungi, and spores at the surface of food and material [24]. The work of Moreau et al. [25] provides the first demonstration of a nonthermal technology allowing mycotoxin destruction and inactivation of their mutagenic activity. They evaluated that the effectiveness of the pulsed light technology for the degradation of mycotoxins. AFB1 was destroyed around 98% by eight flashes of pulsed light.

3. Chemical treatment to degradation of aflatoxins

The use of chemical additives upon the contaminated foods has been one popular method, especially the additives themselves would be used in the foods.

3.1 Ammonia decontamination treatment

Ammonization of maize, rice, barley, peanuts, and cottonseeds to alter the toxic and carcinogenic effects of aflatoxin contamination has been intensely researched by the scientists from government agencies and universities in the world. Several studies have shown that aflatoxin B1 levels were reduced effectively and permanently by 1 hour ammonia treatment. Treatment with either NH_4OH at high temperature or gaseous NH_3 can effectively reduce aflatoxin B1 content sometimes reaching above 99%. But at lower temperature, for example, at 25°C, AF1B level could not be reduced very well. Their study revealed that the moisture level of the product and holding temperature were the crucial factors to have influence upon the efficacy of aflatoxin decontamination [26–29]. The degradation of AFB1 is ammonization of aflatoxin (AFD1), which has been shown to be far less mutagenic than AFB1.

3.2 Hydrochloric acid (HCl) treatment

Aly and Hathout [30] investigated the effect of hydrochloric acid on AFB1 degradation in contaminated corn gluten under different HCl concentrations. The effect of AFB1 degradation by HCl is in a temperature-, HCl concentration-, and time-dependent manner. During the wet milling process, treating with 1 mol/L HCl at 100°C resulted in degradation of AFB1 by 27.6% after 4 hours and reached to 42.5% after 8 hours. When concentration of HCl increased, the degradation of AFB1 increased, and it will completely degrade AFB in the presence of 5 mol/L HCl after 4 hour at 110°C.

3.3 Lactic acid and citric acid treatment

Previous studies have shown that some organic acids have detoxification ability in treatment of aflatoxin-contaminated foods [31]. Mendez-Albores et al. showed that citric acid and lactic acid have efficiency upon aflatoxin degradation. When the acid concentration increased, the amount of B-aflatoxins decreased, and citric acid has more notable effect upon AFB degradation. Lee et al. also found the reduction rates of AFB1 in 1.0 N citric acid and lactic acid treatment for 18 hour could reach 94.1 and 92.7%, respectively [11].

3.4 Ozonation treatment

Ozonation is another commonly used chemical control method. Ozonolysis at a concentration 6–90 mg/L is effective to degrade AFB1 in short-time treatment. As short as 15 min, all molds were inactivated, and *Aspergillus parasiticus* and *Aspergillus flavus* were isolated from dried figs, while AFB1 was degraded in time-dependent manner in dried figs [32]. Aflatoxins in the peanuts at moisture content of 5% (w/w) were sensitive to ozone and easily degraded when treated with 6.0 mg/l of ozone for half hour at room temperature. The detoxification rates of the total aflatoxins and aflatoxin B1 (AFB1) were 65.8% and 65.9%, respectively [33]. Another study also showed that 89.4% AFB1 in the peanuts was decomposed by ozone with a concentration at 50 mg/L, flow rate 5 L/min for 60 hours [34].

4. Biological treatment to degrade aflatoxins

Using microorganisms or enzymes for biodegradation of aflatoxins is one of the well-known strategies to decrease the level of aflatoxins in the foods or feed products. The methods of biologically based interventions are being actively studied because they are efficient, specific, and environmentally friendly as compared with other non-biological degradation methods.

4.1 Soil bacteria

Many bacteria in the soil are able to degrade aflatoxins. *Flavobacterium aurantiacum* NRRL B-184, a kind of bacteria from the soils and water, showed that it can detoxify aflatoxins in high efficiency. The study from Ciegler et al. [35] showed that *F. aurantiacum* NRRL B-184 removed aflatoxin irreversibly from contaminated milk, oil, peanut butter, peanuts, and corns and partially removed from soybeans. The aflatoxins are not only removed away by *F. aurantiacum* NRRL B-184 but also failed to form any new toxic products. The bacteria was also reported that AFM1 could be removed by it from milk [35]. During monitoring the roles of such metal ions as Cu^{2+}, Mn^{2+}, Zn^{2+}, and other chemical materials on AFB1 degradation by the bacteria, they could increase AFB1 degradation by 10–15% [36–38], suggesting enzymatic system was involved in aflatoxin B1 degradation by *F. aurantiacum*. Except *F. aurantiacum*, other microorganisms, for example, *Nocardia asteroides* and *Corynebacterium rubrum*, are able to detoxify aflatoxin [5, 39]. *Mycobacterium fluoranthenivorans* sp. nov. DSM44556, as a single carbon source from soil of a former coal gas plant, could reduce AFB1 concentration to amounts of 70–80% of the initial concentration within 36–48 hours, and no AFB1 could be detected in 72 hours [40, 41], while the cell-free extracts of *M. fluoranthenivorans* sp. nov. DSM44556 degraded AFB1 more than 90% the initial amount of AFB1 at high temperature within 4 hours and fully degraded in 8 hours [41]. Teniola et al. showed that *N. corynebacterioides* DSM20 151 could degrade more than 90% of AF1B after 24 hours treated in cell-free extracts. Alberts et al. [42] examined that AFB1 was biodegraded by *Rhodococcus erythropolis* in liquid cultures. AFB1 was dramatically degraded to 32% of initial concentration by extracellular extracts from *R. erythropolis* liquid cultures. Thus *F. aurantiacum*, *M. fluoranthenivorans*, and *N. corynebacterioides* could be a potential and promising application because of their potent efficient degradation of AFB1 in the food and feed process.

4.2 Fungi

Fungi can not only produce aflatoxins but also degrade aflatoxin. Such four fungal strains *Aspergillus niger*, *Eurotium herbariorum*, a *Rhizopus* sp., and non-aflatoxin-producing *A. flavus* were able to convert AFB1 to aflatoxicol-A (AFL-A); then AFL-A was converted to aflatoxicol-B (AFL-B) by the actions of medium components or organic acids produced from the fungi. Fungi *Penicillium raistrickii* NRRL 2038 could transform AFB1 to a new compound which is similar to AFB2.

Kusumaningtyas et al. found *Rhizopus oligosporus* was able to inhibit synthesis or to degrade AFB1 when cultured together with AFB1-producing fungi *A. flavus* [43].

4.3 Yeasts and lactic acid bacteria

The mechanism of degradation AFB by yeasts and lactic acid bacteria is due to their adhesion to cell wall components. However the role of yeasts and lactic acid bacteria on AFB is controversial. A few study showed there was no effect of yeasts and lactic bacteria upon aflatoxin [44]. The results showed that high levels of aflatoxins in raw maize would not be degraded during the fermentations in the processing of the west African traditional food "kenkey." Other studies reported very efficient aflatoxin reductions after fermentation. Chu et al. [45] reported that AFB1 concentration dramatically decrease during brewing process, which suggested that *S. cerevisiae* yeasts sorb mycotoxin. AFB1 was detoxified into a nontoxic new fluorescing compound corresponding to AFB2a during yogurt-making and dairy product fermentation [46, 47]. Drinking water with *S. cerevisiae* strain showed a positive protection effect on the relative weight of the liver and histopathological and biochemical parameters when giving the diets contaminated with AFB1 [48].

Lactic acid bacteria have been previously reported to possess antimycotoxigenic activities both in vitro and in vivo. The specific strains of lactic acid bacteria will bind selected dietary aflatoxin contaminants. The ability of 12 *Lactobacillus*, 5 *Bifidobacterium*, and 3 *Lactococcus* bacteria strains to bind AFB1 was investigated by Peltonen et al. [49]. Two *Lactobacillus* amylovorus strains and one *Lactobacillus rhamnosus* strain removed more than 50% AFB1 rapidly after a 72-hour incubation period. Another two lactic acid bacteria *Lactobacillus rhamnosus* strain GG (LBGG) and *L. rhamnosus* strain LC-705 (LC705) can significantly and very quickly remove approximately 80% AFB1 from culture media in both temperature- and bacteria concentration-dependent manner [50]. Kankaanpaa et al. [51] found that the binding of AFB1 to *L. rhamnosus* GG decreased its subsequent adhesion capability to Caco-2 cells, thereupon which the bacteria may reduce the accumulation of aflatoxins in the intestine via increasing aflatoxin-bacteria complex excretion.

4.4 Aflatoxin degradation by enzymes

Some specific enzymes to degrade aflatoxins have been purified from microbial systems. Using enzyme to degrade aflatoxins have some merits, such as avoiding to change flavor or impairing the nutritional value. Motomura et al. [52] investigated the ability of degrading AFB1 in cultured supernatants from 19 fungi and purified 1 enzyme with aflatoxin degradation activity from *P. ostreatus* supernatant. The enzyme showed that AFB could make the best degradation of activity at 25°C with a pH of 4.0–5.0. The novel enzyme could cleave the lactone ring of aflatoxin. Another study showed that an intracellular enzyme, named aflatoxin-detoxifizyme, exhibited detoxification activity on aflatoxin B1 and the optimum activity for the enzyme was at 35°C with a pH of 6.8 [53]. Shcherbakova et al. [54] also proved AFB1 degradation by *Phoma glomerata* PG41 strain was stable and reproducible.

4.5 Cold plasma technology to remove AFB1

In the past cold plasma is used for sterilization of sensitive materials. Lately, much attention has been paid to cold plasma as a new microbial decontamination technology in the food industry. It has the advantages of high efficiency and short treatment time, no residue, and low impact on the quality of treated food products [55, 56]. Recently the degradation of mycotoxins by cold plasma was studied.

It was reported that AFB1 could be successfully removed by 5 s of treatment with microwave-induced argon plasma [57]. Nitrogen gas plasma could efficiently bw degraded to 10% of initial concentration within a 15-min treatment [58]. Low-temperature radio-frequency plasma degraded 88% of AFB1 within 10 min [59]. High-voltage atmospheric cold plasma (HVACP) is a novel nonthermal decontamination technology that has the potential to be used in the food industry. HVACP treatment of aflatoxin has been shown to degrade 70% of the total aflatoxin in 12 min [60, 61].

5. Sorbent additives for degradation of AFB1

There is one approach to solve AFB1 contamination is the addition of sorbents in the foods. This process is not the same as the degradation process, because it does not involve destroying or reducing the amount of AFB1 in the foods or feeds. They act as binding agents to prevent AFB1 absorbed from intestinal tract after ingestion. Chlorophyllin added to the contaminated feeds could reduce AFB1-DNA adduct by 37% in rainbow trout which led to a 77% reduction of tumor incidence [62]. Another study observed that chlorophyllin exhibited the reduction of AFB1-DNA adducts, boasting the reduction of AFB1-album adducts by 65% and urinary AFM1 by 90% in rats; chlorophyll also reduces AFB1-DNA adducts, AFB1-album adducts, and urinary AFM1 levels by 55, 51, and 92%, respectively [63].

Clay works similarly to chlorophyll and chlorophyllin. By addition of the clay into the animal feeds, AFM1 level in milk is reduced accordingly with the decrease of AFB1 absorption rate [64]. And no overt toxicities were observed after SD rats were fed with NovaSil clay (NS) for more than half year [65]. For human beings, NS was performed for clinical study, and the side effect were reported in 99.5% of the persons as compared to the control group. After 3 months, the level of AFB1-albumin adduct was significantly decreased in both low-dose group and high-dose group. The level of AFM1 in urine samples decreased 58% in the high-dose group in 3 months. And there was no liver and kidney function or hematological parameter change reported [66, 67]. From these studies, NS diet can be regarded as a safe and effective method to reduce AFB1 toxicity in the foods.

In addition, different types of mineral clays have been tested for their capabilities to bind AF in animal feeds. These absorbents, such as activated carbon (charcoal), zeolite, and saponite-rich bentonite, reduced AFB1 absorption in the gastrointestinal tract [68].

6. Other methods to degrade of AFB1

Recently, some inexpensive, new promising methods on top of conventional methods for decontamination of food and raw materials have been developed. In the beer or wine factories, some fermentation residues were observed to have the ability of degradation of AFB. A group in Italy have shown that biosorption of mycotoxins onto grape pomace may be a reasonably low-cost decontamination method. The theoretical maximum adsorption capacities (mmol/kg dried pomace) were calculated at pH 7 and 37°C; around 1 hour of contact, that pomace could adsorb almost half of initial AFB1 concentration, but it seems the adsorption rate was kept stable within pH ranges [69]. Similarly, Bovo et al. [70] also found AFB adsorption by beer fermentation residue (BFR) ranged from 45.5 to 69.4% at pH 3.0 and from 24.0 to 63.8% at pH 6.0.

7. Conclusion

Among all mycotoxins, the group of aflatoxins has received much attention due to their severe impact on human and animal health. AFB1 is the most potent carcinogenic agent associated with hepatocellular carcinoma. And AFB1 can negatively affect nutrition absorption, growth and development, and immune system function. AFB1 contamination in the food/feed supplies was found in various countries, particularly in Asia and Africa. A lot of methods to remove or prevent AFB1 contamination, degrade AFB1, or inhibit AFB1 absorption have been developed in the last several decades. The efficiency of aflatoxin decontamination is subject to such factors as food conditions (food constituents, moisture content, pH conditions) and decontamination technologies and conditions. The traditional physical methods for separation or dehulling of the contaminated grains are the simple and safe ways without expensive costs to reduce the dietary exposure to aflatoxins; they can be chosen by anyone or in any area, which makes them the best methods for poor or undeveloped area. Decontamination of aflatoxin is one of the significant challenges for the food industry. The treated food should keep their nutrition values or other important desired qualities, and no residues be left or new contaminates be produced. Either most of the physical and chemical approaches for aflatoxin detoxification might affect the nutritional properties of the foods or be unsafe for human consumption; however, gamma radiation, ozone applications, microwave heating, electron beam, pulsed light, electrolyzed water, and cold plasma showed great potentials for future applications. Recently some inexpensive methods showed good perspectives for reducing aflatoxins in beer and wine factory, which are good choice to be adopted in commercial factory. Biological approaches based on removal or degradation of aflatoxins by bacteria and yeasts are of the promising perspectives, although these practices cannot be currently adopted for foods commercially. While applying these new technologies to make decontamination of aflatoxin, it shall be vital to make clear of the mechanisms of aflatoxin detoxification to determine the practical applications of these approaches in food products, especially concerning their impacts upon the food constituents. Furthermore, combination with traditional and novel technologies shall be also considered to improve the efficiency of decontamination and break through the limitations for specific technologies.

Acknowledgements

This study was supported partly by the National Natural Science Foundation of China (Nos. 81860489, 81760502, 81572353,81372639,81472243,81660495, and 81460423), the Innovation Program of Guangxi Municipal Education Department (Nos. 201204LX674 and 201204LX324), Innovation Program of Guangxi Health Department (No. Z2013781), the Natural Science Foundation of Guangxi (Nos. 2018GXNSFAA281043, 2017GXNSFAA198002, 2017GXNSFGA198002, 2016GXNSFDA380003, 2015GXNSFAA139223, 2013GXNSFAA019251, 2014GXNSFDA118021, and 2014GXNSFAA118144), Research Program of Guangxi "Zhouyue Scholar" (No. 2017–2038), Research Program of Guangxi Specially-invited Expert (No. 2017-6th), the "12th Five-Year Plan" Planning Program of Guangxi Education Science (No. 2015C397), the Innovative Program of Guangxi Graduate Education (No. JGY2015139), Research Program of Guangxi Clinic Research Center of Hepatobiliary Diseases (No.AD17129025), and Open Research Program from Molecular Immunity Study Room Involving in Acute and Severe Diseases in Guangxi Colleges and Universities (Nos. kfkt20160062 and kfkt20160063).

Author details

Qian Yang[1,2]

1 Department of Pathology, The Affiliated Hospital of Youjiang Medical University for Nationalities, Baise, China

2 Department of Internal Medicine-Gerontology and Geriatric Medicine, Wake Forest University School of Medicine, Winston-Salem, North Carolina, USA

*Address all correspondence to: yangqian2003@126.com

References

[1] Zain ME. Impact of mycotoxins on humans and animals. Journal of Saudi Chemical Society. 2011;**15**(2):129-144

[2] Nesbitt BF et al. *Aspergillus flavus* and Turkey X disease. Toxic metabolites of *Aspergillus flavus*. Nature. 1962;**195**:1062-1063

[3] Dalvi RR. An overview of aflatoxicosis of poultry: Its characteristics, prevention and reduction. Veterinary Research Communications. 1986;**10**(6):429-443

[4] Carnaghan RB, Hartley RD, O'Kelly J. Toxicity and fluorescence properties of the Aflatoxins. Nature. 1963;**200**:1101

[5] Wu Q et al. Biological degradation of aflatoxins. Drug Metabolism Reviews. 2009;**41**(1):1-7

[6] Gorelick NJ. Risk assessment for aflatoxin: I. metabolism of aflatoxin B1 by different species. Risk Analysis. 1990;**10**(4):539-559

[7] Dickens JW, Whitaker TB. Efficacy of electronic color sorting and hand picking to remove aflatoxin contaminated kernels from commercial lots of shelled peanuts. Peanut Science. 1975;**2**(2):45-50

[8] Matumba L et al. Effectiveness of hand sorting, flotation/washing, dehulling and combinations thereof on the decontamination of mycotoxin-contaminated white maize. Food Additives & Contaminants. Part A, Chemistry, Analysis, Control, Exposure & Risk Assessment. 2015;**32**(6):960-969

[9] Arzandeh S, Jinap S. Effect of initial aflatoxin concentration, heating time and roasting temperature on aflatoxin reduction in contaminated peanuts and process optimisation using response surface modelling. International Journal of Food Science and Technology. 2011;**46**(3):485-491

[10] Raters M, Matissek R. Thermal stability of aflatoxin B1 and ochratoxin A. Mycotoxin Research. 2008;**24**(3):130-134

[11] Lee J, Her JY, Lee KG. Reduction of aflatoxins (B(1), B(2), G(1), and G(2)) in soybean-based model systems. Food Chemistry. 2015;**189**:45-51

[12] Park JW, Lee C, Kim YB. Fate of aflatoxin B1 during the cooking of Korean polished rice. Journal of Food Protection. 2005;**68**(7):1431-1434

[13] Perez-FloresGC,Moreno-MartinezE, Mendez-Albores A. Effect of microwave heating during alkaline-cooking of aflatoxin contaminated maize. Journal of Food Science. 2011;**76**(2):T48-T52

[14] Di Stefano V et al. Mycotoxin contamination of animal feedingstuff: Detoxification by gamma-irradiation and reduction of aflatoxins and ochratoxin A concentrations. Food Additives & Contaminants. Part A, Chemistry, Analysis, Control, Exposure & Risk Assessment. 2014;**31**(12):2034-2039

[15] Applegate KL, Chipley JR. Effects of 60Co gamma irradiation on aflatoxin B1 and B2 production by *Aspergillus flavus*. Mycologia. 1974;**66**(3):436-445

[16] Priyadarshini E, Tulpule PG. Effect of graded doses of gamma-irradiation on aflatoxin production by *Aspergillus parasiticus* in wheat. Food and Cosmetics Toxicology. 1979;**17**(5):505-507

[17] Ogbadu G. Influence of gamma irradiation of aflatoxin B1 production by *Aspergillus flavus* growing on

some Nigerian foodstuffs. Microbios. 1980;**27**(107):19-26

[18] Schindler AF, Abadie AN, Simpson RE. Enhanced aflatoxin production by *Aspergillus flavus* and *Aspergillus parasiticus* after gamma irradiation of the spore inoculum. Journal of Food Protection. 1980;**43**(1):7-9

[19] Zhang ZS, Xie QF, Che LM. Effects of gamma irradiation on aflatoxin B1 levels in soybean and on the properties of soybean and soybean oil. Applied Radiation and Isotopes. 2018;**139**:224-230

[20] Domijan AM et al. Cytotoxicity of gamma irradiated aflatoxin B1 and ochratoxin A. Journal of Environmental Science and Health. Part. B. 2019;**54**(3):155-162

[21] Xiong K, Liu H, Li L. Product identification and safety evaluation of aflatoxin B1 decontaminated by electrolyzed oxidizing water. Journal of Agricultural and Food Chemistry. 2012;**60**(38):9770-9778

[22] Xiong K et al. Differences in fungicidal efficiency against *Aspergillus flavus* for neutralized and acidic electrolyzed oxidizing waters. International Journal of Food Microbiology. 2010;**137**(1):67-75

[23] Fan S et al. Removal of aflatoxin B(1) in edible plant oils by oscillating treatment with alkaline electrolysed water. Food Chemistry. 2013;**141**(3):3118-3123

[24] Elmnasser N et al. Pulsed-light system as a novel food decontamination technology: A review. Canadian Journal of Microbiology. 2007;**53**(7):813-821

[25] Moreau M et al. Application of the pulsed light technology to mycotoxin degradation and inactivation. Journal of Applied Toxicology. 2013;**33**(5):357-363

[26] Martinez AJ, Weng CY, Park DL. Distribution of ammonia/aflatoxin reaction products in corn following exposure to ammonia decontamination procedure. Food Additives and Contaminants. 1994;**11**(6):659-667

[27] Weng CY, Martinez AJ, Park DL. Efficacy and permanency of ammonia treatment in reducing aflatoxin levels in corn. Food Additives and Contaminants. 1994;**11**(6):649-658

[28] Hoogenboom LA et al. Genotoxicity testing of extracts from aflatoxin-contaminated peanut meal, following chemical decontamination. Food Additives and Contaminants. 2001;**18**(4):329-341

[29] Jorgensen KV, Price RL. Atmospheric pressure-ambient temperature reduction of aflatoxin B1 in ammoniated cottonseed. Journal of Agricultural and Food Chemistry. 1981;**29**(3):555-558

[30] Aly SE, Hathout AS. Fate of aflatoxin B(1) in contaminated corn gluten during acid hydrolysis. Journal of the Science of Food and Agriculture. 2011;**91**(3):421-427

[31] Mendez-Albores A et al. Effect of lactic and citric acid on the stability of B-aflatoxins in extrusion-cooked sorghum. Letters in Applied Microbiology. 2008;**47**(1):1-7

[32] Zorlugenc B et al. The influence of gaseous ozone and ozonated water on microbial flora and degradation of aflatoxin B(1) in dried figs. Food and Chemical Toxicology. 2008;**46**(12):3593-3597

[33] Chen R et al. Effect of ozone on aflatoxins detoxification and nutritional quality of peanuts. Food Chemistry. 2014;**146**:284-288

[34] Diao E et al. Ozonolysis efficiency and safety evaluation of aflatoxin B1 in

peanuts. Food and Chemical Toxicology. 2013;**55**:519-525

[35] Ciegler A et al. Microbial detoxification of aflatoxin. Applied Microbiology. 1966;**14**(6):934-939

[36] D'Souza DH, Brackett RE. The role of trace metal ions in aflatoxin B1 degradation by *Flavobacterium aurantiacum*. Journal of Food Protection. 1998;**61**(12):1666-1669

[37] D'Souza DH, Brackett RE. The influence of divalent cations and chelators on aflatoxin B1 degradation by *Flavobacterium aurantiacum*. Journal of Food Protection. 2000;**63**(1):102-105

[38] D'Souza DH, Brackett RE. Aflatoxin B1 degradation by *Flavobacterium aurantiacum* in the presence of reducing conditions and seryl and sulfhydryl group inhibitors. Journal of Food Protection. 2001;**64**(2):268-271

[39] Arai T, Ito T, Koyama Y. Antimicrobial activity of aflatoxins. Journal of Bacteriology. 1967;**93**(1):59-64

[40] Hormisch D et al. *Mycobacterium fluoranthenivorans* sp. nov., a fluoranthene and aflatoxin B1 degrading bacterium from contaminated soil of a former coal gas plant. Systematic and Applied Microbiology. 2004;**27**(6):653-660

[41] Teniola OD et al. Degradation of aflatoxin B(1) by cell-free extracts of *Rhodococcus erythropolis* and *Mycobacterium fluoranthenivorans* sp. nov. DSM44556(T). International Journal of Food Microbiology. 2005;**105**(2):111-117

[42] Alberts JF et al. Biological degradation of aflatoxin B1 by *Rhodococcus erythropolis* cultures. International Journal of Food Microbiology. 2006;**109**(1-2):121-126

[43] Kusumaningtyas E, Widiastuti R, Maryam R. Reduction of aflatoxin B1 in chicken feed by using *Saccharomyces cerevisiae*, *Rhizopus oligosporus* and their combination. Mycopathologia. 2006;**162**(4):307-311

[44] Jespersen L et al. Significance of yeasts and moulds occurring in maize dough fermentation for 'kenkey' production. International Journal of Food Microbiology. 1994;**24**(1-2):239-248

[45] Chu FS et al. Stability of aflatoxin B-1 and ochratoxin a in brewing. Applied Microbiology. 1975;**29**(3):313-316

[46] Megalla SE, Hafez AH. Detoxification of aflatoxin B1 by acidogenous yoghurt. Mycopathologia. 1982;**77**(2):89-91

[47] Megalla SE, Mohran MA. Fate of aflatoxin B-1 in fermented dairy products. Mycopathologia. 1984;**88**(1):27-29

[48] Pizzolitto RP et al. Evaluation of *Saccharomyces cerevisiae* as an antiaflatoxicogenic agent in broiler feedstuffs. Poultry Science. 2013;**92**(6):1655-1663

[49] Peltonen K et al. Aflatoxin B1 binding by dairy strains of lactic acid bacteria and bifidobacteria. Journal of Dairy Science. 2001;**84**(10):2152-2156

[50] El-Nezami H et al. Ability of dairy strains of lactic acid bacteria to bind a common food carcinogen, aflatoxin B1. Food and Chemical Toxicology. 1998;**36**(4):321-326

[51] Kankaanpaa P et al. Binding of aflatoxin B1 alters the adhesion properties of *Lactobacillus rhamnosus* strain GG in a Caco-2 model. Journal of Food Protection. 2000;**63**(3):412-414

[52] Motomura M et al. Purification and characterization of an aflatoxin degradation enzyme from *Pleurotus ostreatus*. Microbiological Research. 2003;**158**(3):237-242

[53] Liu DL et al. Production, purification, and characterization of an intracellular aflatoxin-detoxifizyme from *Armillariella tabescens* (E-20). Food and Chemical Toxicology. 2001;**39**(5):461-466

[54] Shcherbakova L et al. Aflatoxin B1 degradation by metabolites of *Phoma glomerata* PG41 isolated from natural substrate colonized by aflatoxigenic *Aspergillus flavus*. Jundishapur Journal of Microbiology. 2015;**8**(1):e24324

[55] Schluter O et al. Opinion on the use of plasma processes for treatment of foods. Molecular Nutrition & Food Research. 2013;**57**(5):920-927

[56] Thirumdas R, Sarangapani C, Annapure US. Cold plasma: A novel non-thermal technology for food processing. Food Biophysics. 2015;**10**(1):1-11

[57] Park BJ et al. Degradation of mycotoxins using microwave-induced argon plasma at atmospheric pressure. Surface & Coatings Technology. 2007;**201**(9-11):5733-5737

[58] Sakudo A et al. Degradation and detoxification of aflatoxin B-1 using nitrogen gas plasma generated by a static induction thyristor as a pulsed power supply. Food Control. 2017;**73**:619-626

[59] Wang SQ et al. Degradation of aflatoxin B-1 by low-temperature radio frequency plasma and degradation product elucidation. European Food Research and Technology. 2015;**241**(1):103-113

[60] Shi H et al. Structures of degradation products and degradation pathways of aflatoxin B1 by high-voltage atmospheric cold plasma (HVACP) treatment. Journal of Agricultural and Food Chemistry. 2017;**65**(30):6222-6230

[61] Siciliano I et al. Use of cold atmospheric plasma to detoxify hazelnuts from aflatoxins. Toxins (Basel). 2016;**8**(5):125

[62] Breinholt V et al. Dietary chlorophyllin is a potent inhibitor of aflatoxin B1 hepatocarcinogenesis in rainbow trout. Cancer Research. 1995;**55**(1):57-62

[63] Simonich MT et al. Natural chlorophyll inhibits aflatoxin B1-induced multi-organ carcinogenesis in the rat. Carcinogenesis. 2007;**28**(6):1294-1302

[64] Phillips TD et al. Reducing human exposure to aflatoxin through the use of clay: A review. Food Additives & Contaminants. Part A, Chemistry, Analysis, Control, Exposure & Risk Assessment. 2008;**25**(2):134-145

[65] Afriyie-Gyawu E et al. Chronic toxicological evaluation of dietary NovaSil clay in Sprague-Dawley rats. Food Additives and Contaminants. 2005;**22**(3):259-269

[66] Afriyie-Gyawu E et al. NovaSil clay intervention in Ghanaians at high risk for aflatoxicosis. I. study design and clinical outcomes. Food Additives & Contaminants. Part A, Chemistry, Analysis, Control, Exposure & Risk Assessment. 2008;**25**(1):76-87

[67] Wang P et al. NovaSil clay intervention in Ghanaians at high risk for aflatoxicosis: II. reduction in biomarkers of aflatoxin exposure in blood and urine. Food Additives & Contaminants. Part A, Chemistry, Analysis, Control, Exposure & Risk Assessment. 2008;**25**(5):622-634

[68] Giovati L et al. AFM(1) in milk: Physical, biological, and prophylactic methods to mitigate contamination. Toxins (Basel). 2015;7(10):4330-4349

[69] Avantaggiato G et al. Assessment of multi-mycotoxin adsorption efficacy of grape pomace. Journal of Agricultural and Food Chemistry. 2014;**62**(2):497-507

[70] Bovo F et al. In vitro ability of beer fermentation residue and yeast-based products to bind aflatoxin B1. Brazilian Journal of Microbiology. 2015;**46**(2):577-581

Chapter 11

The Toxification and Detoxification Mechanisms of Aflatoxin B1 in Human: An Update

Qun-Ying Su

Abstract

Aflatoxin B1 (AFB1) is the most common carcinogen of aflatoxin, which contaminates many agricultural products in the daily diet of humans. More than 50% of patients with developing hepatocellular carcinoma (HCC) feature AFB1 exposure due to their shared consumption of contaminated food. One of the main mechanisms of AFB1-induced liver carcinogenesis is its biological activation and its interaction with DNA to produce AFB1-E-N7-dG adduct. This product may result in the formation of DNA damage and the mutations of tumor-associated genes such as TP53 and ras. In human, several pathways involving in AFB1 detoxification, including I- and II-type detoxification, DNA repair, have been reported. This study reviewed the detoxification mechanisms of AFB1 in human as well as AFB1 occurrence and toxification. Additionally, we also discussed prevention methods for AFB1 exposure.

Keywords: aflatoxin B1, toxification, detoxification, mechanism

1. Introduction

Aflatoxin B1 (AFB1), an important mycotoxin, is first identified in animal feed in 1961 due to the death of 100,000 turkeys in the UK where these turkeys were feed using the peanut powder with the high concentration of AFB1. Until now, this mycotoxin has proved to come from the secondary metabolites of *Aspergillus* under adverse conditions such as prolonged drought and insect-mediated damage to crops. Growing studies have also shown that individuals having crops contaminated by AFB1 often causes different poisoning. Its high-level exposure will cause acute poisoning and severe cellular damage, even death; whereas its long-term low-level exposure will induce chronic poisoning, genic mutations, even malignant alterations of cells. Evidence from epidemiological and clinicopathological studies displays that AFB1 has strong carcinogenicity, mutagenicity and teratogenicity. For human and animals, AFB1 often induces hepatocellular carcinoma, thus, is classified as one of I-class chemical carcinogen of hepatocellular carcinoma by the International Cancer Research Center [1–5]. Here, we will review the occurrence of AFB1 and its toxification effects on human. Additionally, we will also discuss all known detoxification of AFB1.

2. AFB1 occurrence

2.1 Toxic fungi and their classifications

Toxic fungi often live in the human crops and produce mycotoxins such as aflatoxins. Toxic fungi in crops can be divided into two categories according to whether their mycotoxins are produced before or after crop harvest. The first category is termed as field fungi, which often invade crops and produce mycotoxins before harvest. The another, also called storage fungi, mostly occurs in the storage of crops after harvest. The sources of both types of toxigenic fungi are affected by environmental factors. Crops before harvest, fungi can invade crops to produce toxins by interacting with other organisms, such as insects. The harvested crops are regulated by factors such as nutrients, temperature and humidity in the air, and biological agents (insects, competitive interference). Furthermore, toxigenic fungi can be divided into four types according to their effects on crops: *A. fungi* acting as plant pathogens, such as grass fungi; *b.* fungi producing fungal toxin and stressing plants, such as *Candida* and *A. flavus*; *c.* fungi acting as colonizers (such as *Aspergillus flavus*), which first colonize in harvest plants and subsequently, produce mycotoxin and contaminate crops; and *d.* fungi decomposing plants (such as *Penicillium chrysogenum* and *Aspergillus oryzae*), which often live in the soil [6, 7].

The crop fungi inoculate the growing crop kernels in the field and proliferate in storage under suitable conditions. Among known crop fungi, *Aspergillus*, *Fusarium*, and *Penicillium* have identified as toxin-producing fungi. Although many compounds produced by these toxin-producing fungi are known as their toxins, there have been only five important agricultural mycotoxins until now: deoxycinol, praurone, ochratoxin A, fumarin and aflatoxin. Mycotoxins produced by *Fusarium* include fumonisins, deoxycinol and zerneone. Although *Penicillium* and *Aspergillus* are storage fungi, they can also invade field stress plants and produce toxins. Increasing evidence has shown that *Penicillium* can produce ochratomycin, citrinin and patron, and that *Aspergillus* can produce aflatoxin, citrinin and baturin [8, 9].

2.2 AFB1 occurrence

Several previous reviews have fully summarized the occurrence and biosynthesis of AFB1. Briefly, AFB1 are an important class of mycotoxins mainly produced by *Aspergillus flavus* and *Aspergillus parasiticus*. This term is so named and concerned because of the following several reasons: *a.* this mycotoxin has been identified in the *A. flavus* and regarded as pathologic agent of "turkey X" disease; *b.* this mycotoxin is the first B-type aflatoxin which can produce fluorescent characteristic under UV light; and *c.* AFB1 often display its severe toxic effects on human and animals. Usually, it is synthesized through 18 biological steps under the regulations of a huge neighbor gene cluster consisting of about 60–70 kb in original fungi. This biosynthesis at least involves in the three stages, consisting of the formation of primary product hydroxyversicolorone (the first to eighth step), middle product versicolorin B (the ninth to twelfth step) and ultimate product AFB1 (the thirteenth to eighteenth step). During the biosynthesis of AFB1, several key enzymes, including nicotinamide-adenine dinucleotide, nicotinamide-adenine dinucleotide phosphate reduced form, and 2S-adenosylmethionine, are required for the biosynthesis limitation [3, 10, 11].

3. AFB1 toxification and toxic mechanisms

3.1 The effects of AFB1 on the food chain

A. flavus is widely present in the soil, causing pollution to many crops such as corn, peanuts, rice, etc., and using these crops as a host produces aflatoxin, which in turn contaminates crop fruits. Aflatoxin contamination of food and animal feed has now become a major problem that threatens food safety. Crops can be contaminated with fungi in the field, harvested, and stored, making crop contamination control difficult. The Food and Agriculture Organization of the United Nations (FAO) estimates that 25% of the world's food crops are contaminated with mycotoxins [12]. Aflatoxins, the most harmful toxins, are the most difficult to deal with because they are commonly found in corn, peanuts and their products, cottonseed, peppers, peppers, pistachios and other foods. Studies have shown that the type of mold and its concentration of conidia, as well as the moisture content of corn, play a key role in the process of mold infection, spoilage and AFB1 production in corn. In the field, Aspergillus flavus enters the plant primarily by vaccination or secondary inoculation, which in turn infects the seed to produce aflatoxin. In spring, the source of inoculation of Aspergillus flavus spores is mainly from the propagules in the soil, the plant debris in the soil, and the wintering mycelium, insects or the Aspergillus flavus nucleus in the soil in the litter. In corn fields, spores are mainly derived from the spore-derived sclerotium conidia of Aspergillus flavus. Before the harvest, the insects damage the corn kernels to form the sclerotia. When harvesting, the sclerotia is dispersed in the soil, and the spring conidia are exposed on the surface of the sclerotium. A secondary inoculation source was found in the cotton field, and *A. flavus* was isolated from the leaves, flower buds and leaf discs of cotton, the content was 15, 94, or 56%, respectively. Most of the colonies were mainly distributed on the calyx tablets. Conidia are the main source of secondary inoculation. Fungal spoilage and mycotoxin contamination are major problems in crop contamination. Grains are affected by storage conditions and the environment after harvesting, such as storage containers, oxygen content in the air, water activity, temperature, and insects, all of which are factors of toxin contamination [7]. If stored poorly, it will increase the contamination of mycotoxins. As one of the main crops for human food and livestock feed, corn is planted annually at 120 million hectares and is one of the most polluted toxins. Aspergillus flavus is the main fungus that is infected after corn harvest. The drying and storage conditions of corn before storage are extremely important. Moisture can accumulate from the activity of pests, which provides ideal conditions for the proliferation of fungi and the accumulation of mycotoxins. In order to reduce the effects of mycotoxins on food and feed chains, it is necessary to control pest and fungal contamination [13, 14]. Humidity and temperature have important effects on mold growth and mycotoxin production. Therefore, humid and hot climates in tropical and subtropical regions provide favorable conditions for mold growth. The moisture content of the grain is generally expressed in terms of water content. Pathogenic fungi that invade crops prior to harvest typically require higher moisture levels (200–250 g/kg) to infect, while fungi that can proliferate during storage (130–180 g/kg) require higher moisture levels. Therefore, most feeds with a water content above 130 g/kg are prone to mold growth and formation of mycotoxins [15]. Therefore, the control of the moisture content in the grain becomes particularly important, especially in the control of moisture at the harvesting point, while the drying and storage of the grain before storage and the frequency of grain drying and plowing, as well as the insects and microorganisms in the stored grain are also Factors affecting water activity. It was found to be closely related to climate in the detection of aflatoxin levels after storage of Benin corn. Benin's aflatoxin contamination levels increase in dry and hot conditions in June each year; while the harvest season is affected by climate, the peaks of rainfall or the late planting of corn will increase aflatoxin levels during the rainy season [16]. Limiting the occurrence of AFB1 before crop harvesting can be achieved by reducing drought and temperature, controlling weeds, reducing insect damage, efficient harvesting techniques, and reducing soil Aspergillus spores through crop turnover. Using biological control, a competitive, non-toxigenic strain of Aspergillus flavus is applied to the developing soil to compete with naturally occurring toxigenic strains. Studies have shown that these biological control strategy can aflatoxin. The pollution is reduced by about 80–90%. Control of afb1 sensitive crops after harvest can be achieved by controlling factors that affect fungal growth, such as water activity, temperature, gaseous environment, and the use of pesticides or food preservatives. Harvesting only cereals with a moisture content of around 24% reduces the risk of grain damage and subsequent AFB1 production [17, 18].

3.2 The toxic effects of AFB1 on human and animals

In 1963, Asao et al. completed the structural clarification of AFB1, a member of the aflatoxin family containing a fused difuranyl group [19]. AFB1 is highly toxic to humans and several animals, and has three major characteristics: organophilic, genotoxic, and carcinogenic. Its pro-organism is mainly caused by damage to the liver, which can lead to hepatic hemorrhage and hepatocyte necrosis. The genotoxicity is mainly to induce the formation of AFB1-DNA adduct and the hot spot mutation of P53 gene. The carcinogenicity is mainly caused by hepatocellular carcinoma. The main toxicological effect of AFB1 is to induce DNA damage. AFB1 has been proven to be the main cause of liver cancer in patients with hepatitis B virus infection. It is a genotoxic liver cancer, which may cause cancer by inducing DNA adducts, leading to genetic changes in target cells, leading to DNA strand breaks and DNA base damage. And oxidative damage can eventually lead to cancer. AFB1 is mainly metabolized by the liver, and AFB1 taken from food is mainly metabolized by the cytochrome P450 enzyme to the final carcinogen AFB1-8-9-epoxide (AFBO). When AFBO reacts with DNA, it inhibits gene mutation in P53, a hotspot coding region of exon 249, by interacting with guanine bases, which may lead to HCC. AFB1 is metabolized by the P450 system into a number of hydroxylated products, including AFM1, AFQ1, AFP1, AFB2a [11, 20–25]. After aflatoxin is ingested into the human body, it mainly manifests as an acute or chronic disease. Acute attacks usually involve high concentrations of aflatoxins. For example, 317 cases of acute liver failure occurred in Kenya in 2004. The main reason is the consumption of aflatoxin-contaminated corn, and the case of patients with AFB1 lysine in serum. The adduct concentration was the highest in history. Growth retardation, immunosuppression, and carcinogenicity are chronic effects, and the incidence of chronic attacks in developing countries is higher because of exposure to low levels of aflatoxin intake [26].

3.2.1 Effect of aflatoxin on growth and development

An epidemiological survey was conducted in West Africa to measure exposure to aflatoxins in children between 9 months and 5 years of age, and their growth, development and height were examined against the reference population of World Health Organization (WHO) [27]. Studies have shown a strong association between exposure to aflatoxin in children and dysplasia and underweight. In a field outbreak of aflatoxin, egg production fell by 5% [28]. The study data showed that for every 1 mg/kg of aflatoxin AFB1 in the feed, the growth rate of pigs would be reduced by 16% and broilers by 5% [29].

3.2.2 Immunosuppressive

In these animal studies, AFB1 has been shown to induce immunosuppression. For example, in studies of AFB1 exposed animals, it was found that the activity of B cells and T cells decreased, because T cells were more sensitive to AFB1 toxicity [30]. Research data from GY et al. showed that chicken phagocytic cells were severely damaged during aflatoxosis, and the ability to remove foreign substances from the circulation decreased, which may reduce the ability to process antigenic components. Aflatoxell chickens are more susceptible to infection [31]. In pigs, AFB1 exposure reduces lymphocyte response to mitogens, inhibits large phage migration and delayed skin allergic reactions [32]. Although many data on AFB1 immune effects have been obtained from animal studies, there is little data on the effects of long-term consumption of food contaminated with AFB1 on the human immune system. The effect on the immune system by aflatoxins in the diet of Gambian children found a decrease in sIgA levels in saliva, probably due to the high level of exposure to aflatoxins in the diet [33]. In a study of aflatoxin AFB1 exposure and cellular immune status in 64 Ghanaians, it was found that AFB1 exposure may result in a decrease in the major constituent cell T cells and B cells that cause lymphocyte subpopulations. High levels of AFB1 albumin adducts significantly reduced perforin- and granzyme a levels in CD8+ cytotoxic T cells compared to low levels of AFB1 albumin adduct. In participants with high levels of AFB1, changes in these immune parameters may result in impaired cellular immune function, thereby reducing host resistance to infection [34].

4. Detoxification of AFB1

Since the contamination of aflatoxins in food poses a risk to human health and leads to serious economic losses in crops, we have every reason to implement new methods to ensure the safety of food production. There are two main methods of implementation: (a) prevention of mold contamination and growth; (b) detoxification of contaminated products by opponents. Prevention of mycotoxin contamination can be achieved by storage before or after harvesting of the crop. However, the pollution of toxins is inevitable, and the detoxification pathway for contaminated food after harvest has been the subject of our in-depth research. Detoxification methods commonly used are physical methods and chemical methods. This article will focus on new research on detoxification of harvested contaminated crops.

4.1 Physical method

The most common way to remove AFB1 using physical methods is to heat and use gamma rays. Aflatoxins are highly thermostable. Studies have shown that AFB1 levels are significantly reduced by heating at 100 and 150°C for 90 minutes, respectively, at 41.9 and 81.2%. The AFB reduction rate of the soy milk after cooking was 97.9%, and the AFB1 reduction rate of the steamed soybeans after cooking was 33.6%. And studies have shown that high pressure cooking is better than ordinary cooking to remove AFB1. When the soybean is steamed or steamed in a pressure cooker, the reduction rate of the pressure cooker is about 10% higher than that of the steam. Using autoclave cooking in rice can reduce AFB1 levels by 72–83%. The high-pressure cooking method is low in cost and easy to handle, and one of the challenges it faces is how to ensure the integrity of the food after heating. To ensure the integrity of the food, the use of maximum temperatures is often limited [35, 36]. The gamma ray has a strong penetrating electromagnetic wave that can penetrate the material without leaving any residue, which is its advantage. There have been many reports of the increase, decrease, or even unaffected mycotoxin produced by fungi under different conditions. Studies have shown that the fungal structure on paper with a minimum radiation dose of 16 kGy has been altered to avoid fungal growth. Library and file management staff use gamma radiation protection technology to provide a powerful means for the preservation of ancient books, archives and other paper materials [37]. A dose of gamma radiation exceeding 10 kGy can inhibit the germination of peanut seeds. Therefore, proper drying, packaging and environmental control measures with low relative humidity can reduce the growth of fungi and ensure safe, high quality peanuts [38]. The DI Stefano study showed that a radiation dose of 0.5–15 KGy resulted in a decrease in aflatoxin levels in the feed, while a 15 kGy gamma ray did not completely destroy ochratoxin A and aflatoxin in the test feed, FAO/International The IAEA/WHO Expert Committee on Food Irradiation has concluded in its report that foods with an average radiation dose of 10 kGy will not cause toxicological hazards and that toxicologically tested foods do not require retreatment. It is necessary to irradiate the food with radiation before the mold produces toxins [39].

4.2 Biological treatment

Studies using biotechnology to reduce AFB1 levels in contaminated foods fall into two main categories: one that uses plant extracts to degrade AFB1 and the other that inoculates bacterial strains in food substrates. In recent years, natural plant products have attracted much attention as synthetic antibacterial agents because of their biodegradability, biosafety, effectiveness, and regenerability. At the same time, they are conveniently used as an eco-friendly technology for detoxification. Mycotoxins. Many studies have shown that plant essential oils can inhibit the growth of microorganisms and reduce the production of toxins. Bluma et al. showed that the addition of essential oils in corn kernels has a significant effect on the growth rate, hysteresis and accumulation of AFB1 of aflatoxin molds. Depends on water activity, AFB1 concentration and incubation time [40]. In addition to plant essential oils, water extracts of plants can also be used to dissolve AFB1. Another study by Vijayanandraj et al. also demonstrated the effect of different parameters on the detoxification of AFB1 aqueous extracts from different medicinal plants. They concluded that the leaf extract of Vasaka (*Adhatoda vasica* Nees) showed the greatest AFB1 degradation (≥98%) after incubation for 24 hours at 37°C; the A. vasica leaf extract was heated to 100 by high temperature. Celsius for 10 minutes or autoclaved at 121 degrees Celsius, the detoxification ability is significantly reduced; the A. vasica leaf extract is detected by mass spectrometry to the purified alkaloid, which is believed to be the principle of aflatoxin detoxification [41]. Iram et al. showed that *O. basilicum* leaves extract had significant degradation rates for aflatoxins B1 and B2, and the degradation rates were 90.4 and 88.6%, respectively. The structure of the degradation products was identified by mass spectrometry. Most of the products were passed. Formed by removing the double bond on the terminal furan ring and modifying the lactone group, the degradation property is significantly less toxic than AFB1. The plant extract is easy to obtain, cost-effective and bio-safe, and can be directly sprayed with aqueous plant extracts. Simple, does not involve technical knowledge, is a very good source of detoxification [42].

In another method, inoculation of the bacterial strain is to reduce AFB1 by physical binding or metabolism of the bacterial strain directly to AFB1. The biodegradation of aflatoxins has yielded some successful attempts, although most are carried out in sterile culture. The microbial degradation of aflatoxin is achieved by the activity of the enzyme, which is capable of decomposing the refractory polyheterocyclic molecules of aflatoxin. Brana et al. showed that *Pleurotus eryngii* can degrade AFB1 [43]. Farzaneh et al. showed that the repair rates of AFB1 by *Bacillus subtilis* UTBSP1 in nutrient broth and pistachio were 85.66 and 95%, respectively [44]. Liu et al. used cellulose bacteria to degrade the degradation ability of AFB1 in cottonseed meal. By improving the fermentation conditions, the degradation rate can reach 83.4% [45]. Carolyna and other studies have shown that AFB1 is combined with bacteria through weak non-covalent and acid. Of the bacteria treated, the binding may be intracellular rather than extracellular [46]. It is well known that lactic acid bacteria can degrade aflatoxins. Bueno et al. showed that lactobacillus and *Saccharomyces cerevisiae* can rapidly remove AFB1. The binding of AFB1 with microorganisms is a rapid process (no more than 1 minute), and this binding forms a reversible complex between the toxin and microbial surface without the need for chemical modification of the toxin [47]. Studies by Flora Oluwafemi et al. showed that AFB1 was significantly reduced (44.5%) in 50 ng/g contaminated corn, while AFB1 was the least reduced (29.9%) in 500 ng/g contaminated corn. Because lactic acid bacteria are non-toxic, they have many benefits for human health, and it is also possible to reduce the level of aflatoxin to a lower toxic dose. Lactic acid bacteria have broad application prospects as biopreservatives for food and feed [48].

4.3 Chemical treatment

Mycotoxins can be removed or reduced chemically, and acids, bases, oxidizing agents, and reducing agents have been shown to destroy or extinguish mycotoxins. Acids are a natural part of foods that are added to the industry to add flavor to the food, and even some acids are used as preservatives or antioxidants. Organic acids in foods can degrade AFB1. AIKO et al. tested the degradation of AFB1 by various organic acids and considered that the effect of lactic acid was most effective in the organic acids tested. Since lactic acid is endogenous in the human body and is present in many foods, lactic acid is considered to be safe. Therefore, lactic acid can be recommended for food processing and as a preservative in fermented foods [49]. Rushing and other studies have shown that under acidic conditions, organic acids and arginine can be mixed to treat contaminated foods, and AFB1 can be rapidly converted to AFB2a-Arg within 20 minutes, reducing toxicity [50–53]. Aly et al. showed that HCL can effectively degrade AFB1 during acid hydrolysis [54]. Alkaline cooking is also used in the commercial to remove AFB1 from corn. Amination under high temperature and pressure conditions can also reduce AFB1 in corn. There are also many studies on the degradation of AFB1 in foods using ozone. Ozone has been reported as an antibacterial agent because it has antibacterial effects against spores and bacteria of fungi, bacteria, viruses, protozoa and fungi, and has a wide range of antibacterial agents. Ozone inhibits or microbial growth by oxidizing cell membranes and cell wall complex processes [55]. Diao et al. showed a significant decrease in AFB1 levels in peanut seeds at 13 and 21 mg/l ozone concentrations [56]. Proctor et al. showed that the use of ozone oxidation can degrade AFB1 in peanuts, and at an increased temperature of 75°C, AFB1 degradation rate reached 77% in just 10 minutes [57].

4.4 Sorbent additives

The above method of degrading AFB1 is to destroy or reduce the content of AFB1 in food, and the adsorbent is opposite thereto, which prevents AFB1 from entering the intestinal tract after ingestion by binding to AFB1, so as to prevent hepatotoxicity of AFB1. Novasil clay minerals and aflatoxins are highly affinitive and high-capacity combinations in the gastrointestinal tract. The study of NS has been shown to absorb AFB1 in vitro in both animal models and human studies, reducing the bioavailability of blood toxins, and its use in humans has not affected the utilization of vitamins and trace elements in the body, and has been determined through clinical trials. A safe dose of NS, a NS content of up to 2.0% (w/w) in the diet does not cause significant toxicity [58–62]. Xue and other studies have shown that the enteral nutrient NovaSil can effectively regulate the toxicity and carcinogenicity of co-exposure to AFB1 and fumonisin B1. When the concentration in the diet is as high as 0.5%, liver changes, liver glutathione S The number and size of -transferase (GST-P+) foci were significantly reduced [63]. Another commonly used binder is chlorophyll. Studies in mammals and fish have shown that chlorophyll can inhibit the formation of carcinogens through the combination of AFB1, reduce the bioavailability of tissues, reduce DNA adduction, and reduce the incidence of tumors [64]. Smimonich observed in the study that after adding chlorophyll to the contaminated AFB1 feed, the AFB1-DNA adduct was reduced by 42%, and the AFB1 albumin adduct was reduced by 65%. AFB n7 - guanine Urinary adducts are reduced by 90%. In the same study, it was also shown that chlorophyll reduced the volume of GSTP lesions in the liver by 74% and the mean number of abnormal crypt lesions in the colon by 63%. Studies have shown that chlorophyll can be used as an early biochemical and advanced pathophysiological marker for AFB1 carcinogenesis in the liver and colon [65].

4.5 DNA repair

In China, HCC is a common malignant tumor with a very poor prognosis, accounting for 55% of the world's HCC cases and more than 340,000 cases per year. This area of tumor-prone is mainly concentrated in eastern and southeastern China. Clinical epidemiological studies have shown that exposure to AFB1 and/or chronic infection with HBV and HCV is a major risk factor for liver cancer. Studies on the toxicity of AFB1 indicate that AFB1 damage to DNA plays a central role in the carcinogenic process of HCC associated with this toxin [48, 66]. AFB1 is metabolized by the cytochrome P450 enzyme into a reactive AFB1-8,9-epoxide (AFB1-epoxide), which is covalently bound to DNA to induce DNA damage. AFB1-induced DNA damage includes AFB1-DNA adducts, oxidative DNA damage, and gene mutations. The AFB1-DNA adduct in AFB1-induced DNA damage is 9-hydroxy afb1 (AFB1-N7-Gua), which is the most common type. The formation of the AFB1-N7-Gua adduct is first performed by pre-covalent insertion of the complex electrophilic between the double-stranded DNA and the high-stranded DNA, and then on the imidazole moiety of the formed AFB1-N7-Gua adduct. The charge generates another desired DNA adduct, a ring-opened carboxamide pyridine AFB1 (AFB1-FAPy) adduct. These adducts are capable of forming subsequent anti-repair adducts, dislocations, or lead to error-prone DNA repair, resulting in single-strand breaks (SSBs), double-strand breaks (DSBs), and base pair substitutions. The mutations caused by AFB1 exposure, the current major research and experiments believe that the P53 gene is closely related, there is a common mutation hotspot at 249 of TP53 (AGG to AGT) codon [11, 23, 25, 48]. However, epidemiological evidence suggests that although many people are exposed to the same level of AFB1, only a small percentage of the exposed persons have toxicological effects of AFB1, such as genetic mutations and HCC. The Nucleic Acid Excision Repair Pathway (NER), which has been shown to repair aflatoxin-induced DNA adducts, is the major DNA repair pathway. The repair steps of NER are mainly divided into: damage perception, opening denatured bubbles, cutting damaged chains, transferring damaged oligonucleotides, filling gaps and ligation. There is increasing evidence that genetic polymorphisms in the NER gene are associated with DNA repair capacity and regulate the risk of cancer [66]. In China, molecular epidemiological studies of afb1-related HCC have investigated the association of several genes associated with the NER pathway, such as xeroderma pigmentosum C (XPC) and xeroderma pigmentosum D (XPD). In the oxidative damage of DNA caused by AFB1 exposure, the formation of 8-oxodG is important because it is abundant, highly mutagenic and hepatocarcinogenesis occurs. 8-oxodG lesions are mainly repaired by the BER pathway. The BER pathway promotes DNA repair through two common pathways: a. short patch BER pathway leading to a single nucleotide repair pathway; b. long patch BER pathway, resulting in at least two nucleotide repair pathways. Long et al. first reported DNA repair genes XRCC1, XRCC3, XRCC4, XRCC7, XPD, XPC (including rs25487, rs861539, rs7003908, rs28383151, rs3734091) by analyzing the AFB1-DNA adduct amount, TP53 gene mutation frequency and HCC risk. Genetic polymorphisms of (rs13181, rs2228001) and toxicological effects of AFB1 exposure. Studies have shown that the DNA repair gene XRCC1 gene mutation, XRCC3, XRCC4, XRCC7, XPC, and XPD may increase the AFB1-DNA adduct, the frequency of TP53M, and the risk of hepatocellular carcinoma, genetic mutations with lower DNA repair ability of these genes It should contribute to the toxicological effects of AFB1 and be of a preventive significance by identifying people with low DNA repair capacity [23, 67, 68].

5. AFB1-related legislation

In developing countries, AFB1 contamination of food is inevitable due to poor environmental and technical conditions, and it is not easy to be treated by high temperature, chemical, physical, etc. Humans can directly use contaminated foods (corn, peanuts, sorghum, rice, cashews, walnuts, pistachios, almonds) or animal products such as milk, eggs, etc. produced by using contaminated animals. The primary hazard of mycotoxin contamination in the food supply chain is human health, followed by animal health and productivity [69, 70]. Every country has strict controls on the mycotoxin contamination of food and feed to reduce human and animal exposure. Currently, Developed countries have access to federal regulatory bodies which set food safety standards and inspect domestic as well as imported/exported food products. Additionally, these countries have access to controlled storage conditions, which greatly reduces contamination post-harvest. These factors lead to lower overall contamination rates in developed countries. For example, the United States has reported acceptable AFB1 levels in corn (0–80 μg/kg during 1979–1983) and low daily intake of its citizens (0.34–197 ng/kg depending on the year and region of the country), which is much less than other undeveloped countries [71]. The European Union (EU) has some of the world's most stringent standards for mycotoxins in food and feed. Compared with the rest of the world, the European Union (EU) has the most extensive and detailed AFB1 presence in various foods and feeds provisions. It has been indicated that in many European countries the presence of AFM1 in milk and milk products was in lower range than the Asian and African countries [72, 73].

6. Summary and future direction

AFB1 is a kind of I-type chemical carcinogenic mycotoxin mainly produced by both *A. flavus* and *A. parasiticus* and is known to contaminate most of the world's food supply. AFB1 is the most potent of these compounds and has been well characterized to lead to the development of hepatocellular carcinoma in humans and animals. The contamination of the food chain by AFB1 has a huge impact on human health and economic damage worldwide. The prevention and detoxification strategies of AFB1 have always been the goal of research. Although physical and chemical treatment is currently the main detoxification method, it is easy to lead to the loss of food nutrition. Biotherapeutics is a relatively new detoxification method. Natural plant extracts and plant essential oils are simple to produce, biosafe, and provide an excellent source of toxin detoxification. Studies have shown that individuals' susceptibility, such as genetic polymorphisms in DNA repair genes and/or metabolic genes, play a huge role in the different detoxification and the repair of DNA damage caused by AFB1. Thus, the biofunction supplementary methods which base on this kind of genetic difference may be not only regarded as potential new detoxification methods but served as potential biological markers for predicting the occurrence of such liver diseases as liver damage, liver cirrhosis, and hepatocellular carcinogenesis.

Conflicts of interest and source of funding

The authors declare no competing financial interests. This study was supported in part by the National Natural Science Foundation of China (Nos. 81,860,489, 81,760,502, 81,572,353, and 81,660,495), the Natural Science Foundation of Guangxi (Nos. 2018GXNSFAA281043, 2017GXNSFAA198002 and 2017GXNSFGA198002), Research Program of Guangxi "Zhouyue Scholar" (No. 2017-2038), Research Program of Guangxi Specially-invited Expert (No. 2017-6th), the '12th Five' Planning Program of Guangxi Education Science (No. 2015C397), the Innovative Program of Guangxi Graduate Education (No. JGY2015139), Research Program of Guangxi Clinic Research Center of Hepatobiliary Diseases (No. AD17129025), and Open Research Program from Molecular Immunity Study Room Involving in Acute & Severe Diseases in Guangxi Colleges and Universities (Nos. kfkt20160062 and kfkt20160063).

Abbreviations

Aflatoxin B1 (AFB1)
hepatocellular carcinoma (HCC)
Aspergillus flavus (*A. flavus*)
Aspergillus parasiticus (*A. parasiticus*)
The Food and Agriculture Organization of the United Nations (FAO)
World Health Organization (WHO)
AFB1-8-9-epoxide (AFBO)
Nucleic Acid Excision Repair Pathway (NER)
xeroderma pigmentosum C (XPC),xeroderma pigmentosum D (XPD)
European Union (EU)

Author details

Qun-Ying Su[1,2]

1 Department of Pathology, The Affiliated Hospital of Youjiang Medical University for Nationalities, Baise, China

2 The Centre of Pathology Diagnosis and Research, Youjiang Medical University for Nationalities, Baise, China

*Address all correspondence to: 155373033@qq.com

References

[1] Cole RJ. Etiology of Turkey "X" disease in retrospect: A case for the involvement of cyclopiazonic acid. Mycotoxin Research. 1986;**2**(1):3-7. DOI: 10.1007/BF03191956

[2] Ostry V, Malir F, Toman J, et al. Mycotoxins as human carcinogens-the IARC monographs classification. Mycotoxin Research. 2017;**33**(1):65-73. DOI: 10.1007/s12550-016-0265-7

[3] Bennett JW, Klich M. Mycotoxins. Clinical Microbiology Reviews. 2003;**16**(3):497-516. DOI: 10.1128/cmr.16.3.497-516.2003

[4] Richard JL. Some major mycotoxins and their mycotoxicoses—An overview. International Journal of Food Microbiology. 2007;**119**(1-2):3-10. DOI: 10.1016/j.ijfoodmicro.2007.07.019

[5] Al-Jaal BA, Jaganjac M, Barcaru A, et al. Aflatoxin, fumonisin, ochratoxin, zearalenone and deoxynivalenol biomarkers in human biological fluids: A systematic literature review, 2001-2018. Food and Chemical Toxicology. 2019;**129**:211-228. DOI: 10.1016/j.fct.2019.04.047

[6] Marin S, Ramos AJ, Cano-Sancho G, et al. Mycotoxins: Occurrence, toxicology, and exposure assessment. Food and Chemical Toxicology. 2013;**60**:218-237. DOI: 10.1016/j.fct.2013.07.047

[7] Diener UL, Cole RJ, Sanders TH, et al. Epidemiology of Aflatoxin formation by Aspergillus Flavus. Annual Review of Phytopathology. 1987;**25**(1):249-270. DOI: 10.1146/annurev.py.25.090187.001341

[8] Gnonlonfin GJ, Hell K, Adjovi Y, et al. A review on aflatoxin contamination and its implications in the developing world: A sub-Saharan African perspective. Critical Reviews in Food Science and Nutrition. 2013;**53**(4):349-365. DOI: 10.1080/10408398.2010.535718

[9] Wild CP, Turner PC. The toxicology of aflatoxins as a basis for public health decisions. Mutagenesis. 2002;**17**(6):471-481. DOI: 10.1093/mutage/17.6.471

[10] Trail F, Mahanti N, Linz J. Molecular biology of aflatoxin biosynthesis. Microbiology. 1995;**141**:755-765. DOI: 10.1099/13500872-141-4-755

[11] Wogan GN, Kensler TW, Groopman JD. Present and future directions of translational research on aflatoxin and hepatocellular carcinoma. A review. Food Additives & Contaminants. Part A, Chemistry, Analysis, Control, Exposure & Risk Assessment. 2012;**29**(2):249-257. DOI: 10.1080/19440049.2011.563370

[12] Scholthof KB. One foot in the furrow: Linkages between agriculture, plant pathology, and public health. Annual Review of Public Health. 2003;**24**:153-174. DOI: 10.1146/annurev.publhealth.24.090302.155542

[13] Dorner JW. Management and prevention of mycotoxins in peanuts. Food Additives & Contaminants. Part A, Chemistry, Analysis, Control, Exposure & Risk Assessment. 2008;**25**(2):203-208. DOI: 10.1080/02652030701658357

[14] Munkvold GP. Cultural and genetic approaches to managing mycotoxins in maize. Annual Review of Phytopathology. 2003;**41**:99-116. DOI: 10.1146/annurev.phyto.41.052002.095510

[15] Bryden WL. Mycotoxin contamination of the feed supply chain: Implications for animal productivity and feed security. Animal Feed Science and Technology. 2012;**173**(1-2):134-158. DOI: 10.1016/j.anifeedsci.2011.12.014

[16] Hell K, Cardwell KF, Poehling H-M. Relationship between management practices, fungal infection and Aflatoxin for stored maize in Benin. Journal of Phytopathology. 2003;**151**(11-12):690-698. DOI: 10.1046/j.1439-0434.2003.00792.x

[17] Hell K, Cardwell KF, Setamou M, et al. The influence of storage practices on aflatoxin contamination in maize in four agroecological zones of Benin, West Africa. Journal of Stored Products Research. 2000;**36**(4):365-382. DOI: 10.1016/S0022-474X(99)00056-9

[18] Prandini A, Tansini G, Sigolo S, et al. On the occurrence of aflatoxin M1 in milk and dairy products. Food and Chemical Toxicology. 2009;**47**(5):984-991. DOI: 10.1016/j.fct.2007.10.005

[19] Asao T, Buchi G, Abdel-Kader M, et al. Aflatoxins B and G. Journal of the American Chemical Society. 1963;**85**:1706-1707. DOI: 10.1021/ja00894a050

[20] Applebaum RS, Brackett RE, Wiseman DW, et al. Aflatoxin: Toxicity to dairy cattle and occurrence in milk and milk products—a review. Journal of Food Protection. 1982;**45**(8):752-777. DOI: 10.4315/0362-028X-45.8.752

[21] Habib SL, Said B, Awad AT, et al. Novel adenine adducts, N7-guanine-AFB1 adducts, and p 53 mutations in patients with schistosomiasis and aflatoxin exposure. Cancer Detection and Prevention. 2006;**30**(6):491-498. DOI: 10.1016/j.cdp.2006.10.006

[22] Kensler TW, Roebuck BD, Wogan GN, et al. Aflatoxin: A 50-year odyssey of mechanistic and translational toxicology. Toxicological Sciences. 2011;**120**(Suppl 1):S28-S48. DOI: 10.1093/toxsci/kfq283

[23] Long XD, Zhao D, Wang C, et al. Genetic polymorphisms in DNA repair genes XRCC4 and XRCC5 and aflatoxin B1-related hepatocellular carcinoma. Epidemiology. 2013;**24**(5):671-681. DOI: 10.1097/EDE.0b013e31829d2744

[24] Neal GE. Biochemical and molecular aspects of mammalian susceptibility to aflatoxin B1 carcinogenicity. Human & Experimental Toxicology. 1995;**14**(7):619-620. DOI: 10.1177/096032719501400714

[25] Bbosa GS, Kitya D, Odda J, et al. Aflatoxins metabolism, effects on epigenetic mechanisms and their role in carcinogenesis. Health. 2013;**05**(10):14-34

[26] Azziz-Baumgartner E, Lindblade K, Gieseker K, et al. Case-control study of an acute aflatoxicosis outbreak, Kenya, 2004. Environmental Health Perspectives. 2005;**113**(12):1779-1783. DOI: 10.1289/ehp.8384

[27] Egal S, Hounsa A, Gong YY, et al. Dietary exposure to aflatoxin from maize and groundnut in young children from Benin and Togo, West Africa. International Journal of Food Microbiology. 2005;**104**(2):215-224. DOI: 10.1016/j.ijfoodmicro.2005.03.004

[28] Hamilton PB. A natural and extremely severe occurrence of aflatoxicosis in laying hens. Poultry Science. 1971;**50**(6):1880-1882. DOI: 10.3382/ps.0501880

[29] Dersjant-Li Y, Verstegen MW, Gerrits WJ. The impact of low concentrations of aflatoxin, deoxynivalenol or fumonisin in diets on growing pigs and poultry. Nutrition Research Reviews. 2003;**16**(2):223-239. DOI: 10.1079/NRR200368

[30] Reddy RV, Taylor MJ, Sharma RP. Studies of immune function of CD-1 mice exposed to aflatoxin B1. Toxicology. 1987;**43**(2):123-132. DOI: 10.1016/0300-483X(87)90002-3Get rights and content

[31] Michael GY, Thaxton P, Hamilton PB. Impairment of the reticuloendothelial system of chickens during aflatoxicosis. Poultry Science. 1973;**52**(3):1206-1207. DOI: 10.3382/ps.0521206

[32] Silvotti L, Petterino C, Bonomi A, Cabassi E. Immunotoxicological effects on piglets of feeding sows diets containing aflatoxins. The Veterinary Record. 1997;**141**(18):469-472. DOI: 10.1136/vr.141.18.469

[33] Turner PC, Moore SE, Hall AJ, et al. Modification of immune function through exposure to dietary aflatoxin in Gambian children. Environmental Health Perspectives. 2003;**111**(2): 217-220. DOI: 10.1289/ehp.5753

[34] Jiang Y, Jolly PE, Ellis WO, et al. Aflatoxin B1 albumin adduct levels and cellular immune status in Ghanaians. International Immunology. 2005;**17**(6):807-814. DOI: 10.1093/intimm/dxh262

[35] Lee J, Her JY, Lee KG. Reduction of aflatoxins (B (1), B (2), G (1), and G (2)) in soybean-based model systems. Food Chemistry. 2015;**189**:45-51. DOI: 10.1016/j.foodchem.2015.02.013

[36] Park JW, Kim YB. Effect of pressure cooking on aflatoxin B1 in rice. Journal of Agricultural and Food Chemistry. 2006;**54**(6):2431-2435. DOI: 10.1021/jf053007e

[37] da Silva M, Moraes AML, Nishikawa MM, et al. Inactivation of fungi from deteriorated paper materials by radiation. International Biodeterioration and Biodegradation. 2006;**57**(3):163-167. DOI: 10.1016/j.ibiod.2006.02.003

[38] Oluwafemi F, Kumar M, Bandyopadhyay R, et al. Bio-detoxification of aflatoxin B1 in artificially contaminated maize grains using lactic acid bacteria. Toxin Reviews. 2010;**29**(3-4):115-122. DOI: 10.3109/15569543.2010.512556

[39] Di Stefano V, Pitonzo R, Cicero N, et al. Mycotoxin contamination of animal feedingstuff: Detoxification by gamma-irradiation and reduction of aflatoxins and ochratoxin a concentrations. Food Additives & Contaminants. Part A, Chemistry, Analysis, Control, Exposure & Risk Assessment. 2014;**31**(12):2034-2039. DOI: 10.1080/19440049.2014.968882

[40] Bluma R, Amaiden MR, Etcheverry M. Screening of argentine plant extracts: Impact on growth parameters and aflatoxin B1 accumulation by Aspergillus section Flavi. International Journal of Food Microbiology. 2008;**122**(1-2):114-125. DOI: 10.1016/j.ijfoodmicro.2007.11.050

[41] Vijayanandraj S, Brinda R, Kannan K, et al. Detoxification of aflatoxin B1 by an aqueous extract from leaves of Adhatoda vasica Nees. Microbiological Research. 2014;**169**(4):294-300. DOI: 10.1016/j.micres.2013.07.008 DOI:10.1016/j.micres.2013.07.008

[42] Iram W, Anjum T, Iqbal M, et al. Structural analysis and biological toxicity of Aflatoxins B1 and B2 degradation products following detoxification by Ocimum basilicum and Cassia fistula aqueous extracts. Frontiers in Microbiology. 2016;**7**:1105. DOI: 10.3389/fmicb.2016.01105

[43] Brana MT, Cimmarusti MT, Haidukowski M, et al. Bioremediation of aflatoxin B1-contaminated maize by king oyster mushroom (Pleurotus eryngii). PLoS One. 2017;**12**(8):e0182574. DOI: 10.1371/journal.pone.0182574

[44] Farzaneh M, Shi Z-Q, Ghassempour A, et al. Aflatoxin B1

degradation by Bacillus subtilis UTBSP1 isolated from pistachio nuts of Iran. Food Control. 2012;**23**(1):100-106

[45] Liu J, Song WJ, Zhang NY, et al. Biodetoxification of aflatoxin B1 in cottonseed meal by fermentation of Cellulosimicrobium funkei in duckling diet. Poultry Science. 2017;**96**(4): 923-930. DOI: 10.3382/ps/pew352

[46] Haskard CA, El-Nezami HS, Kankaanpaa PE, et al. Surface binding of aflatoxin B (1) by lactic acid bacteria. Applied and Environmental Microbiology. 2001;**67**(7):3086-3091. DOI: 10.1128/AEM.67.7.3086-3091.2001

[47] Bueno DJ, Casale CH, Pizzolitto RP, et al. Physical adsorption of aflatoxin B1 by lactic acid bacteria and Saccharomyces cerevisiae: A theoretical model. Journal of Food Protection. 2007;**70**(9):2148-2154. DOI: 10.1007/s12602-018-9512-x

[48] Hamid AS, Tesfamariam IG, Zhang Y, et al. Aflatoxin B1-induced hepatocellular carcinoma in developing countries: Geographical distribution, mechanism of action and prevention. Oncology Letters. 2013;**5**(4):1087-1092. DOI: 10.3892/ol.2013.1169

[49] Aiko V, Edamana P, Mehta A. Decomposition and detoxification of aflatoxin B1 by lactic acid. Journal of the Science of Food and Agriculture. 2016;**96**(6):1959-1966. DOI: 10.1002/jsfa.7304

[50] Rushing BR, Selim MI. Adduction to arginine detoxifies aflatoxin B1 by eliminating genotoxicity and altering in vitro toxicokinetic profiles. Oncotarget. 2018;**9**(4):4559-4570. DOI: 10.18632/oncotarget.23382

[51] Rushing BR, Selim MI. Effect of dietary acids on the formation of aflatoxin B2a as a means to detoxify aflatoxin B1. Food Additives & Contaminants. Part A, Chemistry, Analysis, Control, Exposure & Risk Assessment. 2016;**33**(9):1456-1467. DOI: 10.1080/19440049.2016.1217065

[52] Rushing BR, Selim MI. Structure and oxidation of Pyrrole adducts formed between Aflatoxin B2a and biological amines. Chemical Research in Toxicology. 2017;**30**(6):1275-1285. DOI: 10.1021/acs.chemrestox.7b00002

[53] Gomaa MN, Ayesh AM, Abdel Galil MM, et al. Effect of high pressure ammoniation procedure on the detoxification of aflatoxins. Mycotoxin Research. 1997;**13**(1):23-34. DOI: 10.1007/BF02945059

[54] Aly SE, Hathout AS. Fate of aflatoxin B (1) in contaminated corn gluten during acid hydrolysis. Journal of the Science of Food and Agriculture. 2011;**91**(3):421-427. DOI: 10.1002/jsfa.4201

[55] de Alencar ER, Faroni LR, Soares Nde F, et al. Efficacy of ozone as a fungicidal and detoxifying agent of aflatoxins in peanuts. Journal of the Science of Food and Agriculture. 2012;**92**(4):899-905. DOI: 10.1002/jsfa.4668

[56] Diao E, Hou H, Chen B, et al. Ozonolysis efficiency and safety evaluation of aflatoxin B1 in peanuts. Food and Chemical Toxicology. 2013;**55**:519-525. DOI: 10.1016/j.fct.2013.01.038

[57] Proctor AD, Ahmedna M, Kumar JV, et al. Degradation of aflatoxins in peanut kernels/flour by gaseous ozonation and mild heat treatment. Food Additives and Contaminants. 2004;**21**(8):786-793. DOI: 10.1080/02652030410001713898

[58] Afriyie-Gyawu E, Mackie J, Dash B, et al. Chronic toxicological evaluation of dietary Nova Sil clay in

Sprague-Dawley rats. Food Additives and Contaminants. 2005;**22**(3):259-269. DOI: 10.1080/02652030500110758

[59] Afriyie-Gyawu E, Ankrah NA, Huebner HJ, et al. Nova Sil clay intervention in Ghanaians at high risk for aflatoxicosis. I. Study design and clinical outcomes. Food Additives & Contaminants. Part A, Chemistry, Analysis, Control, Exposure & Risk Assessment. 2008;**25**(1):76-87. DOI: 10.1080/02652030701458105

[60] Breinholt V, Hendricks J, Pereira C, et al. Dietary chlorophyllin is a potent inhibitor of aflatoxin B1 hepatocarcinogenesis in rainbow trout. Cancer Research. 1995;**55**(1):57-62

[61] Phillips TD, Afriyie-Gyawu E, Williams J, et al. Reducing human exposure to aflatoxin through the use of clay: A review. Food Additives & Contaminants. Part A, Chemistry, Analysis, Control, Exposure & Risk Assessment. 2008;**25**(2):134-145. DOI: 10.1080/02652030701567467

[62] Wang P, Afriyie-Gyawu E, Tang Y, et al. Nova Sil clay intervention in Ghanaians at high risk for aflatoxicosis: II. Reduction in biomarkers of aflatoxin exposure in blood and urine. Food Additives & Contaminants. Part A, Chemistry, Analysis, Control, Exposure & Risk Assessment. 2008;**25**(5):622-634. DOI: 10.1080/02652030701598694

[63] Xue KS, Qian G, Lin S, et al. Modulation of pre-neoplastic biomarkers induced by sequential aflatoxin B1 and fumonisin B1 exposure in F344 rats treated with UPSN clay. Food and Chemical Toxicology. 2018;**114**:316-324. DOI: 10.1016/j.fct.2018.02.048

[64] Egner PA, Wang JB, Zhu YR, et al. Chlorophyllin intervention reduces aflatoxin-DNA adducts in individuals at high risk for liver cancer. Proceedings of the National Academy of Sciences of the United States of America. 2001;**98**(25):14601-14606. DOI: 10.1073/pnas.251536898

[65] Simonich MT, Egner PA, Roebuck BD, et al. Natural chlorophyll inhibits aflatoxin B1-induced multi-organ carcinogenesis in the rat. Carcinogenesis. 2007;**28**(6):1294-1302. DOI: 10.1093/carcin/bgm027

[66] McCullough AK, Lloyd RS. Mechanisms underlying aflatoxin-associated mutagenesis - implications in carcinogenesis. DNA Repair (Amst). 2019;**77**:76-86. DOI: 10.1016/j.dnarep.2019.03.004

[67] Yao JG, Huang XY, Long XD. Interaction of DNA repair gene polymorphisms and aflatoxin B1 in the risk of hepatocellular carcinoma. International Journal of Clinical and Experimental Pathology. 2014;**7**(9):6231-6244

[68] Long XD, Ma Y, Qu DY, et al. The polymorphism of XRCC3 codon 241 and AFB1-related hepatocellular carcinoma in Guangxi population, China. Annals of Epidemiology. 2008;**18**(7):572-578. DOI: 10.1016/j.annepidem.2008.03.003

[69] Bryden WL. Mycotoxins in the food chain: Human health implications. Asia Pacific Journal of Clinical Nutrition. 2007;**16**(Suppl 1):95-101

[70] Milicevic D, Nastasijevic I, Petrovic Z. Mycotoxin in the food supply chain-implications for public health program. Journal of Environmental Science and Health. Part C, Environmental Carcinogenesis & Ecotoxicology Reviews. 2016;**34**(4):293-319. DOI: 10.1080/10590501.2016.1236607

[71] Rushing BR, Selim MI. Aflatoxin B1: A review on metabolism, toxicity, occurrence in food, occupational

exposure, and detoxification methods. Food and Chemical Toxicology. 2019;**124**:81-100. DOI: 10.1016/j.fct.2018.11.047

[72] Wu F. A tale of two commodities: How EU mycotoxin regulations have affected U. S. Tree nut industries. World Mycotoxin Journal. 2008;**1**(1):95-102. DOI: 10.3920/WMJ2008.x011

[73] Montagna MT, Napoli C, De Giglio O, et al. Occurrence of aflatoxin M (1) in dairy products in southern Italy. International Journal of Molecular Sciences. 2008;**9**(12):2614-2621. DOI: 10.3390/ijms9122614